Massage Therapy

WHAT IT IS
and
HOW IT WORKS

STEVEN SCHENKMAN

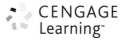
CENGAGE
Learning™

Australia • Brazil • Japan • Korea • Mexico • Singapore • Spain • United Kingdom • United States

CENGAGE
Learning

Massage Therapy: What It Is and How It Works
Author: Steven Schenkman

President, Milady: Dawn Gerrain

Publisher: Erin O'Connor

Acquisitions Editor: Martine Edwards

Senior Product Manager: Philip Mandl

Editorial Assistant: Elizabeth Edwards

Director of Beauty Industry Relations: Sandra Bruce

Senior Marketing Manager: Gerard McAvey

Production Director: Wendy Troeger

Senior Content Project Manager: Nina Tucciarelli

Senior Art Director: Joy Kocsis

For product information and technology assistance, contact us at **Professional & Career Group Customer Support, 1-800-648-7450**

For permission to use material from this text or product, submit all requests online at **cengage.com/permissions**
Further permissions questions can be emailed to **permissionrequest@cengage.com**

Library of Congress Control Number: 2007941007

ISBN-13: 978-1-4180-1233-5

ISBN-10: 1-418-01233-5

Milady
5 Maxwell Drive
Clifton Park, NY 12065-2919
USA

Cengage Learning products are represented in Canada by Nelson Education, Ltd.

For your lifelong learning solutions, visit **milady.cengage.com**

Visit our corporate website at **www.cengage.com**

Notice to the Reader

Printed in United States
1 2 3 4 5 xxx 13 12 11 10 09

Dedication

This book is dedicated to:
My spiritual teacher, Robert C. Sohn
My Amma teacher, Tina Sohn
And of course to my wonderful wife of 33 years, Faye

Table of Contents

Preface

THE MASSAGE THERAPY AND BODYWORK PROFESSION TODAY

Not long ago, the field of massage therapy and bodywork was considered to be an "underground mainstream." When it was finally surveyed, it was discovered that tens of millions of massage therapy and bodywork treatments were being administered by professionals all over the country. They noted that willing consumers, mostly paying one hundred percent out-of-pocket for these services, lined up for treatment and virtually no one was aware of it! These trends have grown stronger still and all the statistics point to continued unprecedented growth. Today it is clear, and no longer any secret, that massage therapy and bodywork has come out from the underground and stepped proudly into the mainstream of our nation's health care system as one of the fastest growing professions in America.

Over the last 30 years my own experience in different facets of this profession—as a licensed practitioner, instructor, college president, massage therapy state board chairman, founding national certification board member and national association president, has stood witness not only to the exponential growth in the numbers of practitioners but also to the incredible diversity of treatment approaches, enhancement of technical skills and abilities of therapists, and the expansion of the field's scope of practice.

WHO THIS BOOK IS FOR

When any profession grows and begins to take hold of the minds and bodies of the population as massage therapy has done, a myriad of other related industries that are necessary for the continued development and support of the field (such as manufacturers of massage tables, oils, crèmes and lotions, other equipment and products, text book publishers), develop around it. This creates an important dynamic that serves the greater massage industry, which in turn allows for and even accelerates continued growth and interest by more and more of the population. As the word spreads, there arises a real need for accurate information and improved education, since more often than not, interest grows faster than the information available. There becomes a growing need for schools and instructors to have access to quality information so they can prepare their students with a foundation built on rock and provide an education that stands the test of time, one that serves as a profound context from which to build the most current skills, knowledge, abilities and attitudes necessary for achieving personal success in the field of massage therapy.

MASSAGE THERAPY: What It Is and How It Works is an excellent text that fills this need. After an extensive review of other massage therapy and bodywork materials, it became evident that although the amount of published resources now available has grown exponentially, there is little that has been written specifically for students and practicing therapists, (even for the lay public as a resource) that presents a comprehensive perspective and overview of this field. The student needs a context from which to help envision the true potential of what is possible to attain in this profession as they begin the journey of a school program. The professional therapist needs to be shown the possibilities of other levels of practice beyond what they may be doing in the present so new pathways of evolution may open before them. And for members of the public looking to understand what they may gain from seeking out a qualified massage therapist, this book can serve as a resource from which to obtain the information they need or desire.

Although not intended to serve as a "career guide," *MASSAGE THERAPY: What It Is and How It Works* can also help to educate and pique the interest of its readers enough to seek training in massage therapy as a full-time or adjunctive career path. This book provides these potential students with a broad perspective of the field helping them to garner the information they need to make an informed decision as to whether or not pursuing a career in massage therapy is right for them.

ABOUT THE BOOK

Due to the growing complexity and widening scope of the field, it is becoming more and more important to have a text that provides an accurate roadmap of possible practice beyond the idea of what hands-on modality or modalities a therapist performs. There was a need for a book that boldly defines the levels and extent of existing and potential practice. Just how far can massage and bodywork therapists take their profession? What are the limits of possibility when it comes to treating and healing using massage therapy? What do practitioners need to know and do to go beyond where they find themselves today?

Section I

Section I of *MASSAGE THERAPY: What It Is and How It Works* elucidates this important discussion in its first four chapters on the "The Three Paradigms" which are: 1) Relaxation and Stress Reduction, 2) Remediation, Therapy, and Pain Relief and 3) Holistic Integration. The Three Paradigms form a continuum of possible practice beginning at the most basic levels of touch leading to the most advanced levels of practice and holistic care. These chapters also include numerous interesting and relevant case histories that showcase, demonstrate and differentiate massage therapy and bodywork practice by First, Second and Third Paradigm practitioners.

Also presented in Section I is another new concept that introduces and explores the idea that there exist Three Levels of Competence that define a practitioner's relationship to their paradigm of practice. The book demonstrates how competence is not simply a product of a therapist's effort *to* practice their modality but rather shows it to be a direct reflection of *how* they practice and their ability to control attention and stay fully focused and concentrated during treatment - a feat not so easily accomplished.

Whereas the Three Paradigms define and describe the possible scope and extent of therapeutic education, training, and practice that exist within the field, the Three Levels of Competence define and describe the level of depth, skill, and overall ability with which massage therapists perform their work, regardless of paradigm.

MASSAGE THERAPY: What It Is and How It Works lays the foundation for students to begin creating their future by providing an understanding of the realm of possibilities in the field. It helps them to envision how far along they may want to go on this path of possible practice. This roadmap also serves as a mirror for therapists enabling them to reflect upon what they have or have not achieved as professionals, what they can still achieve if they wish, and what they need to do to achieve it.

Section II

MASSAGE THERAPY: What It Is and How It Works then moves into a brief history highlighting the beginnings of massage during major historical time periods in different countries or regions of the world up until the present time. This chapter provides a context for understanding the evolution of the important ideas and principles set forth next in the following five chapters of Section II.

Following the history, a new and unique model of the scope of the profession is included to provide an in depth analysis of the existing spectrum of massage therapy and bodywork modalities. It is called "The Continuum of the Four Massage Therapy and Bodywork Levels." When analyzed, the main *intention* of each modality is shown to primarily affect one of the four levels or layers of the energy/matter continuum of a human being. The Continuum of the Four Massage Therapy and Bodywork Levels are 1) Somatic, 2) Somato-Psychic, 3) Bioenergetic, and 4) Energetic.

Within these five chapters 26 of the most popular and effective forms of touch practiced today and generally representative of the field, are detailed and shown to fall within one of the four levels of massage therapy and bodywork. These discussions include a history of the modality and its founder, principles and theories, hand techniques, benefits and contraindications followed by the major underlying principles of assessment used in treatment planning and some of the mechanisms responsible for each modality's efficacy. At the end of each massage therapy and bodywork modality there is information regarding the requirements for practitioner education, licensure, and certification.

In addition, the reader will get a good taste and enjoy a detailed description of what it would be like to experience a treatment in each of the 26 modalities presented. All of this provides the reader with an understanding as to how and why manipulation of the body's tissues and/or energy by the touch of a professionally trained therapist practicing any of these disciplines within the continuum, can garner such positive and healthful responses on so many levels.

After the Continuum of the Four Massage Therapy and Bodywork Levels, a view of the primary practice settings that therapists work in today is included. This chapter takes a good look at employment in private practice, clinics, hospitals, spas, athletic facilities, and in corporations by providing a detailed look at *a day in the life of a massage therapist* in each one of these settings. This true taste of what it's like to actually work in these environments offers students, and practitioners who may be considering changing employment tracks, a real sense of the choices and opportunities available. This chapter also helps the reader to understand the scope of what this field offers in the way of professional services on many levels.

An additional chapter includes the growth, highlights and challenges of the profession and the role of a massage and bodywork therapist within the context of the entire realm of health care today. This important chapter discusses the relationship between the massage and bodywork therapist and the other members of the health care team, including: the patient, the family and significant others, physicians, nurses, acupuncturists, chiropractors, physical therapists, psychiatrists and psychologists.

In this book there is also a glossary and an appendix that includes a detailed reference list, bibliography and additional resources that provides information for those readers who are interested in more in-depth research and study on massage therapy and bodywork.

ABOUT THE AUTHOR

Steven Schenkman, a licensed New York State Massage Therapist since 1984, is an established leader in the field of Complementary and Alternative Medicine. He served as President of The New York College for Wholistic Health, Education, and Research (now known as the New York College of Health Professions) from 1989 through 2001. The college offers associates and bachelor's degree programs in massage and bodywork therapy, master's degrees in acupuncture and Oriental medicine, certificate programs in wholistic nursing and physical arts. Under his leadership the Institution evolved into a premiere college for wholistic education and developed the first associate's degree program in massage therapy in the United States in 1996 and a bachelor's degree in amma therapeutic massage in 1999, the nation's first bachelors degree in bodywork.

Since 2001 Mr. Schenkman has been a consultant and curriculum specialist to career colleges, allied health and business schools and schools of massage therapy. As a consultant he specializes in assistance with accreditation and administration, licensing, internal consulting, reorganization, curriculum and new program development, new business development, marketing & advertising and strategic planning.

Steven Schenkman has also demonstrated leadership and commitment to the profession of Massage Therapy as a founding member of the National Certification Board for Therapeutic Massage and Bodywork (NCBTMB) whose examinations are now used or recognized in statute or rule in 33 states and the District of Columbia. Steven spent five years on that Board. He has also served as Chairman of the New York State Massage Therapy Board for six years and was a member for 10 years. Steven was also a founding member and served as the first President of the American Organization for Bodywork Therapies of Asia (AOBTA) for five years.

Most recently in 2009, Mr. Schenkman has been appointed to the Massage Therapy Body of Knowledge (MTBOK) Project Task Force. This national effort is under the direction of the MTBOK Stewards, representatives from the American Massage

Therapy Association, AMTA-Council of Schools, Associated Bodywork & Massage Professionals, Federation of State Massage Therapy Boards, Massage Therapy Foundation, and National Certification Board for Therapeutic Massage and Bodywork. The Task Force is responsible for defining, developing, and articulating a massage therapy body of knowledge (MTBOK) for the profession. Mr. Schenkman is also a member of the Cengage Learning (formerly Thomson Delmar Leaning) Massage Therapy Advisory Board, the Books of Discovery Advisory Council and he writes a blog for Massage Magazine's web site found under its 'Expert Insights' section.

He has studied and practiced Advanced Amma Therapeutic Massage and was a certified biofeedback specialist and stress management consultant. In addition, Mr. Schenkman was trained in acupuncture using the apprenticeship model and is a master tai chi practitioner and instructor.

To contact the author, call 1-631-659-3090 or go to his website, http://www.schenkmanconsulting.com.

ACKNOWLEDGMENTS

First, and most importantly, a special acknowledgment goes to my student Seung K. Park (known as SK), experienced L.M.T., business owner and aspiring biography writer without whom this book would not have been possible. Having worked with me directly over the last few years, SK was involved from the very beginning of this project and was part of the creation of this text. Many long hours were spent in discussion with SK formulating the structure and content of the book as well as several of the fundamental ideas expounded in this text. SK also contributed greatly to the research and initial writings of the history chapter and all the chapters on the massage therapy and bodywork modalities.

I want to thank my dear wife, Faye Schenkman, M.A., Dipl. in Chinese Herbal Medicine & Bodywork, C.A.T., L.M.T., practitioner in Amma Therapeutic Massage and Oriental Medicine for thirty years, for her contribution to the chapter on Massage Therapy Within the Larger Healthcare/Well Being Team. Faye was also instrumental in organizing, coordinating, writing, editing and working endless hours with me making sure that the ideas and principles discussed in this text were correctly expressed. Without her hard work, dedication and love this book would not have been produced.

I want to thank my student Doug Mandalone, experienced L.M.T., third year acupuncture student and business owner for his contributions to the chapter Practice Settings: A Day in the Life of a Massage Therapist.

I also want to thank my dear friend and colleague Kim Rosado, M.A., Dipl. in Acupuncture & Bodywork experienced L.M.T., L.Ac., who along with SK and Faye, contributed her time, effort and ideas, particularly in the reading, re-reading and editing of the current manuscript as well as refining content and providing her invaluable feedback. Without all of their hard work, dedication and initiative, this book would not have been produced.

I would also like to thank the staff of Cengage Learning for their patience, support and willingness to work with me on finally turning my manuscript into this textbook.

Credits

Figure 1-1: Image copyright 2009, Sabri Deniz Kizil. Used under license from Shutterstock.com.

Figure 1-3: Image copyright 2009, Yakobchuk Vasyl. Used under license from Shutterstock.com.

Figure 1-6: Image copyright 2009, Stephen Coburn. Used under license from Shutterstock.com.

Figure 1-7: Image copyright 2009, Ruben Paz Coburn. Used under license from Shutterstock.com.

Figure 1-8a: Image copyright 2009, Elana Ray. Used under license from Shutterstock.com

Figure 1-8b, 9-7 and 12-8: Image copyright 2009, Salamanderman. Used under license from Shutterstock.com

Figure 1-9: Image copyright 2009, Tatiana Popova. Used under license from Shutterstock.com.

Figure 1-10: Image copyright 2009, Alex Kalmbach. Used under license from Shutterstock.com.

Figure 1-11: Image copyright 2009, Leo Blanchette. Used under license from Shutterstock.com.

Figure 1-12: Image copyright 2009, Sgame. Used under license from Shutterstock.com.

Figure 2-1: Copyright 2009, Dasilva. Used under license from Shutterstock.com.

Figure 2-2, 4-10: Image copyright 2009, Liv Friis-larsen. Used under license from Shutterstock.com.

Figure 2-3: Image copyright 2009, Ana de Sousa. Used under license from Shutterstock.com.

Figure 2-4: Image copyright 2009, Paparazzit. Used under license from Shutterstock.com

Figure 3-1: Image copyright 2009, Andresr. Used under license from Shutterstock.com.

Figure 4-1: Copyright 2009, Yuri Arcurs. Used under license from Shutterstock.com.

Figure 4-2: Image copyright 2009, WizData, inc. Used under license from Shutterstock.com.

Figure 4-3: Image copyright 2009, Garry Wolsey. Used under license from Shutterstock.com.

Figure 4-4: Image copyright 2009, Charles Taylor. Used under license from Shutterstock.com.

Figure 4-5: Image copyright 2009, Kiselev Andrey Valerevic. Used under license from Shutterstock.com.

Figure 4-6: Image copyright 2009, Stephen Strathdee. Used under license from Shutterstock.com.

Figure 4-7: Image copyright 2009, Apollofoto. Used under license from Shutterstock.com.

Figure 4-8: Image copyright 2009, Riekephotos. Used under license from Shutterstock.com.

Figure 4-9: Image copyright 2009, Arne Trautmann. Used under license from Shutterstock.com.

Figure 5-1: Image copyright 2009, Niderlander. Used under license from Shutterstock.com.

Figure 5-8: Image copyright 2009, Paul Prescott. Used under license from Shutterstock.com.

Figure 6-3: Image copyright 2009, Rey Kamensky. Used under license from Shutterstock.com.

Figure 7-1: Image copyright 2009, Leah-Anne Thompson. Used under license from Shutterstock.com.

Figure 7-7: Image copyright 2009, Jonathan Larsen. Used under license from Shutterstock.com.

Figure 7-8: Image copyright 2009, Edw. Used under license from Shutterstock.com.

Figure 8-1: Image copyright 2009, ImageZebra. Used under license from Shutterstock.com.

Figure 8-4: copyright 2009, Oguz Aral. Used under license from Shutterstock.com.

Figure 8-6: Image copyright 2009, AYAKOVLEVdotCOM. Used under license from Shutterstock.com.

Figure 8-7: Image copyright 2009, Szocs Jozsef. Used under license from Shutterstock.com.

Figure 8-8: Image copyright 2009, Patrizia Tilly. Used under license from Shutterstock.com.

Figure 9-4: Image copyright 2009, Orrza. Used under license from Shutterstock.com.

Figure 9-10: Image copyright 2009, Jennifer Sharp. Used under license from Shutterstock.com.

Figure 9-12: Copyright 2009, Tomasz Wieja. Used under license from Shutterstock.com.

Figure 9-14 and 10-3: Copyright 2009, Yanik Chauvin. Used under license from Shutterstock.com.

Figure 10-1: Image copyright 2009, Tara Urbach. Used under license from Shutterstock.com.

Figure 10-2: Copyright 2009, Bruce Rolff. Used under license from Shutterstock.com.

Figure 10-4: Image copyright 2009, Daniela Illing. Used under license from Shutterstock.com.

Figure 10-5: Image copyright 2009, Rgbspace. Used under license from Shutterstock.com.

Figure 10-6: Image copyright 2009, Eduard Härkönen. Used under license from Shutterstock.com.

Figure 11-7 and 11-8: Image copyright 2009, Iofoto. Used under license from Shutterstock.com.

Figure 12-1, 12-3, and 12-4: Image copyright 2009, Monkey Business Images. Used under license from Shutterstock.com.

Figure 12-2: Image copyright 2009, Alexander Raths. Used under license from Shutterstock.com.

Figure 12-5: Image copyright 2009, Mikhail Tchkheidze. Used under license from Shutterstock.com.

Figure 12-6: Image copyright 2009, Cora Reed. Used under license from Shutterstock.com

Figure 12-7: Image copyright 2009, Terry Walsh. Used under license from Shutterstock.com.

Figure 12-9: Image copyright 2009, Gina Sanders. Used under license from Shutterstock.com.

Chapter Opener Images

Chapters 1, 4 to 12: Photography by Yanik Chauvin.

Chapter 2: Image copyright 2009, Stephen Coburn. Used under license from Shutterstock.com.

Chapter 3: Image copyright 2009, Ruben Paz Coburn. Used under license from Shutterstock.com.

Cover Images

Leaf: Image copyright 2009, Italianestro. Used under license from Shutterstock.com.

All other cover images: Photography by Yanik Chauvin.

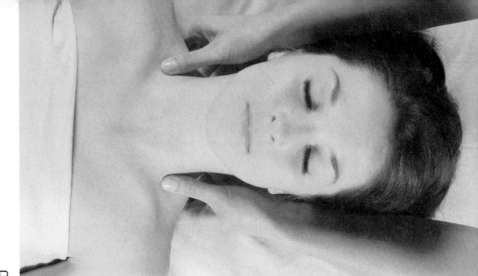

1

CHAPTER

Introduction to the Three Paradigms of Practice

CHAPTER GOALS

1. Define the meaning of the term paradigm.
2. Discuss the meaning and use of paradigms in academic and professional education and training.
3. Discuss the Taoist principle that helps to explain the meaning of the term paradigm.
4. List and describe the Three Paradigms of massage therapy.
5. List and describe the degrees of attention.
6. List and describe the Three Levels of Competence.
7. Discuss the importance of directed attention in the development of a massage therapist.
8. Discuss the evolutionary process of a massage therapist.
9. Explain the importance of compassion and the desire to help others for massage therapists.

INTRODUCTION

The word **paradigm** comes from a Greek word meaning "example," "pattern," or "model." By the mid-seventeenth century, the word was used very specifically as a grammatical term, and from about the 1960s forward, it took on an expanded meaning and began being frequently used in the context of science and other disciplines, referring to thought patterns that sought to understand the limits of human knowledge.

Currently, a paradigm can be thought of as a worldview or a shared way of seeing. It is a philosophical and theoretical framework or perspective through which we see and interpret the world. A paradigm is based upon a core body of knowledge and related underlying theories, principles, and laws that shape our experiences, beliefs, and values. All of this combines to affect the way we perceive reality. Ultimately, the paradigm guides and directs our actions, and these actions have real results in the world.

The term paradigm has many different applications and is often applied to theories of the universe. In this book it is being used to help describe the scope of the "universe of possible practice" of the field of massage therapy. This framework defines and explains the range and limits of education and technical training of therapists whose work is rooted in one, two, or all three of the paradigms that comprise the profession of massage therapy.

The Three Paradigms are

1. Relaxation and stress reduction
2. Remediation, therapy, and pain relief
3. Holistic Integration

This chapter also presents the idea that related to each paradigm there are Three Levels of Competence that can define a practitioner's relationship to their paradigm of practice. These levels are characterized by personal effort and degree of attention. Whereas the Three Paradigms define and describe the possible scope and extent of therapeutic education, training, and practice that exist within the field, the Three Levels of Competence define and describe the level of depth, skill, and overall ability with which massage therapists perform their work, regardless of paradigm.

PARADIGMS IN ACADEMIC AND PROFESSIONAL EDUCATION AND TRAINING

There is always a paradigm at the root of any field or health profession. Different levels or degrees of academic and professional education and training are a direct expression of the extent to which a specific paradigm has been encompassed, that is, studied and put into practice. The fields that have larger bodies of information and skills to study and master often have a continuum of defined levels in which students can choose to either finish their training and education at a certain point along the continuum or move through all levels to attain the highest degree of training in a particular field. These levels or degrees are usually defined by the length, depth, and detail to which a subject, content area, or entire field has been mastered. In an academic environment, successful completion of these levels is recognized by awarding certificates, diplomas, associate's degrees, bachelor's degrees, master's degrees, and doctoral degrees (Figure 1-1).

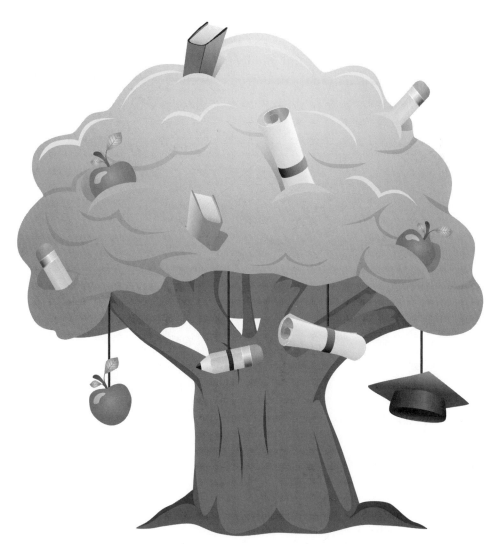

Figure 1-1 Composed of the trunk, main branches, and many sub-branches and leaves, "The Paradigm Tree" reflects a whole that is greater than the sum of its parts.

Image copyright 2009, Sabri Deniz Kizil. Used under license from shutterstock.com.

For example, this can be seen in the nursing profession—the associate's degree-level nurse is the licensed practical nurse, or LPN. The four-year bachelor's in nursing is the registered nurse, or RN. There is also the graduate-level nurse and/or nurse practitioner, or NP which is often taught at the master's degree level, and, finally, the doctoral degree nurse, or Ph.D. Each of these degrees suggests a different level of scope of practice and reflects that part of the paradigm or continuum of education the training has encompassed. A scope of practice describes the limits of professional practice, including the procedures, actions, and processes that are permitted for practice by law (Figure 1-2).

Many of the allied health and medical professions today, including massage therapy, now encompass numerous specialties and subspecialty areas of practice that require continued education and training. With greater

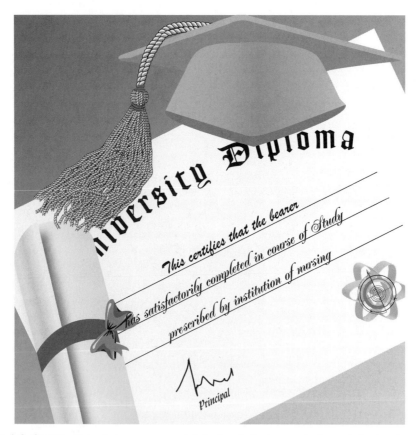

Figure 1-2 Certificates, diplomas, associate's, bachelor's, master's and doctorate degrees encompass increasingly larger parts of The Paradigm Tree.

education and training usually comes greater responsibility, greater technical skills and abilities, and a much deeper and broader level of understanding of the field itself. The assumption is also that a practitioner's competence level has increased as a result of the more prolonged personal efforts made to encompass more of the paradigm by completing longer, more involved, and more complex programs of study.

At this time there are no national standards for the educational requirements of massage therapists and the laws that govern the practice of massage therapy vary from state to state. Educational requirements may vary from 300 to 1000 hours of training depending upon the state one is training in. Programs that offer an associate's degree are usually somewhere between 1200 and 1300 hours when the 60 or more credits are transposed into hours. The **National Certification Board of Therapeutic Massage and Bodywork** (NCBTMB) recommends a minimum of 500 hours of classroom training. The current trend is moving towards a minimum of 600 hours and more. NCBTMB guidelines recommend that the subjects included in massage training should be anatomy, physiology, pathology, business practices, massage technique, and ethics.

Understanding Paradigms through Taoism

In **Taoism,** an ancient Chinese philosophy, there is a fundamental principle that helps to explain the idea of paradigms. It is the principle that *Li* (pronounced "lee") precedes *Qi* (pronounced "chee"). It means that Li, the underlying notion or idea of anything, must first come into existence before it can become manifest into material being through Qi, the energy or vital force used to bring it into reality. In short, idea precedes manifestation. For example, before a skyscraper can be built it first comes into existence as an idea (Li) in the mind of its architect, who then puts all the detail down on paper to create blueprints of the building. The blueprints are then brought to life through the energy (Qi) of the builders, who turn it into a three-dimensional physical reality (Figure 1-3).

So in a sense the Li of anything is really like an invisible blueprint. This parallels very closely the idea of paradigms and how ultimately what manifests through a massage therapist's hands will be a reflection of how well they have developed the Li of understanding their paradigm of practice.

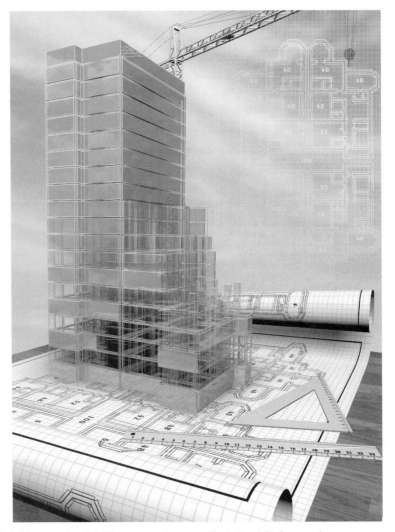

Figure 1-3 Li precedes Qi. Idea precedes manifestation! Before a skyscraper can be built, it first comes into existence as an idea in the mind of its architect, who then creates detailed blueprints of the building. *Image copyright 2009, Yakobchuk Vasyl. Used under license from shutterstock.com.*

As massage therapy students evolve into professional practitioners, they absorb and then integrate their training and practical experiences into a kind of blueprint of understanding. With the right attention and efforts, this understanding grows into a comprehensive framework or paradigm that equals the efforts they have made to embrace their education and hone their technical skills. In the end, it's the clients and patients who become the fortunate recipients of the paradigm of practice that emanates as intention (or Li) through their massage therapist's hands (Figure 1-4).

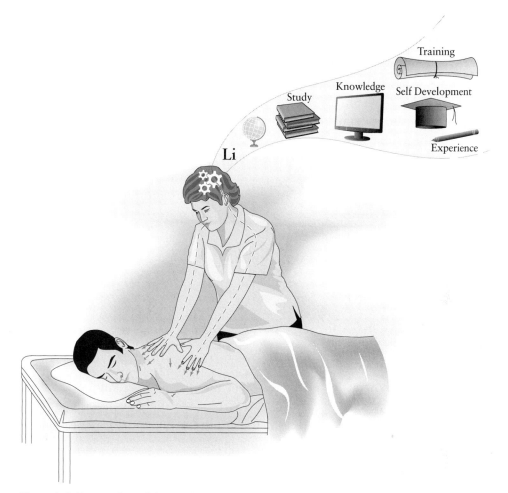

Figure 1-4 Expression of the understanding of one's Paradigm reflecting through the hands of a skilled massage therapist.

In the United States, 43 of the 50 states and the District of Columbia regulate the practice of massage therapy. Depending on the state where a practitioner resides, additional requirements beyond school and examinations may be necessary in order to receive a license to practice. Do not confuse an academic certificate, diploma, or degree that one has earned through the successful completion of a rigorous course of study at an accredited academic institution with a license to practice that profession in a state. State licensing is concerned primarily with public safety, not academic excellence. Its role is to assure the public that those who are licensed to practice a profession in their state are trained to minimal competence and to do no harm.

THE THREE PARADIGMS OF MASSAGE THERAPY

In the second part of this book, specifically Chapters 6 through 10, the broad spectrum of massage therapy and bodywork approaches is discussed, providing a new and unique model for organizing and understanding the existing modalities practiced today. Twenty-six of the most popular and effective approaches have been detailed and grouped within one of four levels. This model is based upon the concept that humans, just like the universe we live in, are composed of a continuum of layers of energy and matter. It demonstrates how the main intention of each massage modality is primarily to treat and affect one of the four levels or layers of the energy/matter continuum of the human mind-body (see Figure 6-3).

The Four Layers are

1. Somatic
2. Somato-psychic
3. Bioenergetic
4. Energetic

Organizing the many varied disciplines and modalities of massage and bodywork therapy into four separate layers provides an easy way to comprehend the *breadth* of the field of the massage and bodywork therapy profession. In order to properly present the scope, or *depth*, of the field of massage therapy and bodywork, it is necessary to begin the important and more philosophically oriented discussion of the Three Paradigms from which massage therapy can be practiced.

The Three Paradigms together form an overlapping continuum of potential practice and treatment, beginning at the most basic levels of touch and leading to the most comprehensive and advanced levels of therapeutic treatment and holistic care practiced in bodywork today. A proper understanding of the paradigms provides comprehension and insight into the full scope of massage therapy practice and its many positive, healthful benefits and outcomes.

The idea of different paradigms in massage therapy is one that is intimately bound to the length and depth of successful education and training, continuing education, and the extent of a therapist's practical experience in treatment (Figure 1-5).

The First Paradigm—Relaxation and Stress Reduction

The most basic level of practice is described by the **First Paradigm**—Relaxation and Stress Reduction. At this level the aims and goals of all education and

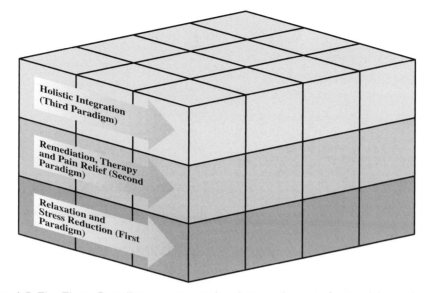

Holistic Integration
(Third Paradigm)

Remediation, Therapy
and Pain Relief (Second
Paradigm)

Relaxation and
Stress Reduction (First
Paradigm)

Figure 1-5 The Three Paradigms as an overlapping continuum of potential practice and treatment, beginning at the most basic and leading to the most advanced levels of practice.

training, regardless of the particular approach of massage therapy studied, are taught within a context that views bodywork as a personal consumer service. This level of treatment is based on the well-researched need for non-threatening, nurturing touch and is not targeted toward treating or healing specific conditions (Figure 1-6). Regular massage and bodywork therapy treatment that is geared toward First Paradigm relaxation and stress reduction lends itself well to preventative health care programs designed to restore, maintain, and help slow down the overall physical and mental degeneration that humans naturally experience and that can often lead to a state of disease. First Paradigm hands-on work is noninvasive, relaxing, pleasurable, and stress reducing.

In the 2008 Massage Therapy Consumer Survey Fact Sheet, sponsored by the American Massage Therapy Association, 59 percent of those surveyed indicated that they were more stressed then the year prior. The economic situation was cited as the source of most stress for 45 percent of Americans, according to the survey. Fifty-five percent of those ages 25 through 34 were "greatly stressed" by the current economic situation and 51 percent of women of all ages agreed. The survey also indicated that Americans are seeking out massage therapy treatment for relaxation and reduction of stress more than in

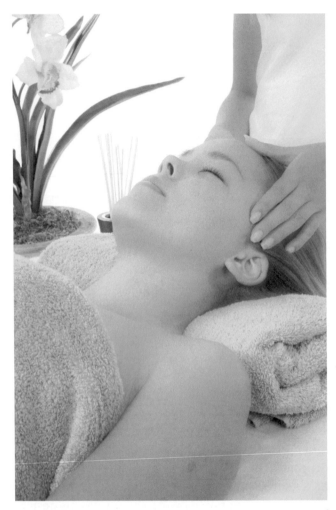

Figure 1-6 Woman receiving First Paradigm massage therapy treatment for relaxation and stress reduction in a spa setting. *Image copyright 2009, Stephen Coburn. Used under license from shutterstock.com.*

past years. Also expressed in the survey was another important statistic stating that 36 percent of the American public had received massage therapy for the specific purpose of stress relief and relaxation, compared to the 22 percent reported the year before. The survey also indicated that 38 percent of Americans considered the possibility of seeking out massage therapy treatment for the purpose of managing their stress (AMTA, 2008). Amazingly these statistics occurred despite the collapse of the housing and financial markets that occurred in that year.

Some of the primary physical and emotional benefits of relaxation and stress reduction include, but are not limited to

- satisfying the client's need for caring, nurturing touch.
- relieving stress and aiding in relaxation of the mind-body complex.
- helping reduce mental stress.
- calming the nervous system of the body.
- relieving tired, aching muscles, muscle tension and stiffness.
- increasing joint flexibility.
- increasing range of motion.
- reducing headaches related to muscle tension and stress.
- promoting deeper and easier breathing, which helps to increase overall vitality.
- improving circulation of blood and movement of lymph fluids.
- improving posture.
- promoting restful sleep.
- fostering peace of mind.
- improving the ability to better focus and concentrate the mind.
- reducing chronic pain.
- reducing levels of anxiety.
- increasing awareness of the mind-body connection.

These extremely positive benefits, accomplished at the level of First Paradigm treatment, require minimal training in the basics of western science, assessment, treatment principles, technique, knowledge of scope of practice, and knowing when to refer to another health care practitioner, such as a physician, chiropractor, or psychologist. Generally speaking, the average 500-hour training program covers the First Paradigm of massage therapy practice and often can begin covering the education and training necessary for Second Paradigm practice—remediation, therapy, and pain relief.

The Second Paradigm—Remediation, Therapy, and Pain Relief

This level of practice is described by the **Second Paradigm**—Remediation, Therapy, and Pain Relief. At this level the aims and goals of all education and training, regardless of the particular massage therapy approach studied, are taught within a context that views massage therapy and bodywork as a

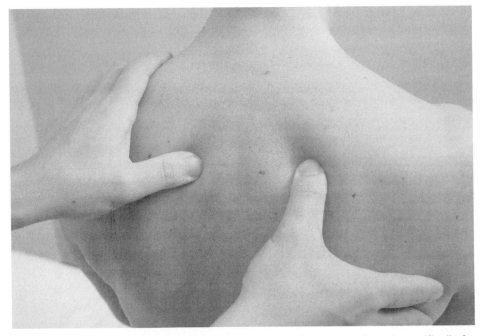

Figure 1-7 Man receiving Second Paradigm massage therapy treatment specifically for pain due to a shoulder injury. *Image copyright 2009, Ruben Paz Coburn. Used under license from shutterstock.com.*

means toward the correction of human dysfunction and remediation of pain (Figure 1-7).

Although the range of conditions treated and the methods and techniques used by different approaches may vary, the following is a general and brief list of specific conditions that Second Paradigm practitioners may treat:

- Back pain
- Sprains or strains
- Injuries
- Sports injuries
- Post-operative or post-traumatic adhesions
- Restricted range of motion
- Pain due to postural imbalances
- Muscular imbalances
- Headaches

- Menstrual disorders
- Digestive difficulties, constipation, irritable bowel syndrome (IBS)
- Arthritic joint pain and stiffness
- Sleep disorders

Millions of Americans suffer from pain, resulting in increased visits to physicians and other health care practitioners. The effects of pain can result in the repeated loss of sleep and the ingestion of all sorts of toxic pain medications in addition to exhaustion, irritability, and the buildup of stress from having to endure the pain throughout one's working day.

According to the 2008 Massage Therapy Industry Survey commissioned by the American Massage Therapy Association, the country's largest professional association of massage therapists, more people than ever are seeking massage for the purpose of remediation therapy to manage and relieve their pain. The survey indicates that almost one-third of the adult American population reported that they have used massage therapy at least once for pain relief. It also indicates that of Americans who have had at least one massage in the last five years, 30 percent reported that they did so specifically for health conditions such as pain management, injury rehabilitation, migraine headache control, or overall wellness. And when asked, 87 percent of those surveyed agreed that massage can be effective in reducing pain.

The same survey also indicated that research over the last five years has found that there are therapeutic benefits of massage therapy for cancer related fatigue, chronic low back pain, osteoarthritis of the knee, post surgical pain, and decreasing the symptoms of carpal tunnel syndrome. The survey also stated that more people recognize massage therapy as an important element in their overall health care regimens (AMTA, 2008b).

Other clinical research on the efficacy of massage for the treatment of pain management has also shown that it can

- be more effective for chronic back pain than other complementary therapies.[1]
- promote relaxation and alleviate the perception of pain and anxiety in cancer patients.[2]
- reduce post-traumatic headaches better than cold-pack treatments.[3]
- lessen pain and muscle spasms in patients who have undergone heart bypass surgery when part of hospital-based surgery treatment.[4]
- stimulate the brain to produce endorphins.[5]

In addition, the 2008 Massage Therapy Industry Fact Sheet reported a 30 percent increase in the number of hospitals using massage therapy from 2004 to 2006 and that 67 percent of those hospitals use massage therapy for pain management.[6]

Given that the primary purposes and goals of Second Paradigm treatment are for the remediation of pain, its practice therefore requires a more advanced level of knowledge of the western sciences, as well as increased training and skills in hand techniques, assessment, treatment principles, and evaluation of client conditions. In addition, more advanced training specific to the modality being used is also necessary. For example, if the Second Paradigm practitioner is using **shiatsu**, a form of Asian bodywork, an in-depth study of Asian **anatomy** and **physiology**, including a thorough understanding of the energetic channels and point system, a series of stimulating and sedating hands-on techniques, and a variety of specific treatment patterns must be studied in order to provide remediation of various conditions.

The average 500-hour training program will begin to introduce the knowledge, skills, and abilities necessary for the Second Paradigm of massage therapy practice. Depending on which particular massage therapy modality is being taught, the program may even provide some of the more advanced training necessary for competence at this level. In addition, since educational standards in U.S. schools have been rising beyond the 500-hour minimum, to anywhere between 600 to 1000 hours, even two-year associate's degrees (more than 1200 hours) in which the increased hours are used for additional massage theory and technique training practitioners at Second Paradigm levels has become more common.

The Third Paradigm—Holistic or Integrative

This level of practice is described by the **Third Paradigm**—Holistic or Integrative. At this level of practice the aims and goals of all education and training, regardless of the particular approach of touch therapy studied, are taught within a context that views massage therapy and bodywork as a means of preventive and proactive health care. The focus here is on a more overall approach to enhancing, balancing, and transforming the quality of life of the patient.

A *holistic* practice is one that affirms the need to understand human health from a broad perspective and incorporates the principles of holism, a philosophy which emphasizes the fundamental idea that "the whole is greater than the sum of its parts." It expresses the unity of mind and body and understands that people are not simply a collection of different parts, but represent something far more complex and profound, integrating numerous complex systems that result in a living human being. A holistic approach to health care uses many complementary and integrative therapies as part of its arsenal of healing.

Generally speaking, when a recipient is being treated by a practitioner of the Third Paradigm, relaxation, stress reduction, and remediation of pain—the primary aims and goals of the first two paradigms—are often byproducts of the overall transformation that the patient experiences through Third Paradigm treatment. Third Paradigm practice requires the most extensive training and years of experience in the field (Figure 1-8).

Although primarily focused on massage and bodywork therapies, professionals practicing the **Holistic** or **Integrative paradigm** are more likely to seriously incorporate the use of nutritional counseling, vitamins, supplementation, herbs, exercise, movement, meditation and mind-body integration into their practices. Clearly then, there is a need for additional education and training. It is not uncommon to find Third Paradigm massage therapy practitioners holding dual licensure in other professions, as well as other certifications in adjunctive forms of manual therapy. For example, many nurses (RNs) have become very skilled licensed massage therapists, expanding their scope of practice by integrating their knowledge, skills, and abilities of both worlds and becoming nurse massage therapists (NMTs). There is a national organization called The National Association of Nurse Massage Therapists whose membership is specifically for nurses that practice massage. Many massage therapists who practice Asian bodywork as their main form of touch also become licensed in **acupuncture** and/or nationally certified in Chinese herbal medicine, covering the bases of health care from an Asian medical point of view. More and more personal trainers, who are experts in fitness and exercise and sometimes also in nutrition and supplementation, are becoming practitioners of massage. From this vantage point, these professionals offer a wide array of services to their patients, often bringing their services right into their patient's home.

While there are numerous possible professional combinations, the point to be stressed is that Third Paradigm practitioners usually have an arsenal of adjunctive services, techniques, methods, and ways of assisting their clients to improve their health, prevent disease, and maintain a balanced body with a healthy state of mind. In a way, it can be said that these practitioners bring more to the table for their clients than simply massage and in doing so broaden their market and potential for success. However, being a Third Paradigm practitioner does not in any way guarantee success or that such a practitioner will make more money than a First Paradigm therapist working in a busy, high-end clinic or spa.

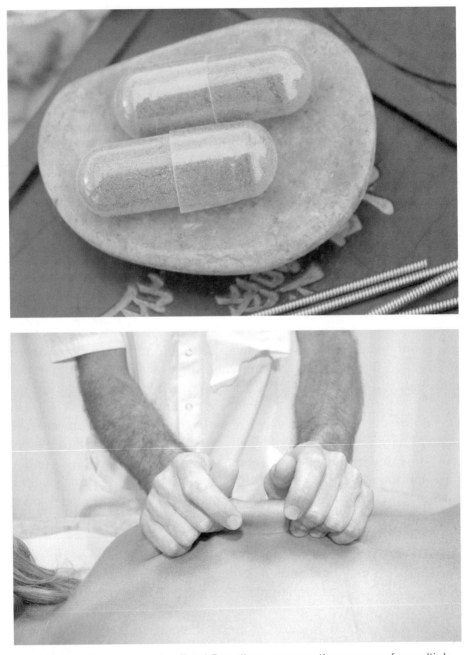

Figure 1-8a & b Woman receiving Third Paradigm massage therapy care for multiple sclerosis (MS), an autoimmune disease that attacks the central nervous system, using a combination of tuina, acupuncture, herbs, vitamins, and supplements. *Image copyright 2009, Elana Ray. Used under license from shutterstock.com. Image copyright 2009, Salamanderman. Used under license from shutterstock.com.*

Depending upon the treatment approach used, practitioners of the Third Paradigm may appear very different in what they actually do for their patients. However, at this level it is not so much what is specifically done or what type of massage therapy techniques are utilized but rather the outcomes the practitioners are seeking for their patients.

Third Paradigm practitioners are better prepared and generally more able and willing to take on more serious cases. Therefore, they often will treat more complex conditions. Along with this level of responsibility and commitment there must also be a willingness on the part of these therapists to take responsibility for their patients by consistently following through with them even outside of the treatment room when necessary. Often this may include phone calls to their patients to see how they are doing; contacting other health care professionals for assistance or more information; and researching their patient's condition, looking up medications, herbs, supplements, and vitamins the patient may be taking for any possible side-effects, interactions with other medications, and **contraindications** for treatment. This may also include preparing patients for doctor visits by providing them with pertinent questions related to their conditions so that they are better able to make educated decisions.

Unlike most practitioners in the First Paradigm, who generally treat the same client only once or very infrequently, the patients of Second and Third Paradigm massage therapy practitioners are often regular clients, placing their health, at least in part, under the care of Second and Third Paradigm massage therapists. Such practitioners must always be aware that another human being's health has been entrusted to them. This must be regarded with great seriousness.

Taking responsibility for patients must also include a practitioner's ability to maintain all professional boundaries and emotional objectivity. At the same time, these therapists must work to reach deep inside to manifest empathy and compassion as they reach out to understand the suffering, pain, and difficulties that are being experienced by their patients.

Personal opinions, viewpoints, judgments, or any expression of negative emotion have no place in the therapist–patient relationship. This of course generally applies to practitioners across the board of any paradigm, but becomes an area of greater concern for therapists in the Second and Third Paradigms of practice. These practitioners tend to see the same patients regularly, sometimes for years and for far more serious conditions, and often become privy to the most intimate details of their patient's lives. Sometimes, however, such therapist–patient relationships can begin to seriously break down.

As more and more boundaries are crossed, the tendency toward manifesting less-professional behavior patterns becomes greater, and the important foundation of that therapeutic relationship is lost. Here the old saying that "Familiarity breeds contempt" rings very true!

In addition, it often becomes the role of the Second, and even more so, the Third Paradigm massage practitioner, to suggest, encourage, and cajole, if necessary, to assist patients in making the changes that their treatments and health care programs necessitate. In order to effectively do this, practitioners must be cultivating themselves as role models for their patients. They should never require their patients to follow a regimen that they themselves have not tested or have thoroughly researched. Practitioners must maintain objectivity and never judge their patients for their lifestyle or inability to make changes, for example in diet or exercise. Practitioners need to manifest the utmost patience and concern, gently and consistently nudging their patients in the proper direction. Second and particularly Third Paradigm practitioners form partnerships with their patients through which patients are educated to better understand their condition and are taught to value their health. Practitioners must see themselves in their patients, "stand in their patients' shoes," in order to develop true compassion and self-cultivation.

It is important to emphasize that defining The Three Paradigms in massage therapy is for the purpose of describing the continuum of practice that exists today. The field has evolved dramatically over the last 30 or so years and continues to transform at quite a rapid pace. Describing what lies along the continuum of practice does not imply that practicing from one paradigm or point on the continuum is better or worse than practicing from another. The term *level,* sometimes used interchangeably with *paradigm,* may give the impression that one mode of practice is higher or lower than the other, and mistakenly may be understood to mean better or worse. However, a therapist's level or paradigm of practice really concerns the portion of the continuum of education and training practitioners have encompassed within their particular massage therapy and bodywork discipline. Without any judgment, the description of the continuum of practice simply reflects a view of the field and provides a road map for students, practitioners, clients, and patients to locate where they stand within the context of the entire massage therapy profession. It also provides a direction for those who wish to continue their evolution in the profession, helping them to envision a goal to be attained.

As you will see next, what defines a therapist's true level of competence and quality of professional practice has most to do with the *ability to pay attention* than with which one of the Three Paradigms he or she may practice from or what particular massage therapy and bodywork techniques are used.

PARADIGM COMPETENCE

Having completed their training, therapists need to focus on the quality of their techniques and their level of competency. Simply having gone further along the continuum of education (i.e., more hours of training) does not mean that practitioners are more competent. Prospective students and practitioners should also try to avoid the tendency for their training and practices to be "a mile wide and an inch deep." This occurs often because many institutions develop training programs that include a multitude of short courses in different modalities in the hope and mistaken belief that this will somehow have a positive outcome for the graduate and for the school. Although it may look appealing and exciting to an uneducated, prospective enrollee (as in "look at all I'm going to learn if I enroll in this program"), it more often than not produces a program that turns out graduates weak in the fundamentals and the technical competencies of treatment. Certainly, it's not simply the amount of hours of training or the number of different massage techniques learned that make competent practitioners. The focus of this chapter will now turn to the characteristics that do.

There are basically Three Levels of Competence of practice. Each one of these competence levels can be directly characterized by a different degree of attention. The more focused, concentrated and directed a practitioner's degree of attention, the greater and more profound his or her competency. The advanced stages of practice within any of the three paradigms of massage therapy are impossible without focused attention. Therefore before we can get to the detailed explanations of 'The Three Levels of Competence' listed below, an understanding of different attention levels is necessary.

The Three Levels of Competence are

1. Practicing *Without* a Paradigm
2. Practicing *From* a Paradigm
3. *Being* the Paradigm.

It's a Matter of Attention

When massage therapists' attention is weak and scattered, their treatments will also be weak and scattered, regardless of the techniques being used or the paradigm they are practicing from. When massage therapists' attention is strong, directed, and concentrated, their treatments will be strong, directed, and concentrated as well and will produce profound results. Treatments from a therapist who is focused and present and whose intention is clear will invariably result in quicker and more definitive physical and psychological benefits for his or her clients and patients.

What is most significant in this context is the therapist's internal world. When massage therapists become so wrapped up in their own personal considerations during treating—be they positive or negative—there isn't much room for the client or indeed anything else. The more therapists practice being present in the moment, learn how to direct their attention, and are able to put aside their personal issues during treatment times, the more they can begin to see and hear unfiltered reality from the quietness of their inner state.

This translates into

- increased sensitivity because therapists are able to feel much more going on when they palpate and treat the body without their own emotional interference.
- gathering necessary and more accurate information about each patient prior to treatment.
- making more accurate assessments.
- developing more effective treatment plans.
- having greater access to the knowledge and principles of their paradigm of practice to draw upon when the mind is calm and free from distraction.

Basic attention can generally be divided into degrees: zero, drawn, and directed attention. Zero and drawn attention are more the "normal" states of attention. That is to say, they occur naturally and automatically, requiring no effort of will or mind. Directed attention, on the other hand, is not a given state of attention, although we like to think it is. It must be cultivated through consistent effort and practice. Directed attention requires an effort of both will and mind.

The Three Degrees of Attention

1. Zero
2. Drawn
3. Directed

Zero Attention and Massage Therapy Practice

People often go through their daily lives with very little attention to what is happening around and inside of them. Occasionally an individual really pays attention to some event, train of thought, or conversation with another person. Quite often, however, after having just finished "listening" to a person talk one may realize one did not hear a word that was uttered. Everyone has had the experience of reading several paragraphs, perhaps even pages in this book, and then "waking up" and realizing that, although every single word had been read, they could not recall any meaning of anything on those pages. This degree of attention is called **zero attention**. It is a state in which the mind wanders from place to place, like a feather blowing in the wind, while the physical body goes through the external motions of carrying on the appearance of paying attention, as in the example above—reading a book, eyes moving across every sentence, turning the pages, but having no awareness of anything read.

When massage therapy practitioners are functioning from this state of attention while treating their clients, regardless of what paradigm they are working from, very little is taking place other than the fact that their bodies are mechanically going through the motions of treating. This is not unlike reading the pages in a book word for word but never really being present enough to know what was read. So like a well-trained machine doing what it does, the practitioner, without really being present, performs all the techniques, converses when necessary with the client, makes recommendations and suggestions, sets up another appointment, and goes through all the motions to complete the session.

Many clients may not notice the difference, though often those who have been treated by different therapists at more advanced levels of competence will most certainly notice that something was missing from the treatment and more than likely will choose not to return.

Drawn Attention and Massage Therapy Practice

Drawn attention is the state of attention that is drawn or pulled to a particular object, event, or task. *Pulled* is the operative word; the implication is that the person is not in charge of his or her attention. Rather, attention is being drawn or pulled to the object of attraction like a magnet. This degree of attention has a strong emotional involvement related to whatever the object of attention may be. In this state of emotional involvement, there really is not much freedom to attend to anything other than what the draw is. The problem is that it *feels* like we are choosing to pay attention or deal with whatever we wish. In fact, in those moments it is difficult to attend to anything other than what and where the mind is being pulled by the emotions of the moment.

Personal likes and dislikes generally become the major determining factors responsible for where and in which ways attention is drawn. Some common examples of drawn attention are reflected in expressions such as "I stayed up all night watching television, even though I had to get up early this morning, because I was *glued* to the TV screen"; "The time passed so quickly because I was so *immersed* in what I was doing"; " The boxing match was great, *I could not take my eyes off it*." All these statements describe a strong emotional attraction and pull toward a particular object or event, suggesting that there is something involuntary about this common state of attention that often dominates the mind.

For the massage therapist this degree of attention is a double-edged sword. On one hand it plays a necessary part in a practitioner's evolution. It fuels the attraction, the reason, the draw, and is the result of the emotions behind why a person has decided to become a massage therapist in the first place. It certainly plays a positive and important role in continuing to drive and evolve a massage therapist's relationship to and love of the art. Most often, drawn attention will support the aims and goals of therapists allowing them to joyfully embrace and focus on their paradigm and be encouraged to practice by evolving their ability to direct and concentrate attention, thus becoming a superior practitioner.

However, drawn attention left to the whims of personal likes and dislikes of the moment can cause a loss of objectivity and a breach of ethics in which the practitioner crosses the boundaries of the client–therapist relationship. This can lead to inappropriate behavior on numerous levels, such as when a sexual attraction occurs and a therapist forgets the professional boundaries that must be maintained, or in the case of an aversion (negative attraction) to a client in which the therapist allows repulsive feelings to dictate and overrule the professional code of ethics. This can result in poor treatment and client neglect. Other forms of drawn attention that are common occur when a therapist's emotional and personal issues, relationship difficulties, financial stresses, or any other disturbances draw the attention away from what should be the practitioner's primary focus— the therapeutic aim, goal, and execution of the treatment of the moment.

Directed Attention and Massage Therapy Practice

The real control of attention means being able to direct attention at will. It is the ability to choose to focus on any object or activity, idea or topic, word or phrase, or body part, without being pulled or drawn away by intruding emotions, thoughts, or any outside activity. Unlike zero and drawn attention, **directed attention** has a more developed and stronger level of intention behind it. For example, by desiring and striving to become an attorney, Olympic athlete, neurosurgeon, business executive, or massage and body-work therapist, there is a purpose in directing the attention to the enormous amount of study, learning, memorization, training, and skill development required to accomplish the goal. A great deal of energy is required to attain the goal, although the person would probably like nothing more than to relax or pursue trivial pleasures.

For massage and bodywork therapists, directing attention is the primary means of attaining their treatment goals, regardless of what paradigm they practice from. In spite of how much there is inside an individual that opposes focusing and holding attention on an object of concentration, in the case of massage therapy treatment, practitioners must have and hold an *aim* for what they wish to accomplish for their patients. Then they must willfully and repeatedly direct and return their attention over and over again to that aim. This is the means that leads to success. Since attention automatically tends to wander, massage therapy practitioners must recognize that unless they can purposefully direct and redirect their attention, they will be unable to truly attain their goals.

Now that we have an understanding of the different types or degrees of attention, we can further explore how they correlate to the Three Levels of Competence.

First Level of Competence: Practicing *Without* a Paradigm *(Zero Attention)*

A declaration of "Practicing *without* a Paradigm" is really another way of saying that the massage and bodywork practitioner is in a state of disconnect from the goals and principles of the paradigm. It is a reflection of zero attention. In this state of zero attention, massage therapy treatment is being done in a vacuum, without a relationship to the foundations of one's education and aims in treating. Therapists practicing from a zero state of attention are generally functioning like good machines, without intention, going through all the motions but with no one really present to direct in the moment.

Most often this level or stage of competence is where novice practitioners, that is, recent graduates, find themselves. Some never leave this level while others pass through it on their way to greater levels of competency. It is a normal transition for motivated beginner practitioners who struggle with transforming all they have learned into technical expertise expressed through their hands. These practitioners make concerted efforts to remain aware of and build upon the foundations of what they were taught. They integrate and infuse their practice with new insights, experience, and continued education to move past the beginning level. These efforts require an inner struggle to direct attention to the paradigm and aim. If a beginning practitioner strives to think about, ponder, remember, and apply all of this in their ongoing practice, they will grow and move into the next stage of competence relative to their paradigm.

Practicing *without* a paradigm can also be the result of a loss of focus due to "burnout." Seasoned practitioners can and often do experience stress and exhaustion from pushing themselves to treat more and more clients, sometimes running from place to place and ignoring their own health needs. When this takes place the joy and love of the art previously infusing a practitioner's treatments is turned off like a faucet, leaving practitioners dry and with nothing more to give to their clients. At this point dealing with clients' complaints and concerns as well as treating them becomes an imposition and a burden. Once this happens there is a loss of purpose and connection to the paradigm. This may be a good time for a well-deserved vacation or for enrolling in a continuing education seminar to reinject therapists with the joy and love of the art. This will remind them why they became massage and bodywork therapists to begin with.

Every massage therapist, regardless of their paradigm of practice, forms habits and patterns of treating after doing what they have done for years. Therapists can easily become fixed in their method of treatment and reach a point of stagnation. This doesn't mean that practitioners are not doing a good job overall. Many have reached a high level of skill and consistently get wonderful results. However, if nothing is done to continue to cultivate their skills, then they will begin to lose what they have gained. What's worse is that often therapists may not even realize they are stagnating until they begin to notice that their practice is dwindling.

Brushing up on old knowledge and techniques after years of experience will often lead to greater and deeper insight into what practitioners already know and do. Seeking to continually perfect their treatments, like an artist evolving into a master, will have a wonderful effect on their practice and will immediately reflect positively in their treatments. Expanding one's knowledge and technical base with training in new specialty areas is another powerful way to enhance levels of skill and breathe new life into practice. The trends in the massage field are changing rapidly. Therapists getting stuck in old patterns and habits may think that they know enough or that they are good enough run the risk of being quietly left behind. The speed at which the therapeutic massage and bodywork profession is moving is so fast that therapists must really work to keep up!

Without at least drawn attention to fuel the desire to continue to evolve in whatever way the therapist chooses, very little will change. A massage and bodywork therapist can take hundreds of hours of continuing education and spend thousands of dollars, but if it is done from that same empty, unmotivated, aimless place of zero attention, then little benefit will be gained except perhaps another certificate and the necessary continuing education credits to maintain certification and licensure. Within a short period of time, any newly gained enthusiasm and skills to grow and improve quickly wanes as the therapist slips quietly back into old treating patterns and habits, integrating little or nothing taught during any seminar or workshop.

Massage therapy and bodywork practitioners owe it to themselves as professionals to continue learning and training in their chosen profession. It is vital that all therapists hold a view that it is their personal and professional responsibility to seek continuing education in order to keep growing in their knowledge, skills, and abilities. Most of all, practitioners owe it to their clients and patients who depend on them for the best and most effective treatments possible, regardless of the paradigm or particular approach used. Therapists should make it their personal commitment to seek self-improvement and continue to serve their clients and patients with compassion, safety, and competency.

Second Level of Competence: Practicing *From* a Paradigm (*Drawn Attention*)

When therapists are "Practicing *from* a Paradigm" it usually indicates that they are more present and engaged in the process. In such a state there is a positive emotional or drawn component of their attention being pulled to the ideas, techniques, and principles of their paradigm and there is a joy in practicing. They are making concerted efforts during the treatment process to bring to bear and integrate in the moment what they have studied, learned, and experienced thus far. These therapists may have even signed on for further study with a mentor, a teacher of high skill, who they can apprentice with and get regular correction and direction. Since each patient is different in body and mind, often seeking different outcomes from the treatment process and usually presenting with a different set of symptoms or conditions, it becomes obvious that the therapist will have to dig deeper into his or her experience and paradigm, even seek out the experience of a mentor or expert, to always be able to provide patients with what they need and want.

It should be clear that there is a big difference between the First and Second Levels of Competence. Practitioners and their clients alike should be clear that this difference represents a pathway of potential and profound depth that therapists can and should evolve toward in their practice of massage therapy and bodywork, whatever their particular modality and regardless of their paradigm of practice.

Since what is being described here are levels of competence, it is important to remember that practitioners functioning from this competence level may also be at different places in the process of their evolution. However, what is clear is that as their evolution within this level begins to grow and deepen, they often touch on places, states, and experiences in the treatment room that border on the transcendental as they begin to enter into the third and highest level of competence, "*Being* the paradigm."

Third Level of Competence: *Being* the Paradigm (*Directed Attention*)

Massage therapy and bodywork practitioners realize the third and highest stage of paradigm competence when the distinction between their paradigm of practice and themselves as therapists dissolves. In other words, the therapist and the paradigm have become one. At such a point in their evolution the intention, compassion, experience, knowledge, skills, and abilities of these therapists have been fully integrated. These practitioners can be said to have truly embodied their paradigm of practice.

At the highest levels of this stage of *Being* the Paradigm, some therapists evolve into true healers, where the level of their attention, intuition, understanding, and sensitivity, no matter what approach and paradigm of practice they are using, has become a powerful, penetrating, almost laser-like force that is manifested and transmitted at will through touch. More often than not, it is this special and high quality of touch channeled through their own personal work and growth that accomplishes the "miracles" both small and large, that we sometimes hear about in this hands-on profession.

When practitioners at the Second Level of Competence begin to enter into this third level of accomplishment, it is most likely a result of long-standing efforts to direct their attention. This is more easily accomplished by having a teacher or mentor to both aspire to and to be critiqued by. As therapists grow and persevere through personal challenges they begin to evolve an overall heightened awareness and sensitivity that can often develop into special healing abilities. This might include a state where the compassion and empathy for their patients have become so focused and integrated with knowledge of their paradigm that they begin to intuitively understand and treat their patient's conditions. In other words, they instinctively and intuitively know what is wrong and what to do and their hands just begin to do it without any real need to specifically refer back to the details, knowledge, or principles of their paradigm. They have transcended knowledge into understanding. It's all present. This most closely expresses the true meaning of "*Being* the Paradigm." Such practitioners could easily be classified as masters or healers in their particular form of practice.

Rare though it may be, some people are born with such abilities and sensitivities already fully developed. Others, however, must move through these Three Levels of Competence and evolve such gifts through years of intense and dedicated practice.

EXERCISES FOR THE DEVELOPMENT OF DIRECTING ATTENTION

The following are three basic exercises for the practice of directed attention. They are presented in an increasing order of difficulty. The first is the simplest and easiest to accomplish, and the last is the most difficult. The degree of difficulty of each exercise is connected mostly to the area or place where the attention is focused. In the first exercise, the attention is focused on an external object. In the second exercise, the attention is focused on a part of the body, requiring that you *sense* it with your mind. In the third exercise, an imaginary object is created and held in the mind. Although these exercises may appear to be very simple, do not be fooled. You will note during practice that they require a consistent effort of will to direct and hold your attention. Accomplishing this will yield great benefits by helping you generally strengthen all mental activities and processes.

Candle Gazing

Place a lighted candle a few feet away from you so that it is in full view. Make sure it is at eye level. Look directly at the flame. Keep your eyes open, allowing them to blink naturally, while thinking and focusing only on the flame. Your attention should be directed and fixed as completely as possible on the flame. When your attention wanders, bring it back immediately to the flame. Try to do this for five minutes. Practicing this exercise will strengthen your ability to direct your attention (Figure 1-9).

Focusing Attention on a Part of the Body

Close your eyes and focus your attention on any body part (e.g., left ear, right hand, lips, nose, eye, solar plexus). Try to feel the area with your mind by bringing all of your attention to that part of your body. You may begin to feel strange sensations, tingling, or even warmth in that area. That is fine and is often a sign of increased energy (Qi) and circulation to that body part. As in the other exercises, once you take note that your attention has wandered off for one or another reason, return it immediately to the body part you are focusing on. Try to hold your attention on the chosen body part for five minutes (Figure 1-10).

Focusing Attention on an Internal Image

Concentrate in your "mind's eye" on a pencil. A pencil (or any simple neutral object) is good to use as a focus of attention because it generally has no particular draw or significance. Look at the clock and make a mental note of the time. Tell yourself that you are going to keep the pencil's image

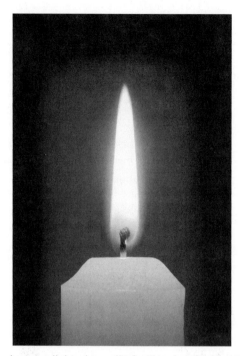

Figure 1-9 Practice staring at a lighted candle for the development of directed attention. *Image copyright 2009, Tatiana Popova. Used under license from shutterstock.com.*

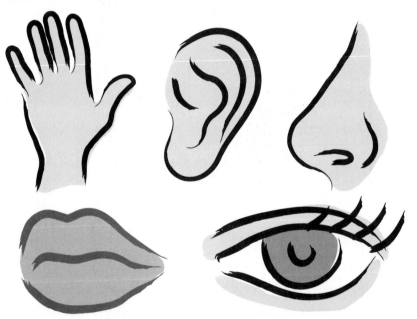

Figure 1-10 Practice internally focusing on a body part for the development of directed attention. *Image copyright 2009, Alex Kalmbach. Used under license from shutterstock.com.*

in your mental focus for five minutes. Prior to beginning, take a real pencil and examine it closely so that you notice the size, shape, color, texture and its various parts. Then close your eyes and create the image of the pencil. Keep your attention fixed on that image. Only the pencil should occupy your attention. Do not think about the time, but make a note of it. After a while you will probably realize that you are thinking of something else. Open your eyes and note the time and then return immediately to holding the image of the pencil. Return immediately to the pencil's image each time you note that your attention has wandered off. Avoid any judgment or self-criticism. Just concentrate (Figure 1-11).

A more advanced aspect of the pencil exercise is learning to trace the cause of your repeated loss of attention. Once you have noted that your attention has wandered, try to find the cause of this. Was it due to a drift in your thoughts beginning with lead, wood, the eraser, or any of the hundred direct associations you made to the pencil? Was it due to the intrusion into the mind of bodily discomfort, disturbed breathing, sensory perceptions through hearing, sight, smell, or touch? Was it due to wondering about something,

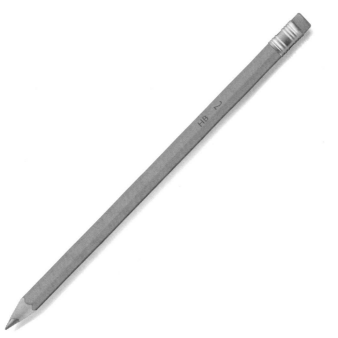

Figure 1-11 Concentrate on an internal image in the mind's eye of a pencil for the development of directed attention. *Image copyright 2009, Leo Blanchette. Used under license from shutterstock.com.*

anxiety, hurt pride, anger, fear, discontentment, worry, or anything of this kind? Whatever it was, work your way backwards to the pencil by following the exact train of thought, in reverse, that took you away from your focus in the first place. In doing this, you will also begin to familiarize yourself with your underlying attitudes, inner patterns, and habits of thought and feeling. This will contribute to developing a clearer understanding of how you take in and alter perceptions.

The above exercises can be done individually or in sequence. It is recommended that if you are a beginner you should work on and master the candle and body-part exercises before moving on to the pencil exercise.

In addition to these exercises, the regular practice of **Tai Chi Chuan, Qi Gong**, or traditional **Hatha Yoga** will build directed attention by using the mind to direct the movements, the breath, and the isolation and relaxation of the muscles. These are profound forms of self-cultivation that can develop directed attention, a calm and peaceful spirit, and an increased sensitivity and healing ability.

THE EVOLUTIONARY PROCESS OF A MASSAGE THERAPIST

There is an evolutionary process that takes place through the Three Levels of Competence, moving from basic proficiency to expert, as therapists grow and embody their paradigms of practice.

Briefly, the process progresses something like this:

1. Large amounts of information and technical skills are taken into the surface of the student practitioner's mind as he or she begins to learn and practice the art and science of massage therapy and bodywork, most often while attending a school for that purpose.

2. The information and techniques are then valued, studied, pondered, practiced, and integrated over time. The results of that integration process move deeper within the practitioner's mind and body and begin transforming into real knowledge and practical expertise—experience.

3. After years of continued, intense, and directed study (often as an apprentice with the guidance of a mentor or master) as well as actual practice, this *knowledge* and *experience* begin to unite and transcend into a level of *true understanding*. At this stage of development a practitioner stands apart from other massage and bodywork therapists because he or she is now truly a living expression of the paradigm of practice. The massage therapist becomes the conduit through which understanding of the paradigm is

expressed through the hands. When a practitioner has reached this level, any of his or her patients can rest assured that they are literally in "good hands." This is an advanced stage of practice that some truly dedicated practitioners aspire to, and even fewer people are born into—that is, the level of the master or healer.

This kind of evolutionary development is a function of the voluntary dedication of therapists to their paradigm of practice and not an automatic, involuntary given of the profession. It is not inherent in the level of the paradigm itself. Instead, growth through these successive levels of competence and passage through the inevitable plateaus that therapists will experience on the way depend on the cumulative development of each practitioner's ongoing efforts to direct his or her attention, integrate the essentials of the paradigm studied and practiced, and his or her willingness to accept correction and guidance from a teacher.

Although this may seem obvious—that is, to study what you are taught in school, apply it well, and pay attention while you practice—it is not uncommon for massage practitioners to fall into the routine of habitually and robotically performing the same or similar treatment over and over again, without paying attention and giving little thought to modifying the treatment to better suit the complaints and needs of their clients and patients. The uneducated client may not even notice, since it still "feels good," and despite the basic nature of such treatment, it may even do some good for the client because of the general benefits that manual therapy brings. Usually, this level of treatment is performed by a beginner in any paradigm who has yet to evolve beyond the first stage of competence. Ideally, in time most such novice practitioners will grow way beyond this form of treatment. Unfortunately, however, there are practitioners who have been in the field for years that have not made the efforts to grow past this point.

As in any health profession, there will be those practitioners who take their studies to more advanced levels than others. Also, there will always be those practitioners who stagnate and never really mature in their fields. In the case of the massage therapy and bodywork profession, such practitioners never grow beyond being a good "machine" or technician. This is not intended as a moral judgement or statement; rather it is a reflection of the developmental level of the practitioners themselves regarding the art and science of massage therapy and its impact on the quality of treatment the practitioner is able to provide. It is important to note from the clients' standpoint that should they want a more serious form of massage therapy care, practitioners who have moved beyond the first level of competence into the second and third levels are more appropriate and more likely to meet their needs.

What it takes for massage therapists to evolve to the third and highest level of competence in any one of the paradigms is the commitment and determination to really think about and pay attention to what they have learned; to integrate it into an organic working body of practical knowledge; and then to constantly apply, correct, and modify their assessments, treatments, point and technique selections, and patient recommendations. Over time, such practitioners will find that as they do this they will become more and more conscious in their paradigm until they fully embody it. As a result, their competence level dramatically increases to the point where massage professionals find themselves healing their clients more and more by doing less and less.

COMPASSION AND THE DESIRE TO HELP OTHERS: AN ESSENTIAL INGREDIENT

It should be noted and understood that critical to any positive outcomes in the health care professions are a practitioner's compassion and desire to help and heal others (Figure 1-12). There is much that could be said about how the great hands-on healers, through simple, uneducated laying-on of the hands, can translate and transmit deep compassion and unconditional love through touch, resulting in miraculous healings. Books have been written about these kinds of people, but such pure beings and healers are the exception and not the rule. For the masses of students who are less gifted to start with but who wish to become professional healers in their own right, the serious study of the techniques, theory, and science of massage and bodywork therapy must be undertaken. Eventually, seeking a mentor to help further development is recommended. It is through this process of study and the experience over time of treating people from all walks of life with different problems that a practitioner begins to learn the deeper meaning of compassion. Often, the presence of this important and powerful ingredient on the part of the therapist can make all the difference in the results of the treatment.

SUMMARY

The purpose of this chapter is to introduce the Three Paradigms of Practice that exist within the massage therapy and bodywork profession. A knowledge of the continuum of the three paradigms helps to more clearly define and describe the possible scope and extent of therapeutic education and training. This chapter also introduces and explores the idea of the Three Levels of

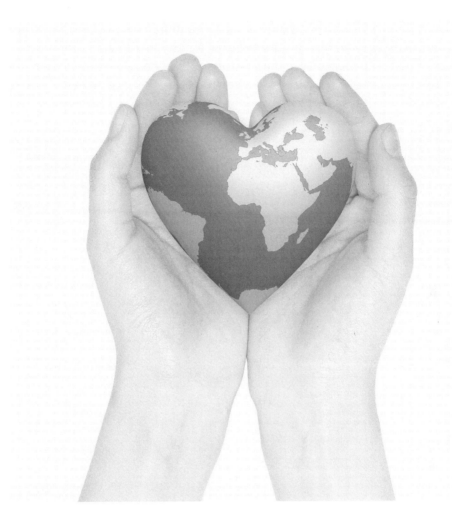

Figure 1-12 Compassion. *Image copyright 2009, Sgame. Used under license from shutterstock.com.*

Competence within each paradigm. These three stages, characterized by individual efforts and degrees of attention, define and describe the level of overall competence through which massage and bodywork therapists perform their work. The most advanced practitioners learn to integrate their education, training, and ongoing experience into a dynamic body of understanding, sensitivity, and technical ability.

The chapter also discusses how the framework of the Three Paradigms of Practice and the Three Levels of Competence provides a good way for potential clients and patients to understand the scope of treatment they can expect from a particular therapist. Understanding this can also help them form the right questions to ask prior to making an appointment. In addition, the chapter also describes the evolutionary process of massage therapists as they grow from beginner to expert and also points out how for any health care practitioner, including massage therapists, compassion and the desire to help others are essential character traits that factor positively into the healing process.

CHAPTER REFERENCES

1. Cherkin, D. C., Eisenberg, D., Sherman, K. J., Barlow, W., Kaptchuk, T. J., Street, J., et al. (2001). Randomized trial comparing traditional Chinese medical acupuncture, therapeutic massage, and self-care education for low back pain. *Arch Intern Med., 161*(8), 1081–1088.
2. Ferrel-Tory, A., & Tand Glick, O. J. (1993). The use of therapeutic massage as a nursing intervention to modify anxiety and the perception of cancer pain. *Cancer Nurse, 16*(2), 93–101.
3. Jensen, O. K., Neilson, F. F., & Vosmar, L. (1990). An open study comparing manual therapy with the use of cold packs in the treatment of post-tramatic headache. *Cephalalgia (Norway), 10*(5), 241–250.
4. A pilot study conducted at Cedar-Sinai medical center in Los Angeles, CA.
5. Kaard, B., & Tostinbo, O. (1989). Increase of plasma beta endorphins in a connective tissue massage. *Gen. Pharm., 20*(4), 487–489.
6. From 2008 massage therapy industry fact sheet survey commissioned by AMTA.

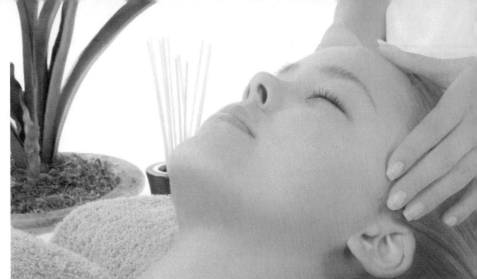

2

CHAPTER

First Paradigm—Relaxation and Stress Reduction

CHAPTER GOALS

1. Develop an understanding of the First Paradigm of practice.
2. Distinguish the Second and Third Paradigms of practice from the First Paradigm of practice.
3. Understand the First Paradigm of practice as primarily relaxation and stress reduction in its scope of and approach to treatment.
4. Understand the basic principles and underlying mechanisms of the stress response.
5. Gain a knowledge of the most common stress-related symptoms.
6. Understand as a practitioner of the First Paradigm of practice the nature of the relationship between therapist and client.
7. Understand the importance of developing the knowledge, skills, and abilities most necessary, useful, and relevant for this level of practice.
8. Gain an appreciation for First Paradigm practice through becoming familiar with some actual case histories that accurately demonstrate this level of practice.

INTRODUCTION

When we take a look at the continuum of the Three Paradigms of practice, it is only natural to think in terms of levels—of a hierarchy of better and worse. However, the idea of levels when referring to the paradigms simply describes how far along the continuum of professional education and training practitioners have gone, rather than implying any negative or positive judgment about them. This is important to understand, because the extent of practitioners' training and education becomes the foundation from which they treat, as well as the primary factor that defines and limits how far and how deep they can take their scope of practice.

Perhaps an interesting way of illustrating this is by looking briefly at the stages and levels along the continuum of the **western medical paradigm**. Good examples are the clinical medical assistant (CMA), the physician assistant (PA), and the physician (MD). Clinical medical assistants are trained to perform routine clinical and clerical tasks, including taking medical histories and recording vital signs, drawing blood, removing sutures, explaining treatment procedures to patients, preparing patients for examinations, and assisting physicians during examinations. They also collect and prepare laboratory specimens and sometimes perform basic laboratory tests on the premises, dispose of contaminated supplies, and sterilize medical instruments.[1] Some medical assistants are trained on the job, but many complete one-year or even two-year associate's degree programs.

Physician assistants train for several years and provide health care services under the supervision of physicians and surgeons. According to the U.S. Department of Labor, Bureau of Labor Statistics, Occupational Outlook Handbook, "PAs are formally trained to provide diagnostic, therapeutic, and preventive health care services, as delegated by a physician. They work as members of the health care team, take medical histories, examine and treat patients, order and interpret laboratory tests and x-rays, and make diagnoses. They also treat minor injuries, by suturing, splinting, and casting. PAs record progress notes, instruct and counsel patients, and order or carry out therapy. In 48 States and the District of Columbia, physician assistants may prescribe some medications."[2] Physician assistants are trained to do all of the above and yet they are not doctors (Figure 2-1).

The scope of practice of a PA as just described encompasses a much smaller core of knowledge of the western medical paradigm than that from which a physician practices; however, it is much greater than that of a CMA. If a PA wanted to continue to study and become a medical doctor, many more years of schooling and training would be involved. As a result, the PA's scope of practice would be enormously enhanced by encompassing the greater body of knowledge and skills of the western medical paradigm. In this illustration of a continuum of practice, the CMA can be viewed as a First Paradigm practitioner, the

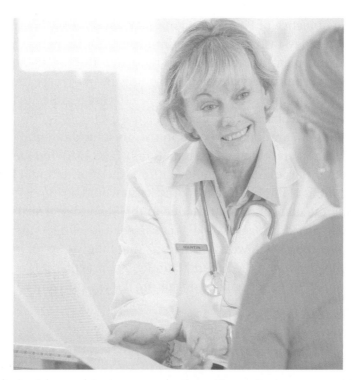

Figure 2-1 A physician assistant communicating with a patient. *Image copyright 2009, Dasilva. Used under license from shutterstock.com.*

PA as a Second Paradigm practitioner, and the physician as a Third Paradigm practitioner, all by virtue of their education and training.

By extension, this analogy can be applied to an understanding of the Three Paradigms of massage therapy and the continuum of knowledge and practice that defines the entire framework of the massage therapy profession today.

THE WAY OF THE FIRST PARADIGM: THE FOUNDATION

First Paradigm massage therapy practice is either a stage that every massage professional passes through on his or her way to studying and practicing more complex and involved treatment levels (regardless of what form or techniques they practice), or it is a choice made on the part of practitioners to offer massage treatments for the sole purpose of providing relaxation and stress reduction for their clients.

The main objective of First Paradigm practitioners is to relax their clients and reduce their day-to-day stress by administering treatments that are non-invasive, relaxing, pleasurable, and stress reducing. The specific intent here is to provide warm, compassionate touch to soothe the body, ease the burdens of the mind, and contribute to clients' overall health care regimen to help restore and maintain health and prevent disease (Figure 2-2).

Since the First Paradigm is rooted in the most fundamental practices of massage education and training, it can naturally be considered the basis upon which the other paradigms are built. Without the foundational knowledge, skills, and abilities of this paradigm of practice, it would be impossible to move further along the continuum of practice to the Second or Third Paradigms. There is really no skipping possible because each level depends on the one before and lays the groundwork for the one that follows. So for practitioners to competently move into the Second Paradigm of practice, it is assumed that they have gained the experience of mastering the First and are willing to take

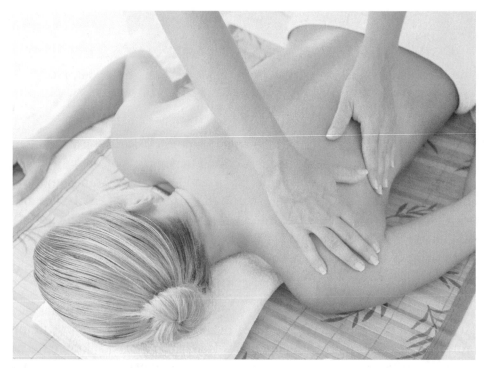

Figure 2-2 A woman receiving First Paradigm massage therapy treatment for general relaxation and the reduction of day-to-day stress. *Image copyright 2009, Liv Friis-larsen. Used under license from shutterstock.com.*

on the greater responsibilities that come with expanding and moving along the continuum. Similarly, it is the same for those practitioners wishing to move from the Second to the Third Paradigm.

The fact that many professional massage therapists choose to remain First Paradigm practitioners bears no reflection on their ability, competence, intelligence, or any other attribute that good professional massage therapists embody. Mostly, it is simply a personal preference—a choice that practitioners make relative to the kind of work they wish to perform. Quite often, after years of practice, First Paradigm practitioners decide to undergo more intensive training in order to move on and practice in the realms of the Second Paradigm and beyond.

The overriding point here regarding paradigms of practice is that together they make up a living, breathing whole—an organic body of knowledge that provides a great roadmap of the range of possibilities of this field. Students and practicing therapists alike should be aware that the path is broad, diverse, and filled with opportunities, and it is really up to each individual to choose what part of the whole they wish to embody. Clients and patients can also use a basic understanding of the Three Paradigms to help them identify the kind of treatment they wish to receive and the level of practitioner they want to work with in order accomplish their specific health care goals.

Relaxation and Stress Reduction

In order to understand the impact of this Paradigm, it is necessary to know a little more about its scope of practice—relaxation and stress reduction. Knowledge of stress and how it negatively affects the human mind-body complex and what role treating stress plays within the continuum of therapeutic massage is fundamental. Also knowledge of the extremely powerful and beneficial effects of competently performed massage therapy on alleviating the suffering of human beings from stress and stress-related disorders are essential to gaining a broader comprehension of massage therapy provided at the First Paradigm level.

Understanding the psychology and physiology of the stress response mechanism is a must for First Paradigm massage therapists to fulfill the goals of their work with most clients. Identifying the signs and symptoms of stress, creating and administering flexible treatment plans, targeting stress and its symptoms, and making basic, healthful recommendations to help clients alleviate and gain control over their stress is the primary role of the First Paradigm massage practitioner.

Stress and the Mind-Body Complex: It's Really a Matter of How We See

Stress can be defined as the buildup of physical and psychological tensions that are created by the way in which we perceive and interpret the challenges and difficulties of the world around us. In other words, the events of our daily life can act as catalysts that ignite the stress response—an automatic and instinctive reaction that initiates a cascade of physiological changes in the body. Often, the results of these changes lead to the negative emotional states that we commonly refer to as "stress" (Figure 2-3). If not too intense, stress may simply and quickly pass on its own. That is normal. However, when stress becomes **chronic** and left unresolved, it results in a continuous physiological state in which the body's natural rhythms and functions are accelerated and left in a constant state of "on." Without the necessary opportunity for rest, this persistent stress often leads to a myriad of serious, degenerative conditions such as high blood pressure, ulcers, depression, fear, anxiety, and so on. It can have a hugely negative effect on our overall outlook on life, which will continue to fuel the stress response. This underscores the importance of regular First Paradigm massage therapy treatment to help prevent or break the cycle

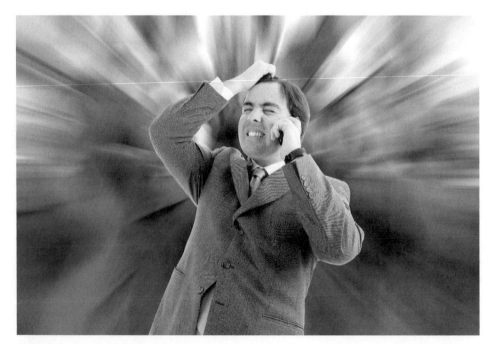

Figure 2-3 Stressed-out business man reaching his limit and exploding in frustration and anger. *Image copyright 2009, Ana de Sousa. Used under license from shutterstock.com.*

by alleviating any buildup of stress, which can have damaging and far-reaching consequences. First Paradigm massage therapy enables the complete relaxation of the body, mind, and emotions, revitalizes the spirit, and promotes the body's inner healing mechanisms. Also, many clients of First Paradigm practitioners use these treatments as a way to relax into meditative states.

Since the beginning of humanity's time on earth, the innate **stress response** has evolved as a self-protective means of survival by preparing the human body to appropriately deal with the real and accurate perception of dangerous or life-threatening situations. However, whether or not the mind accurately or mistakenly perceives an event threatening to itself, an automatic barrage of nervous and hormonal activities is catalyzed by the involuntary part of the autonomic nervous system, known as the sympathetic nervous system, in order to ready the body to deal with the "danger."

Under stress, the heart rate intensifies and begins to speed up. Breathing quickens and becomes shallow, while **glucose** enters into the bloodstream making larger amounts of oxygen and energy available as the stress response readies the body for increased physical output. Blood pressure increases, providing more circulation and distribution of essential **hormones, enzymes,** oxygen, and other nutrients for the body's defenses. Overall consciousness of one's surroundings is heightened as all the senses become more acute. Even blood-clotting factors are made more available in the blood stream to help limit the potential loss of blood in the case of injury. Perspiration increases, muscles tense up, and digestive processes halt to conserve energy as **adrenaline** is poured into the blood stream, readying the body to fight off or flee from the perceived "enemy."

This automatic, self-protective mechanism is a carryover from days long ago when existence was far less complex and the moment-to-moment dangers threatening survival were real and constant. In those times, men had to hunt in order to eat and live and were always either on the run from or fighting off predators to survive. This instinctive mechanism, deeply integrated in humanity's animal nature, served our ancestors well. Although the **"flight or fight response"** is still at times appropriate, we no longer live in a world faced with the same kinds of challenges, and therefore it most often serves no purpose at all; in fact, due to the chronic stress that so many people experience, it has become a major factor in the exponential spread of **degenerative** and stress-related conditions and disease.

Recognizing the Symptoms of Stress

Each person experiences the results of the stress response differently, and so it is important for massage therapists to understand the fundamental mechanisms of stress and to be aware of how the most common stress symptoms manifest in their clients. First Paradigm practitioners can help their clients become more aware of their cycle of stress while also helping them begin to effectively manage it through regular massage therapy treatments. Therapists can also provide some basic and simple tools that will allow clients to better handle the moment-to-moment events of their lives.

Following is a list of common stress symptoms. Clients who have been experiencing several of these symptoms on a frequent basis are likely to be suffering from chronic stress.

Fear or panic	Tension and being on-edge
Difficulty sleeping	Change in eating
Diarrhea/constipation	Sweaty palms
Upset stomach or pain	Lack of interest in life
Inability to focus	Poor memory
Chronic fatigue	Apathy
Cold extremities	Fear of losing control
Shortness of breath	Constant "butterflies"
Muscle tension	Heart palpitations
Loss of self-confidence	Headaches
Sudden pessimism	Feeling under pressure
Short temper	Chronic worry

Short-Term Stress and the Relaxation Response

There are two kinds of stress: short-term stress and long-term stress (or chronic stress). It is essential that a First Paradigm professional understand the difference between the two. **Short-term stress** is benign, natural, and easily dealt with by the mind-body complex. This type of stress is also known as "healthy" stress and is the body's appropriate response to a catalyst that is perceived without distortion. Short-term stress generally results in immediate and rational action and resolution. This is the same instinctive response that human beings naturally share with the animal kingdom. Once the appropriate action has been taken and the catalyst is neutralized, both the mind and the body relax and return to their normal state of functioning. This process of returning to normal, of coming back down from a heightened state, is called the "**relaxation response.**" It is controlled by the **parasympathetic nervous system,** a division of the **autonomic nervous system** and also the counterpart to the **sympathetic nervous system.**

AN EXAMPLE OF SHORT-TERM STRESS AND THE RELAXATION RESPONSE

A pilot of a jet airliner announces that he has to make an emergency landing due to failure of one of the aircraft's engines. Naturally, there's an immediate activation of the stress response in everyone aboard. This heightened state of fear for one's life keeps the stress response activated, including all the bodily physiological changes that are part of the response. However, once the plane touches ground safely and all signs of danger are gone, there is an immediate release of emotion and tension accompanied by a normal, gradual movement back to a baseline state of relaxation. The relaxation response is activated, bringing the mind and body back to normal.

Long-Term Stress and Disease

Since short-term stress naturally resolves itself, the real threat to health is **long-term** or **chronic stress**, which has become the scourge of modern humanity. Left untreated it leads to numerous mental and physical problems. Because chronic stress lingers unresolved, it slowly over time increases the damage to the emotional and physical nature of its victims. Chronic stress is most commonly catalyzed by conflicts that seem to have no end in sight or are not being properly dealt with and resolved. For example, family and relationship problems, unemployment or difficulties on the job, and financial woes, are the kinds of things that can often persist for long periods of time without resolution and slowly wear down a person's mental and physical state of being.

The continuous state of an intensely aroused physiology produced by long-term stress is experienced in the body as though it were under constant threat of danger. This may be felt as ongoing states of worry, anxiety, frustration, fear, and tension. Interestingly, more often than not, chronic stress goes unnoticed. Like a fish in water, humans can become so used to a level of mental and physiological agitation that it fades from their awareness. Hence a patient's surprise when the doctor takes his blood pressure and finds that it is very high. Stress can become so habitual that even when in a non-stressful situation our bodies can remain tense and defensive without any recognition of its state. Living in such a state of physiological excitation, without the natural balance of the relaxation phase that automatically and naturally occurs after a short-term stress response, eventually leads to physical disease and mental breakdowns.

The good news is that massage therapists can easily detect this state of muscular and emotional tension through palpation and the sense of touch.

Once these areas of stress are located, it is the responsibility of therapists to bring it to their clients' attention, treat them to dissolve and release this tension, and work with them at least until they have begun to take the right steps toward resolution of their stress. In some cases, therapists may need to refer their clients to psychological counseling so that a professional skilled in emotional treatment can teach them the necessary skills for coping and resolving their problems.

AN EXAMPLE OF LONG-TERM STRESS

The CEO of a company, having to answer to his board of directors, is feeling the effects of the downturn in the economy. Besides growing competition eating into his company's profits and market share, he is also being pressured by an employee management crisis. In addition, his financial matters have become more and more difficult to manage, while the demands of his family have increased as well. He is worried about his son's growing behavioral problems, he is deeply concerned about his spouse's poor health, and he is troubled by his own lack of wellbeing since he is overweight and a heavy smoker. In addition, his family history places him at a high risk for heart disease, which he is well aware of—another reason for worry and concern. He has not been able to relax or get a good night's sleep for quite some time, mostly because he constantly replays in his mind all the things which are bothering him. Unfortunately this brief biography is not an exception to the rule. Sadly, it has become very common.

Chronic Stress and Disease

Understanding what triggers the cycle of stress can help massage therapists assist their clients manage stress better by providing relaxation and support on mental, emotional, and physical levels. If chronic stress is not dealt with properly, even the smallest source of stress can easily become the negatively tinted veil through which people see and interpret the world, ensuring that the stress cycle continues unabated. This of course wastes tremendous amounts of energy and puts enormous strain on the mind and body. As a result, the body's adaptive mechanisms begin to wear down, leading to physical and emotional illness and in some cases even premature death.

While First Paradigm massage therapy treatment requires the least amount of education and training, massage therapists practicing this work play an important function in relieving many of the tensions and pains of day-to-day living that are often induced by stress. By doing so, these professionals play a major role in preventative health care.

Chronic stress can lead directly, or indirectly as a contributing factor, to one of the following conditions:

- High blood pressure
- Heart disease
- Headaches, including migraines and tension
- Cancer
- Asthma
- Gastritis, ulcers, colitis, Crohn's Disease
- Nervous system diseases, e.g., multiple sclerosis
- Chronic common skin conditions, including eczema, dermatitis, hives
- Weakening of the immune system, which can lead to increased vulnerability to flu, colds, and infection by bacteria and viruses
- Chronic backache
- Overeating due to stress, leading to obesity
- Vertigo

And this is by no means an exhaustive list.

RELATIONSHIP BETWEEN FIRST PARADIGM PRACTITIONERS AND THEIR CLIENTS

When compared to therapists practicing the Second and Third Paradigms, practitioners of the First Paradigm affect a relatively small portion of their clients' lives. This is due primarily to two main reasons. Firstly, clients of First Paradigm practitioners are usually transient. Some come and go as they please, most often based on their own assessment of their health, while others only come in for treatments while on vacation once or twice a year. Because of this, these clients are simply not around enough for therapists to consistently influence their well-being. Secondly, practitioners at this level do not handle major health concerns. It is important to note that while the treatments administered by First Paradigm practitioners are extremely beneficial to both mind and body, therapists at this level are not equipped to handle more serious conditions and because of this, First Paradigm practitioners' relationships to those they treat are largely as clients—not as patients.

The relationship between First Paradigm practitioners and their clients usually begins and ends with the treatment. This differs greatly from the relationships between Second and Third Paradigm therapists and their patients, which are much more involved and complex and extend well beyond the timeframe of the treatment itself. This distinction between clients and patients will be more fully addressed in Chapters 3 and 4.

THE PRIMARY WORKPLACE OF FIRST PARADIGM PRACTITIONERS

By far the most prevalent place of practice or work setting that First Paradigm massage therapists are found in are the thousands of spas located all around the world. More recently, a number of successful massage therapy clinic franchises, many with spa-like qualities and features, have begun to appear and spread throughout the country. These generally employ large numbers of First Paradigm professionals. In addition, First Paradigm therapists also enjoy practicing in the corporate environment, where they can positively impact the lives of stressed-out corporate and office employees by providing onsite seated or chair massage. This type of massage has gained increasing popularity in recent years.

Spas

In 2007, the International SPA Association (ISPA) released its figures on the U.S. spa industry, indicating that in the United States alone there were 14,615 spas and that it has become a 9.4 billon-dollar industry. Day spas accounted for the largest category with the most locations in the United States. Resort/hotel spas are the second largest group, followed by medical spas, club spas, mineral springs spas, and destination spas, which came in third. There were approximately 110 million spa visits made in the United States in 2006 and most were for massage therapy treatment. This industry growth points to the enormous and still-evolving role of First Paradigm practitioners that continues to spread throughout this country. These statistics also suggest that there has been a profound and positive impact on the health of the American people by massage practitioners quietly helping to relax and reduce their stress (Figure 2-4).

In many of these different spa settings, First Paradigm massage therapists can be found working alongside estheticians, cosmetologists, hairstylists, manicurists, and other members of the beauty and wellness industry. The often trendy and tranquil environments these spas offer are a perfect backdrop for a relaxing and stress-reducing massage. Great care is often paid to the ambience with

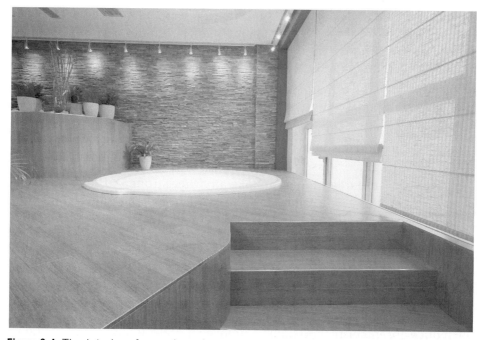

Figure 2-4 The interior of a modern day-spa. *Image copyright 2009, Paparazzit. Used under license from shutterstock.com.*

soft lighting, relaxing music, and treatment rooms that are warm and inviting in order to soothe and appeal to the senses of their clients. In contrast, the work settings for Second and Third Paradigm therapists are often more clinical in appearance, with anatomical charts and diagrams adorning the walls.

Since the spa setting is most often the place where people have their first full-body massage experience, practitioners of the First Paradigm have the unique responsibility to make a first and lasting impression. As individual ambassadors for the entire field of massage therapy, they have the opportunity to manifest a strong and competent professional image and demonstrate what is possible through the power of touch.

Seated Massage at Corporate Offices

For people working in a busy corporate environment or a bustling office setting, taking the time for a conventional, full-body massage may be impractical and expensive as a regular way to relax, reduce stress, and resolve the minor aches and pains that come with sitting behind a desk all day. Fortunately for them, more and more businesses have been creating opportunities for massage therapists to offer what is known as on–site seated **chair massage** to their busy office staff and other employees.

As a result, **seated massage** has become a very popular modality of professional touch for many First Paradigm practitioners. There are no oils or lotions used and it is performed directly over a client's clothes on a very comfortable and **ergonomic massage chair** (Figure 2-5). Often, these treatments are conducted in a private setting within the workplace. Besides large corporations and other businesses, therapists offering **chair massage** can also be found practicing in airports, shopping mall kiosks, convention centers, dentist offices, sporting events, and hospitals (to name only a few).

In the workplace, sessions can be scheduled for weekly, biweekly, or monthly visits, and treatments can take anywhere from 5 to 20 minutes per person (but can be scheduled for longer) so that they can easily be fitted into a lunch hour or morning or afternoon coffee break. The cost is relatively inexpensive and may be fully financed by some employers as a well-appreciated perk. Other employers may split the cost with interested employees or they may simply provide the space, time, and opportunity for willing staff to pay out of their own pockets for the service.

Regular seated massage has been shown to increase employees' productivity, reduce absenteeism, and boost employee morale. It has also been shown to help employees increase alertness, relax and to reduce their stress.[3] More specifically, seated massage, like full-body massage therapy, can help relieve other minor stress-related conditions such as tension headaches, stiff necks,

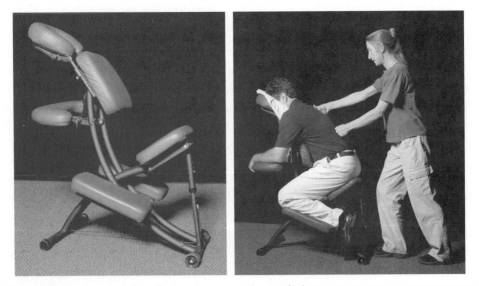

Figure 2-5 A man receiving chair massage at the workplace.

tight shoulders, and sore backs that arise from working on a computer all day and from long drives to and from the workplace. It can also help relieve and resolve repetitive motion injuries such as carpal tunnel syndrome.

THE TREATMENT

From a First Paradigm perspective, a long and involved client assessment is not necessary prior to treatment so this process is often over in just minutes. In the Second and Third Paradigms, client assessment is generally a greater portion of the patient–practitioner interaction. It is where much time can be spent deciphering the exact nature of a patient's condition and deciding on the appropriate treatment plan to follow. In First Paradigm treatments, however, the focus is much more general. As opposed to having patients fill out an in-depth case history form and go through an involved interview and assessment process, First Paradigm professionals may simply ask a few basic questions to be sure that there aren't any contraindications and that it is safe to proceed with the treatment. They will then find out about any painful areas, where clients feel stressed, and what they would like to get out of the session before moving into the treatment itself.

Second and Third Paradigm therapists have a more thorough plan of action for each patient, and it often must be adjusted as they continue to treat and work with the same patient over time. The framework that these massage therapists practice from requires that they look beyond the surface and begin to connect physical issues that present with other factors including lifestyle, diet, lack of exercise, and so on. In the First Paradigm, therapists are largely concerned with the most immediate aches and pains—the symptoms that clients complain about. Other factors that could be contributing to client's current state of health such as posture, emotional issues, lifestyle, and medical history are not heavily explored.

While therapists practicing at this First Paradigm level can utilize just about any form of massage and bodywork for their purposes, there are certain modalities that lend themselves well to certain paradigms. Swedish massage, for one, will likely be the most prevalent form of massage practiced in this category. While advanced **Swedish massage** techniques can certainly be used in the Second and Third Paradigms of treatment for more specific therapeutic purposes, this modality lends itself greatly to muscular relaxation and is the most commonly performed technique in First paradigm treatment. It is also the primary modality of treatment taught in most all basic, entry-level massage therapy programs.

Many First Paradigm therapists who practice seated massage use variations of more advanced Asian bodywork modalities such as **acupressure, shiatsu, or tuina.** (See Chapter 9, The Bioenergetic Layer of the Massage and Bodywork Therapy Continuum for more on acupressure, shiatsu, and tuina.) These complex forms of treatment have been reworked into quick and focused stress-relieving massage sessions for employees at the workplace that are too busy to leave their desks. During these sessions, practitioners manipulate the soft tissue, following the energy channels, and press the same points that are needled in acupuncture to obtain the healthy benefits. This is intended not only to relax tense and aching muscles but also to release and balance the energy (Qi) system in order to invigorate both mind and body. Using acupressure, shiatsu, or tuina, therapists can easily focus on treating muscles in the back, arms, hands, shoulders, neck, and head while their clients let go and relax into the comfortable massage chair. This form of treatment is of course very different from traditional full-body Swedish massage. Seated massage therapists use their hands, thumbs, and even their elbows to knead, pull, and stretch their clients' muscles and manipulate the energy channels and points.

Seated massage is also used by Second and Third Paradigm therapists as an additional way in which to accomplish some therapeutic goals with their patients. In this case, much more involved assessments are made and treatments are tailored to address each patient's major complaints. Essentially, for the Second and Third Paradigm practitioner, the use of the massage chair is a tool more suited for particular clients who are better positioned in the massage chair for the specific treatments they need or for those who are unable to lie down on a massage table due to their condition.

The way in which massage therapists allocate their treatment time can also be vastly different from paradigm to paradigm. In Second and Third paradigm treatment, the entire session may be geared for treatment of just one or two key areas of the body with an eye toward getting to other areas and issues in upcoming sessions. In the First Paradigm, in contrast, treatment time is spread almost evenly throughout the whole body unless specifically requested by the client. A few extra minutes may be spent on certain areas that the client is having specific problems with, but in general the session will be mostly global, covering the entire body. When clients are treated in the workplace with chair massage, session times are usually much shorter than those given in the spa environment and treatments are performed primarily on the posterior of the client's body as they relax and let go facing into the massage chair.

Following the treatment, First Paradigm therapists may offer simple, easy-to-remember instructions that will benefit their clients, such as "drink lots of water," or "remember to take time to relax and stretch." And because treatments are often booked back-to-back (particularly in the spa industry) there may be little time for much else. This is usually the point where the client–practitioner interaction will end in a First Paradigm setting and the practitioner will often never see that client again. In the other two paradigms, this post-treatment phase can be a lengthy process filled with discussions of treatment findings as well as follow-up conversations to prepare for the next phase of treatments. Significant time may also be devoted to making recommendations on dietary changes, herbal and vitamin supplements, lifestyle modifications, and exercise programs.

CASE HISTORIES OF FIRST PARADIGM THERAPISTS AT WORK AND WITH CLIENTS

The following case histories provide an overview and insight into how and where most First Paradigm massage therapists practice. They include some description of the work settings, the nature of basic therapist–client interactions and the general state of being of clients who sought out and are receiving the care of First Paradigm practitioners. In each of the examples the client is being treated generally for relaxation, stress reduction, and the relief of minor aches and pain due to stress.

First Paradigm Treatment at a Spa

CASE HISTORY

ALLIE

Working at a spa in an upscale gym in the Upper East Side of Manhattan, Janice sees a variety of very affluent, international clients. Her last client has just returned from his family's home in South Africa and her next client is in international finance. Although their work pays for a lavish lifestyle, their bodies have taken a toll. However, because of the gym atmosphere in which Janice works, most of her clients are used to working out and are in fairly good shape. If she was working in a more clinical setting, she would see a much greater diversity in the condition of the clients walking through the door. In fact, some may not even be able to walk without assistance. In this environment, however, clients **debilitated** to that degree are a rarity.

The spa at the gym offers a full line of services, including massage therapy, skin care, facials, and body waxing. It offers a variety of massage therapy services, including **aromatherapy,** hot stone treatments, shiatsu, **Thai massage**, deep-tissue massage, and of course the classic Swedish massage. The spa is also situated right next to a full-service hair salon that the gym also owns. This range of services offered by the gym is quite attractive for the busy lives that its members lead.

Here, Janice works three 6-hour shifts throughout the week. Like many of her friends and colleagues, she works at several different locations, including another upscale spa in Union Square and another spa right down the street. They each offer similar services and cater to a similar clientele. The only real difference between the locations is the environment. The spa treatment rooms in the gym are done quite nicely and have stone floors with drains and Vichy showers that allow for a wide range of hydrotherapy spa, skin care, and wellness treatments. They also have washbasins inside each room, personal heaters, hydroculators, and the ability to control music levels. At some of the other locations, there is less control over the room environment. For example, in the more basic spa down the street, the only dividers between the rooms are curtains. Although the fabric goes almost all the way up to the towering ceiling, they still allow only a fraction of the privacy that the other locations offer. The spa in Union Square is decorated in an all-white theme with a wide, long corridor that leads to a plush lounge in the back where the spa can host parties and guests. Champagne can be served there, lunch can be delivered, and the whole place can be rented out for the right price.

At the spa in the gym each client is met in the softly decorated waiting area, which acts as a sort of decompression chamber from the outside world. Just beyond the doors in one direction are a bustling waiting area and three floors of well-equipped gym space. On the other side is a dimly lit corridor lined in stone with soft music washing over the entire space. This is where Janice emerges from to greet her client.

With a warm hello and a handshake, Janice takes Allie to one of the seven treatment rooms that she'll be using for that day. The rooms are always prepared prior to greeting clients so that the moment clients walk in they can begin to unwind and relax. As they walk, Allie tells Janice about being very stressed from having to travel so much for work these days. She says her back and neck have been killing her so she made an appointment to see Janice as soon as she landed. She'll be leaving later in the week again to her employer's sister company in England.

Janice shows Allie the room and instructs her to disrobe and lie face down on the table underneath the large draping towels. She leaves the room to allow her some privacy. Janice only has a few moments to think about how to approach the session before needing to re-enter and commence with the treatment. A minute later she knocks on the door and quietly enters. Allie's breathing is much more relaxed as she lies under the covers with her neck and upper back exposed. As soon as Janice starts to work on Allie, she can feel all the tell-tale signs of tension. She begins to immediately massage Allie's neck in order to ease her way into the tightly wound musculature. She builds the pressure gradually and checks several times to make sure that it's not too much for Allie, who says the pressure feels good, so the treatment continues.

Janice's strokes move over Allie's entire neck and back and then she begins work on her legs. Allie combats her high-stress job by going to the gym as often as possible. She has an affinity for the stair-climbing machine, which Janice can feel in the tight and swollen muscles on the back of Allie's legs. With long, firm massage strokes, she attempts to soften and relax these muscles. In Allie's calves she can feel a more pronounced tension that's like a knot of hard clay. She goes over all of this with the gliding motions of Swedish massage, passing over the muscles again and again so that they'll begin to let go and relax. Before turning Allie over, Janice spends a few moments treating her feet, which Allie seems to greatly appreciate as evidenced by her sighs of relief.

With Allie on her back now, Janice spends more time treating her neck and shoulders to make sure any tensions there have been massaged away. Having recently come back from a trip herself, Janice vividly remembers the havoc that a plane ride can wreak on the body. The strokes extend from neck to shoulder, shoulder to arm, arm to hand, and all the way back up again to the shoulder in one continuous flow without ever breaking contact. She does a few mild stretches to Allie's neck while instructing her to breath deeply before moving down to work the legs.

Now, nearing the end of the session, Janice comes back to the head to massage the scalp—a secret hiding place for a lot of stress and tension. People are often surprised at just how much tension this area can hold. As she closes the massage, Janice quietly holds a few points at the base of Allie's head. Slowly, she breaks contact and with a voice just a few degrees above a whisper, informs her that the treatment is over. Allie takes a huge breath and exhales loudly before saying thank-you—obviously very relaxed. Janice leaves the room for her to dress and she waits outside with a small cup of water in hand.

Allie takes her time to gather herself, and when she opens the door Janice notices that a sleepy smile that wasn't there before has crept onto her face. Allie says she feels wonderful, that her neck and back pain has diminished greatly, and that it was exactly what she needed. Janice tells her to make sure to drink lots of water to flush out the toxins that get released after a massage and suggests that she come back as soon as she returns from her trip next week.

First Paradigm Treatments at a Corporate Office with Seated Massage

MARY

Mary is the human resource director for a large Fortune 500 company in New York City. She's actually the one who arranged for the onsite seated massage program for the employees. Mary has been taking advantage of it since the beginning and reports that she has gained great benefit from weekly treatment.

To receive her treatment she eagerly takes a seat in her therapist Mike's ergonomic massage chair. The well-cushioned massage chair places the client in a supported, kneeling position with both feet tucked underneath. It also supports the chest and forearms while the face relaxes gently against a soft cushioned face cradle. Mary said at first that it felt a little unusual, although relaxing. As always, Mike begins to work on her very tense neck and shoulder muscles with his hands and thumbs. Mike uses a firm pressure with his techniques,—but checks in with her often to see if he is being too rough. Mary explains that it feels a bit painful, but in a good way and without being too uncomfortable.

Instead of the slow, oil-based gliding strokes of a full-body Swedish massage, this treatment is energetic, fast, and invigorating. Mary wouldn't have expected to feel so relaxed from this kind of movement. As Mike works his way down Mary's spine, he uses both his fingers and thumbs and alternating with his elbows to ease her tense and knotted muscles. He continues working down to her hips. He finishes her treatment by massaging her hands, wrists, forearms, and fingers.

Afterwards Mary feels a bit light-headed, almost as if she is floating on air. Mike offers her a bottle of water in order for her to hydrate herself. She feels so relaxed that she could fall asleep. Feeling refreshed and rejuvenated, she heads back to her office while still on break to just sit and dwell in her relaxed state before having to get back into the grind of her busy work day. Mary has become a big proponent of seated massage in the workplace, especially as a quick and convenient way of helping employees of the company release their pent-up stresses, relax their aching muscles, and improve their work performance.

ALLEN

Allen is 35 years old and works in the marketing and sales department of a large Los Angeles firm. It is a busy, fast-moving office in which staff members make important decisions and have to handle a great deal of ongoing responsibility. On top of that stressful and intense work environment, Allen is a "Type A" individual. These people, who are also often "workaholics," tend to drive themselves really hard and are highly competitive and often aggressive in their behavior. The main thing that a Type A individual has the most difficulty doing is relaxing. Allen describes his work environment as "**manic**" but feels massage helps him to keep moving and stay on top of things.

Fortunately for Allen, his company offers weekly onsite seated massage as one of the company's many benefits to help combat stress. Allen also has a one-hour drive to and from work each day and looks forward to unwinding during his seated massage treatments. He readily admits that if the chair massage therapists didn't come to him in the workplace, he would never take the time out himself to find a practitioner and get regular massage. He loves the convenience of the weekly chair massage sessions where he gets to just relax and rest his mind in the privacy of his office. He remarks that it helps to clear his mind and put things into perspective and that he is always noticeably more pleasant and more productive after treatments.

SUMMARY

The main purpose of this chapter was to present a detailed description of the First Paradigm of practice and, in doing so, lay the basic groundwork for the Second and Third Paradigms. During this chapter, it was explained how the scope of practice of First Paradigm massage therapy and bodywork therapists is rooted in the effort to help clients they treat to relax, to reduce their stress, and to relieve their minor aches and pains. On the continuum of growth and development of a massage therapist, this level of practice reflects the essential foundation upon which all massage therapy and bodywork is built.

This chapter also discusses the fact that many practitioners choose this level of treatment as their primary work and derive great satisfaction from helping their clients to relax and reduce their stress. It also points out that many of these practitioners eventually decide to move on along the continuum of practice to become competent Second and Third Paradigm professionals. The chapter also underscores the importance for First Paradigm therapists to have a good working understanding of the underlying principles, mechanisms, and physiology of stress and that they need to know its signs and symptoms in order to recognize it and to help their clients manage it.

In addition, this chapter included a brief discussion of some of the most common massage modalities that lend themselves to First Paradigm treatment, including full-body Swedish massage, which is the most common technique performed in spas, and variations on some Asian bodywork modalities (including acupressure, shiatsu and tuina) used in onsite seated massage in the corporate workplace as well as other settings. A few brief case histories were also presented to help provide an understanding of and appreciation for this paradigm of practice.

CHAPTER REFERENCES

1. Bureau of Labor Statistics, U.S. Department of Labor. *Occupational outlook handbook, 2008–09 edition, Medical assistants.* Retrieved August 20, 2008, from http://www.bls.gov/oco/ocos164.htm
2. Bureau of Labor Statistics, U.S. Department of Labor. *Occupational outlook handbook, 2008–09 edition, Physician assistants.* Retrieved August 19, 2008, from http://www.bls.gov/oco/ocos081.htm
3. Field, T., Ironson, G., Scafidi, F., Nawrocki, T.,Goncalves, A., Burman, I., et al. (1996). Massage therapy reduces anxiety and enhances EEG pattern of alertness and math computations. *International Journal of Neuroscience, 86*, 197–205.

3

CHAPTER

Second Paradigm—Remediation, Therapy, and Pain Relief

CHAPTER GOALS

1. Develop an understanding of the Second Paradigm of practice.

2. Distinguish the First and Third Paradigms of practice from the Second Paradigm of practice.

3. Understand the Second Paradigm of practice as primarily remediation, therapy, and pain relief in its scope of and approach to treatment.

4. Recognize the evolution of a client into a patient.

5. Understand the changes that occur in the relationship between therapist and patient when a practitioner moves from the First Paradigm of practice into the Second Paradigm.

6. Understand the importance of developing knowledge, skills, and abilities of some of the most useful and relevant adjunctive therapies that can be integrated into treatment plans and treatment in order to help remediate injury and reduce or resolve pain.

7. Gain an appreciation for Second Paradigm practice through becoming familiar with some actual case histories that demonstrate integrative thinking and problem solving.

8. Illustrate how beginning to integrate massage therapy with other adjunctive modalities increases a Second Paradigm practitioner's ability to help remediate injury and reduce or resolve pain.

INTRODUCTION

Achieving the primary goals of treatment for Second Paradigm practitioners—remediation, therapy, and pain relief—requires a strong commitment and a level of study beyond a First Paradigm education. The education provided by First Paradigm training will most likely not be adequate for graduates to be competent enough to practice at this level, but should certainly serve as a solid foundation for the next stage of learning necessary for Second Paradigm practice.

Second Paradigm practitioners must have a firmer grasp of the body's structures, functions, limitations, and potentials and of assessment and treatment principles than First Paradigm practitioners. In addition, they must also be armed with a broad range of treatment strategies and techniques that can serve as part of a more comprehensive arsenal for this level of practice.

Conditions treated by Second Paradigm practitioners include, but are not limited to:

1. sprains, strains, post-operative or post-traumatic adhesions, restricted range of motion, pain due to postural and muscular imbalances, arthritis, headaches, menstrual disorders, digestive difficulties, joint and muscle pain and stiffness
2. fibromyalgia, sleep disorders
3. sciatica, and all sorts of muscle and joint injuries, including sports injuries.

Treating these conditions require that therapists have strong and well-developed clinical intentions and are able to determine the specific nature of their patients' pain through testing and evaluation. They must also be able to construct an effective treatment plan from the information gleaned through careful analysis and assessment, as well as guide and direct the patient through the healing process.

Second Paradigm massage therapists practice well as part of a clinical team alongside chiropractors, acupuncturists, physical therapists, and other allied health care professionals working in concert for the purpose of remediation, therapy, and pain relief for their patients (Figure 3-1).

These therapists may also come into contact with patients who have more serious ailments like cancer, AIDS, and diabetes, and who are on many medications. Although therapists practicing at this level may not be knowledgeable enough or have the skills to properly care for and directly affect patients with these conditions, as most experienced Third Paradigm practitioners, they should still have a realistic and clear picture of how much their treatments

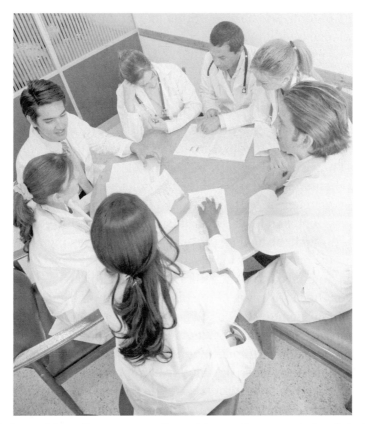

Figure 3-1 Second Paradigm massage therapists practice as part of a clinical team alongside chiropractors, acupuncturists, physical therapists, and other allied health care professionals. *Image copyright 2009, Andresr. Used under license from shutterstock.com.*

can help these conditions while remaining aware of their limitations and any contraindications that may exist. It is now a well-established fact that massage therapy, even in its most basic practice, can still yield some important positive health benefits to even the sickest of patients.

THE WAY OF THE SECOND PARADIGM

In order to practice as Second Paradigm massage therapists, practitioners must begin taking on many new roles and responsibilities than those of the more basic practices of therapists of the First Paradigm. These professionals must begin to more seriously extend their skills and abilities into the domains of education and counseling. Second Paradigm practitioners need to grow and become a source of knowledge and information concerning exercise, stretching, proper breathing, meditation, and basic nutrition and supplementation. This expansion of knowledge is vital to a successful Second Paradigm practice and will begin to lay the groundwork for the more advanced training necessary to acquire the knowledge, skills, and abilities to evolve into a Third Paradigm massage therapy professional.

A fully matured Second Paradigm practitioner is able to competently and professionally handle a large, diverse patient load, providing much-needed remediation and pain relief from a broad range of conditions. Like guides that have greater knowledge of the terrain, Second Paradigm practitioners are not only able to encompass the work of the previous paradigm but also to delve into territories generally inaccessible to First Paradigm therapists. With careful analysis, assessment, and focus, Second Paradigm therapists guide and direct their patients through the healing process, which can often include referrals to physicians to rule out more serious health concerns. This level of practice is a dramatic shift from relaxation and stress relief to health care and healing.

In addition, because many of the pains and ailments people suffer from contain emotional elements, Second Paradigm therapists must also be able to recognize and help redirect their patients' patterns of thinking toward new and more healthful ways. These practitioners should be able to make appropriate and helpful recommendations and always be supportive. Of course, this does not replace the genuine need that some patients have for professional counseling. Second Paradigm therapists working at this level must stay within their scope of practice and know when the patient will be better served by seeking help through other sources. A **clinical psychologist** or **psychotherapist** should be part of a practitioner's network so that patients can be referred to a qualified health care practitioner if necessary.

EVOLUTION OF THE THERAPIST AND CLIENT RELATIONSHIP INTO THERAPIST AND PATIENT

In the Second and Third paradigms, clients are often referred to as patients. This seemingly small change significantly shifts the dynamics of the patient–therapist relationship. One way of explaining the difference is that Second and Third Paradigm massage practices, given their focus, provide mostly medically oriented care. Often, in fact, this massage care is delivered to a patient with a medical necessity under the direction of a prescribing physician or other health care practitioner and usually paid for by a third party if the patient's medical insurance policy covers these services. First Paradigm treatment is viewed more as a personal service to consumers upon their request and is delivered to clients who in turn pay for the service themselves. (Obviously, practitioners from all three paradigms treat people who pay out of pocket—one of the financial benefits of working in this field.)

Some practitioners make this distinction simply on the basis of where the person came from. They use the term "client" for those who self-refer and come through promotion of their practices or from other practitioners, while the term "patient" is reserved for those who are doctor referred. Some practitioners are adamant about not using the term "patient" because they feel it belongs only to the realm of doctors ("patients are people that doctors see") and may open them up to legal issues such as practicing medicine without a license. This is also why it is rare that the word "diagnosis" is ever used by a massage therapist. Massage therapists are trained to and can make assessments but cannot diagnose. Doctors diagnose. In some states because of how the scope of practice guidelines are written, the use of the term "patient" for massage therapists is not permitted. Yet many other health care workers other than doctors use the term patient for those they treat and care for such as nurses, physical therapists, physical therapy assistants and various others in the healthcare field such as radiology and ultra sound technicians. Many of those have a 2 yr degree and others have less education. It is also not uncommon to see the term 'client/patient' used in both literature and written into the language of some state laws to allow the use of both terms and somehow cover the gamut of usages and also not to cause offense. In the Second and Third paradigms, therapists assume a more authoritative position because their greater levels of education and experience have shown them that treatment may need to take a certain path for reasons that are not always obvious to the patient. **Trigger points**, for example, send burning, tingling, or numbing sensations to different areas. A trigger point in the neck may be felt in the chest, back, or forehead. However, from an Asian bodywork perspective, an energetic excess pattern of "stomach heat" can also give rise to frontal headaches. Thus, discerning the source of the issue is vital to resolving the complaint. Working directly in these remote areas where the pain is felt may alleviate it temporarily, but because the root of the problem hasn't been addressed, the pain will likely return.

Establishing a relationship in which patients heed and respect the advice of their practitioners requires that a certain rapport be established. This is created not only in part by the therapists' knowledge and education but also by how these practitioners conduct themselves. For example, having a positive and friendly relationship with patients is good, but if it becomes too casual, therapists are in danger of diminishing their main objective—to help their patients achieve a greater level of health and wellbeing. Out of friendship, therapists may hold back on telling their patients something that they may not want to hear. Similarly, patients may also stop giving their therapists' suggestions as much weight if they think of them as just friends with faults and frailties of their own, rather than a professional health care practitioner.

This does not mean that therapists should be standoffish or noncompassionate. Warm, friendly, and caring relationships can greatly influence healing potential. However, practitioners must intentionally establish professional boundaries in order to retain their ability to create positive change in their patients' lives. This healthy relationship can be shaped by many factors, including punctuality, dress, manner of speaking, questions asked, topics discussed, and the maintenance of a professional barrier between patient and therapist. Clearly, socializing with patients would cross this therapeutic boundary. Done correctly, therapists should be warm and friendly while still maintaining the professionalism necessary to be effective caregivers.

With the focus first and foremost on patient care, the more aware and wise therapist does not allow personal desire to interfere with the patient's therapeutic time. Issues that arise amongst people who are familiar with one another such as the tendency to be agreeable, the need to be liked or steering the conversation toward things that they would rather converse about is not recommended. Such may be said of the First Paradigm as well, but here it is mentioned because of the more severe effect it could have on patient compliance to practitioner recommendations and the trust necessary for the best possible therapeutic outcome at this level of care.

PATIENT RESPONSIBILITY: THE EDUCATION OF BOTH THERAPIST AND PATIENT

In the course of the training to become a Second Paradigm practitioner, therapists have likely gone through a longer massage therapy training program and have at least several relevant continuing education courses under their belts. However, even though these practitioners will generally have a greater number of techniques and modalities at their disposal, it is not until they have acquired the right kind of experience that they can truly be considered practicing at the Second Paradigm stage. Once they have attained this degree of skill and understanding, which generally only comes with time and years of experience treating, massage therapists may begin to more freely borrow from other systems and begin to utilize and integrate techniques, methods, and principles that lie outside the borders of massage and bodywork. Such areas of additional training include nutrition, physical therapy, yoga, pilates, personal training, tai chi, qi gong, and so on. Finding and working with a mentor who practices from the Second or Third Paradigm is a wonderful way to gain the necessary knowledge and experience.

Usually this kind of expansion occurs naturally as therapists grow in their understanding and ability because they come to see that there are other factors in their patients' lives that are contributing to their current state of health. Certain foods may be inflaming their arthritis or causing heartburn and indigestion. Lack of movement and exercise may be a cause of poor circulation, fatigue, pain, and even constipation. For the betterment of their patients, therapists who desire to practice on a Second Paradigm level begin to seek out new ways to evolve their practice so that they can properly educate and care for patients with more serious conditions—conditions that require assistance beyond what First Paradigm massage therapy treatment can provide. At this point, practitioners may recommend specific dietary changes, lifestyle modifications, stretches, exercises, and basic nutritional supplements that target specific conditions and imbalances and greatly assist in expediting recovery.

Unfortunately, these recommendations are not always easy to follow and may even go against patients' personalities. This is when patient education becomes of particular importance. Even though patients may not want to make certain changes, therapists must somehow impart their knowledge in a digestible and meaningful way that will inspire their patients to begin making better decisions. Many times, when patients are shown clearly how their current habits are creating their "dis-ease" they are often much more likely to at least try their therapists' recommendations. In addition, when therapists can impart this information neutrally by educating their patients rather than seeming judgmental, chances are much greater that these recommendations will be valued and taken much more seriously.

NEW RESPONSIBILITIES AND THE WORKPLACE

As the capabilities of Second Paradigm practitioners deepen and expand, so too do their responsibilities. While First Paradigm practitioners have little work and responsibility outside of the treatment itself, the work of Second Paradigm practitioners involve keeping treatment records, researching treatment protocols, cultivating an ongoing therapeutic relationship with their patients, and studying additional modalities that support the goals and scope of the Second Paradigm.

As these massage therapy professionals evolve and mature into the world of the Second Paradigm, it becomes more and more self-evident that they can be an integral link in their patient's health and that it is necessary for them to start thinking in terms of taking on the responsibility of becoming role models. Practitioners should try to become models of health care for their own sake, as well as for their patients. Through education and guidance patients are encouraged to make changes in lifestyle that enable them to become active players in their own health care evolution. When practitioners and patients work together, their minds and energy fields connect and interact to maximize patients' health care potential. Massage therapists moving into this stage of development need to be educated as to what health care really means so that it becomes possible for them to provide more of a meaningful and valuable way to ensure a successful outcome for their patients and for their own practices. In this way, too, patients become catalysts for their therapists, who need to work on taking their own responsibility to grow towards and achieve optimal health. Patients help to make their therapists role models.

As practitioners approach Second Paradigm levels, a closer alliance naturally begins to form with their patients in order to help heal and restore their balance. At this stage practitioners must begin looking beyond their particular technique and see their patients with bigger eyes so that they can develop the ability to sense **somatic** and/or energetic imbalances with their hands. And, they need to begin to get in touch with the more advanced state of intuiting with their "hearts," an ability that comes more easily and sometimes even naturally to advanced Third Paradigm practitioners.

Second Paradigm practitioners can sometimes be found working alongside medical doctors and nurses in medical clinics. However, most often they can be found either working privately or in multidisciplinary clinics with their closest allies in the complementary health care field, chiropractors and acupuncturists. These kinds of allegiances provide therapists with the added advantage of being able to discuss cases and work together with other like-minded professionals. Working in these settings can also provide more employment opportunities to work for oneself. In contrast, First Paradigm practitioners are more often employed or contracted by spas.

Also, whereas the surroundings of the First Paradigm practice are generally concerned with comforts of the senses (dim lights, soft music, etc.), the atmosphere for Second Paradigm practitioners will usually be more clinical, with décor often serving a more functional purpose. Charts and diagrams of muscles, nerves, and energetic points and pathways are commonly found adorning the walls. Tools, books, and other supplies may be more prevalent as well.

THE INTAKE, ASSESSMENT, AND TREATMENT PHASES

The intake, assessment, and treatment phases in the Second Paradigm of practice are considerably more involved and detailed than that of the First Paradigm. They also differ vastly depending upon the style of bodywork performed. A sports massage therapist may concentrate on the patient's range-of-motion or body mechanics as they throw a ball, run, or swing a club. Practitioners of Amma therapeutic massage, a form of Asian bodywork, may look to the tongue and pulse as their primary means of assessing the Qi of the channels, or meridians, of the energy body, while the practitioner of shiatsu, another form of Asian bodywork, may primarily palpate the *hara* (abdominal region) to assess the same underlying energetic layer of the patient. A Rolfer, on the other hand, may utilize a detailed postural analysis to help determine the correct course of treatment.

The initial interview and intake process depends mostly upon the purpose and intent of the treatment. This underscores the difference between what a First Paradigm practitioner needs to know versus that for a Second or Third Paradigm Practitioner. An interesting way of visually seeing this difference in "need to know" can be viewed in the differences between the sample of a brief client intake form used by a First Paradigm practioner and the more comprehensive patient health history intake form used by Second and Third Paradigm practitioners shown in Figures 3-2 and 3-3.

As previously stated in Chapter 2, a concise client history by First Paradigm professionals may include a few basic questions to be sure that there aren't any contraindications and that it's safe to proceed with the treatment. At most, a brief client intake form should be filled out. Through this process practitioners will be able to discern any painful areas, where in the body clients feel stressed, and what they would like to get out of their session before moving into the treatment itself.

In the case of Second and Third Paradigm practitioners, a lengthier interview is necessary after the patient has filled out a much more comprehensive health history form. From these forms, practitioners can glean an enormous amount of useful information about their patients' physical, physiological, psychological, and social condition and how it all relates to their health complaints.

Client Intake Form

Name _____ Today's date _____

Address _____ Phone _____

City-State-ZIP _____ Email Address _____

Date of birth _____ Age _____ Sex _____

Do you currently have any muscle pain, stiffness, or tension?

If so where?_____

Are there any areas of the body where you would like extra treatment time spent?
(neck, shoulders, low back. . . .)

_____

What physical activities do you participate in? _____

Do you suffer from any conditions such as diabetes or high blood pressure?_____

Do you have any allergies?_____

Do you have trouble sleeping?_____ Are your bowels regular? _____ Have you had

any recent surgery?_____

Are you pregnant?_____ If so due date:_____

Are you wearing: Contact Lenses?_____ Hearing Aids?_____ Dentures? _____

Please Indicate and List Any Other Medical Problems or Conditions That You Feel We
Should Be Aware Of

In case of emergency notify _____ Phone _____

Relationship _____

I understand that the massage services are designed to be a health aid and are in no way
to take the place of a doctor's care when indicated. I am aware that the massage therapist
does not diagnose disease nor prescribe medications. Information exchanged during any
massage session is educational in nature and is intended to help me become more aware
and conscious of my own health status and is to be used at my own discretion.

Client signature _____ Date _____

Figure 3-2 Client intake form.

A good patient medical history form will ask for information regarding past
and present medical conditions, medications, vitamins, supplements, surgeries, bowel habits, traumas (such as car accidents or falls), allergies, family
history, and so on. Some may ask for information regarding patients' dietary
habits as well. Good **intake forms** will also include a simple diagram of the
body so the patient can indicate areas of pain, stress, and concern. The intake

Client Health History

Name _____ Today's date _____
Address _____ Home phone _____ Other phone _____
City-State-ZIP _____ Email address _____
Date of Birth _____ Age _____ Occupation _____
Who were you referred by or how did you find out about our services? _____
What is the reason for your visit to our office? _____
_____
What results would you like to achieve with our work? _____
Have you seen a doctor or another health practitioner regarding this or similar
conditions? _____
List their names and phone numbers. Do I have your permission to contact them? _____
_____
When did you first notice the condition and what started it? _____
What makes it worse? / better? _____
Please indicate any of the following conditions that apply to you. Mark any current
conditions with an "X" and past conditions with an "O."

__ Chronic pain, where   __ Asthma   __ Learning difficulties
    _____   __ Fatigue   __ Depression
__ Joint pain, where   __ Frequent respiratory   __ Trouble sleeping
    _____   illness   __ Trouble concentrating
__ Muscle pain, where   __ Lung or respiratory   __ Memory loss
    _____   condition   __ Hearing problems
__ Other pain, where   __ Cold hands or feet   __ Vision problems
    _____   __ Swollen ankles   __ Contacts
__ Headache   __ Varicose veins   __ Paralysis
__ Numbness, where   __ High blood pressure   __ Nervous system
    _____   __ Low blood pressure   conditions
__ Broken bones, where,   __ Lymphedema   __ Allergies
    when _____   __ Heart condition   __ Rashes
__ Sprains/strains, where   __ Indigestion   __ Skin conditions
    _____   __ Loss of appetite   __ Tumors/cancer
__ Arthritis   __ Diarrhea   __ Shingles/herpes
__ Osteoporosis   __ Constipation   __ Pregnancies
__ Bursitis   __ Gas/bloating   __ PMS
__ Tendonitis   __ Ulcers   __ Hysterectomy
__ Scoliosis   __ Digestive condition   __ Menopause
__ Bone disease   __ Bowel condition   __ Birth control
__ Dizziness   __ Eating disorders   __ Prostate
__ Difficulty breathing   __ Panic attacks/anxiety   __ Reproductive concerns
__ Sinus conditions   __ Hyperactivity

Explain any conditions noted above. _____
_____

Figure 3-3 Patient health history form.

(Continues)

Infectious and childhood diseases (list what and when) _____

Congenital or acquired disability (describe) _____

Surgeries (list what and when) _____

Injuries or accidents causing injury _____

List any other medical or health condition not listed _____

List, including frequency of use, all medications, remedies, herbs, and supplements you use. _____

Do you use any of the following? List frequency and amount.

Caffeine _____ Nicotine _____ Alcohol _____

Sugar _____ Recreational drugs _____

List stress-relieving activities you participate in. Include type and frequency; that is, exercise, massage, hobbies, sports, etc. _____

List any other concerns or comments regarding you health status or well-being. _____

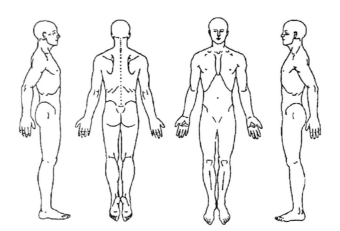

On the above diagram, indicate any areas in which you experience pain with an X and circle any other areas of concern.

To the best of my knowledge, I have disclosed all of my past and current health conditions. I will inform the therapist of any changes in my health status.

Client signature _____ Date _____

Figure 3-4 Patient health history form.

Release of Medical Information Form

Client's name _____ Phone _____

Address _____ City _____ State ___ ZIP _____

I hereby authorize _____(Practitioner's Name)_____ to release to any physician or health
care practitioner directly involved in my care any medical records or other personal
health information necessary for the purpose of receiving physician's recommendations
and approval, or sharing concerns regarding my health and well-being.
This authorization remains valid for the period of _____ to _____ or
for the time period that I am seeing the above-named practitioner.

Signed _____ Date _____

Figure 3-5 Medical Information Release Form.

form should also ask for information and permission to contact patients' physicians and any other health care providers they may be seeing. Patients of Second and Third Paradigm practitioners will need to sign a "**Release of Medical Information**" form. This will give their practitioners permission to share their personal information with other health professionals (Figure 3-5).

Besides providing essential information that will help shape the treatment plan, the interview and intake process provides practitioners with important information regarding whether to proceed, refer out to another health professional, or perhaps make a call to a patient's physician for further information and clarification before beginning treatment.

This evaluation is of the utmost importance because it will determine the direction and goal of each session. During this phase, therapists are seeking to understand the exact nature of what their patients are experiencing. Often what they will find is a combination of physical ailments and pent-up emotional issues that may require looking beyond the obvious. These practitioners must listen carefully not only to what their patients say but also to the more subtle cues and clues that are expressed nonverbally. These may come in the form of an inflection in the voice, the skin's appearance, the way they walk, or simply how they breathe. These factors can help therapists gauge the pressure, style, and intent for each treatment. This initial assessment process can take anywhere between 10 and 30 minutes before the treatment, but may continue throughout the entire session.

Another major difference that separates the First and Second Paradigms is that the treatment itself becomes much more specialized. Full-body sessions will become rarer simply because of the focus, time, and energy that are needed to really treat an injury or ailment. This doesn't mean that therapists will always focus on one area for the entire session or that they will neglect the rest of the body. It just means that some areas may need more work than others at specific times. That said, most forms of Asian bodywork will always utilize the full-body treatment to address the injured area.

The length of each appointment can range anywhere from 20 to 90 minutes depending on the approach, treatment plan, and condition being treated. In Second Paradigm practice, there is often a greater number of shorter treatments; however, the frequency of treatments may increase to two or three times a week.

To the outside observer, a Second Paradigm treatment may not look all that different from a First Paradigm session. Oftentimes, similar techniques will be employed; however, the application will be more precise and the end results will be completely different. This is because the driving force behind each technique will be different as well. Each technique applied by the Second Paradigm practitioner will be infused with greater knowledge and intent and will often be used in conjunction with an array of other bodywork techniques that support it.

These applied massage techniques build on one another and move the session in a more focused and specific direction. Yet, even as their technical skills become more effective, Second Paradigm practitioners will begin to rely less solely on their own efforts as they become more experienced. To really take their treatments in the direction they want to go in, their patients may in fact need to become active participants in the treatment process.

In this paradigm, patients are not always passive receivers as they often are at the First Paradigm level of practice. The dynamics are quite different here. Interactions are generally more involved because patients may be asked to engage in the treatment process by talking about their issues, breathing into areas that are constricted, participating in active muscle testing and **range-of-motion assessments**, or simply observing what their bodies are doing. Through this process, patients can gain valuable awareness and insight. Most people are unaware of what's happening internally and do not have a real sense of how their bodies operate and their energies (Qi) move. Through these kinds of interactions during treatment, patients often realize that they habitually hold tension in specific areas. By remembering to relax those areas or simply breathing more fully, they can undo a lot of the tensions experienced on a daily basis. This also helps therapists take the treatment deeper and further than they would be able to do on their own.

CASE HISTORIES

This brief compilation of Second Paradigm case histories provides an insight into the way a massage therapist practices at this stage. They include histories of patients who were under the care of experienced Second Paradigm practitioners as they were treated for pain, physical ailments, and a wide variety of other issues that fall within the scope of this paradigm.

Case histories presented in this format can provide opportunities for students, therapists, and patients alike for integrative thinking and problem solving, although each for different reasons. They are written here to teach students how to think and solve problems and to demonstrate the profound kinds of outcomes possible through massage treatment; for practitioners to demonstrate what's possible to others regarding the integration of different techniques, methods, and adjunctive disciplines in the planning and treating of their patients; and to give some good examples for patients themselves of what is available and possible in the world of massage therapy to help what ails them.

In general, writing up case histories is actually a good practice for both students and therapists because it requires that they describe what they see, what they feel, and what they do. And by having to explain to ourselves, in some form or another, what it is we do, we can learn to better evaluate, correct, adjust, and perfect how we do it. To respect privacy, names, and at times gender, were changed in writing these brief histories to disguise any patient identification. However, the essential facts remain intact.

CASE HISTORY

Frozen Shoulder—Right Shoulder and Arm Pain Due to a Car Accident Treated with Deep Tissue Massage using Trigger-Point Therapy and Full-Body Swedish Massage

Amy, a member of her high school tennis team, complained of a condition called "frozen shoulder." Ever since a car accident three months ago, she has gradually been losing mobility in her right arm and shoulder. She says her right shoulder hurts a lot and the arm feels "stuck" when she tries to lift it up. When testing her arms for range of motion, there is a clear difference between the left and right arms. Even just raising her arms horizontally into a "T" position is difficult. Her left arm points straight out to the side while her right arm shakes and tilts downward. Testing the muscles for strength reveals that her right shoulder is considerably weaker than her left.

This condition that Amy exhibits is not uncommon, especially after an accident. In these types of traumatic events, the muscles suffer small tears. As the torn muscles become inflamed, the surrounding musculature tightens and restricts movement as an instinctive form of protection to the area. This does brace the area and prevent further injury, but it also traps metabolic wastes and decreases the vital flow of nutritive blood and lymphatic fluid to the injured area that help to heal the damaged tissue.

The first session of deep tissue massage and trigger point therapy lasted 30 minutes, and the entire time was spent on the shoulder and associated musculature. Much work was done to the rotator cuff (a group of muscles that attach the arm and shoulder blade) as well as to the shoulder, neck, and upper back.

Afterwards Amy felt much less pain, her range-of-motion was increased somewhat, and her strength improved a little as well. She was given home stretches, which she has been doing every day and has come for treatments twice a week for two months. As Amy's motion was restored more and more, she was given full-body Swedish massage treatments for one of her biweekly sessions, mostly to increase the circulation throughout her body, relax her, and to help set the deep tissue and trigger point work more permanently. She no longer exhibits the weakness that she did before and her range of motion has almost completely returned. Presently, she only comes for regular Swedish massage treatments twice a month as part of an overall maintenance program.

Carpel Tunnel Syndrome Treated with Shiatsu Therapy

Robert is a police officer who spends most of his time behind the desk working on a computer. About a year ago he started having pain in both wrists and hands, as well as tingling, burning, weakness, and some numbness. He was diagnosed with carpal tunnel syndrome. His condition became so severe that he ended up having surgery on one wrist, but the pain hasn't really let up. This unfortunate result has left him hesitant to have an operation on the other wrist, his original plan, even though the pain and other symptoms are getting worse.

Since he had exhausted the treatment methods that western medicine had to offer, including pain and **anti-inflammatory** medications, splints and braces, and because his first surgery did not seem to help that hand, he began to look elsewhere for treatment options. Robert checked out the Internet and found that there had been similar cases to his own and found some solid research in which a batch of regular massage therapy treatments had successful outcomes.

He did some further research to find the right massage therapist and set up his first appointment. The massage professional Robert visited was an experienced shiatsu practitioner who put him through his detailed intake process, including some testing. Shiatsu, a form of Asian bodywork, was a good choice because the treatment offered the benefits of both the soft tissue manipulation as well as direct pressure to specific acupuncture channels and points that would have a really deep energetic and unblocking effect. The therapist explained to Robert what exactly he thought would be the best course of treatment for his problem. Robert agreed and then proceeded to get his first in a series of shiatsu treatments.

The shiatsu routine consisted primarily of stroking and manipulation of moderate to deep pressure from the fingertips to the elbow. It also included treatment to Robert's shoulders and neck helping to open up the circulation to those areas and reduce any buildup of tensions stemming from the original problem in both hands. In addition, Robert's treatment included the practitioner's pressing and holding a series of acupuncture points on the affected channels in those same areas. After a block of 10 regularly administered treatments, 3 each during weeks one and two, and 2 treatments each during the following two weeks, the symptoms of carpal tunnel were diminished greatly, including in the hand that had been operated on. The shiatsu treatments not only helped to reduce the pain, tingling, and numbness but they also increased Robert's grip strength.

In addition to treatments, Robert was given a regimen of shoulder, arm, and hand stretches to practice daily and was advised to make changes to his diet, particularly to eliminate foods that are inflammatory. He was also given breathing techniques to help him become aware of and relax the unconscious tensions that he holds during work, mostly while typing on his computer. Robert was also counseled on the correct posture to reduce stress on his wrists and forearms while working at his desk.

Joint Pain Treated with Reiki

Lawrence, a 38-year-old male postal worker, had pain in almost every joint in his body. He had received an entire battery of tests done by a rheumatologist and surprisingly they all turned out negative for arthritis. He was taking a few different medications that had helped relieve the pain at first but the effects were wearing off. It appeared that he built up a tolerance to the medication, not an uncommon problem. After one year of conventional medical treatments, Lawrence had exhausted all efforts at treating his condition from the western perspective, so he decided to try **Reiki** on the recommendation of a friend. Although he had no real idea of what Reiki was and tended to be a bit skeptical, he was desperate for help and decided to go with the friend's referral. His pain and discomfort were making it harder and harder for him to do his work for the Post Office. And as is usual with pain syndromes, it was also taking its toll on him emotionally.

After the first few treatments by a Reiki Master, Lawrence began to feel a very clear relief, even though he did not really understand why or how. The essential work of the Reiki practitioner is to boost the amount of life force within the body and balance it within an individual. By increasing the amount of the fundamental substance (Qi) flowing through an individual, the skilled Reiki practitioner can often dramatically improve many functions of the body and mind.

The treatments are conducted through a series of hand positions, usually beginning from the top of the head and down either to the feet or to the pelvis. Most positions are directly on or over the major energetic centers along the midline of the body, known as chakras, and each position is held for three to five minutes. Lawrence began experiencing some relief after the first few treatments, and now after several months of weekly treatment, his joint pain has resolved. During this time, Lawrence's therapist also helped him improve his diet, which was a major contributor to his painful joint condition. Working at the Post Office has once again become easier and his freedom from pain has also allowed him to begin using personalized gym workouts for further rehabilitation.

Lower Back Pain Treated with Full Body Swedish Massage integrated with Deep Tissue and Myofascial Release Techniques

Sylvia, a 73-year-old woman with good energy and in good shape for her age, recently started having low-back pain that became so severe she had to start walking with a cane. Although she usually was accustomed to a youthful vibrancy, she said that she felt much older as of late. She saw her physician, who ruled out more serious conditions as a potential cause and recommended that she try a series of massage therapy sessions. She was referred to a massage therapist by her son.

After each Swedish massage session, her back felt better, but invariably the pain would return—often the very next day. So the therapist decided that she needed to do some deeper work to get to the root of Sylvia's problem. She was originally trying to avoid having to go much deeper due to Sylvia's advanced age. However, Sylvia was in fairly good physical shape and agreed to let her therapist do some deeper work after it was explained what needed to be done. The therapist then proceeded to integrate some deep tissue and myofascial techniques in alternating sessions. As a result, Sylvia was getting longer lasting periods free from pain.

At one of the earlier sessions, the therapist noticed something about the way Sylvia got up from her chair. She seemed to be hurting herself by the way she leaned forward and used her lower back to lift the entire weight of her upper body. After some questioning, it was discovered that it was motions like these (getting up from sitting or from lying down) that gave her the most discomfort. After evaluating the movement, Sylvia and her therapist spent time reorganizing the way she used her body. Instead of leaning forward when getting up, she was taught to keep her back straight and use the muscles of her legs to stand straight up. It was a little difficult at first because she wasn't used to this motion, but it was immediately obvious that she could do it without pain. She was given a series of exercises to develop strength in both legs and was directed to practice this new motion every time she stood up from sitting. The therapist restructured the way Sylvia got up step-by-step so that she was able to perform the action without hurting herself in the process.

A very diligent woman, Sylvia has been doing her exercises every day and has practiced her new movements whenever she had the chance. As a result of the combination of treatment and consistently practicing the exercises she was taught, the pain has almost completely resolved and she no longer needs a cane. Since then, she has continued to come in every other week for her massage therapy treatments, which are adjusted each time based on how she is feeling. Sylvia reports that these treatments are crucial to helping maintain her vitality, relaxed state and pain-free lower back.

Migraine Headaches—Treated with Amma Therapeutic Massage and Craniosacral Therapy

Michael, a 32-year-old carpenter, had long suffered from migraines. They were so severe that they interfered with his work and had become more prevalent lately to the point where it was affecting his income from days lost simply lying at home in a darkened room. He had tried all the western medical approaches, including a battery of neurological tests and prescription medication, which he was not happy about because of its negative side effects. After talking to a number of his business associates and doing his own research on the Internet, Michael decided to take a more natural approach by seeking out a massage therapist who had experience and success with treating headaches, especially migraines. When he arrived at the therapist's practice, she immediately noticed that he looked fatigued and that one eye, his left one, was a bit less open than the right. Also, both his shoulders were elevated. The therapist suggested a series of Amma therapeutic massage treatments. Amma is a form of Asian bodywork that focuses on acupressure points and deep manipulation of the energy channels of the body. Michael reluctantly agreed. He was unfamiliar with this form of bodywork and was expecting the most common form of massage therapy, Swedish massage.

After his first visit, Michael didn't notice feeling anything different, but admitted that he did sleep better that night—actually better than he had in a very long time. Over the next week, Michael found that his digestion, energy levels, and general tension headaches, which regularly plague him, had significantly improved. He thought that perhaps the treatment was more beneficial than he previously realized. Although he suffered a migraine, it was not one of his worst ones, a very hopeful sign.

Michael returned for another visit and this time the therapist commented on his left eye and recommended alternating Amma treatments with **craniosacral therapy** to help alleviate the imbalance manifesting in his eye, as well as further work on the migraines from this approach. The treatment is a series of gentle holding patterns that did not feel like much to Michael, but through these treatments he began to recall some past experiences. In one instance he recalled being shunned by his brother. In another, he remembered being hit in the head with a kickball. Each time, as per the therapist's suggestion, Michael spoke of his past experiences and the therapist noticed a freeing of his sphenoid and temporal bones of the skull. At the end of the treatment, Michael arose, amazed at how light he felt. As he fixed his hair in the mirror preparing to go, he was astounded to see that his left eye was just as open as his right.

Michael's massage therapy practitioner also made many nutritional recommendations, specifically related to staying away from the foods that are known to catalyze migraine headaches. Michael had come across some of this same basic information during his own research on the Internet and was really shocked to find this out—and more so that his physician never mentioned making any dietary changes. As a final recommendation, his therapist suggested that he look into biofeedback and locate a certified practitioner in the area to learn how to control the physiological processes involved in migraines. Biofeedback training is widely known for teaching chronic migraine sufferers how to control and eventually end these painful migraine syndromes. In the ensuing weeks, as he returned for alternating Amma and craniosacral therapy treatments, Michael's migraines began to disappear. He no longer misses days of work or time with his family.

Herniated Discs in the Lower Lumbar Region Treated with Deep Tissue Massage and Full Body Swedish Massage

Gerald, a 38-year-old male, has bulging (herniated) discs in his lower lumbar area that was aggravated by a car accident 15 years ago. Recently, the pain had begun to increase, catalyzed by some heavy gardening work in his backyard. He was also experiencing shooting pain down the front of his thighs to his knees. It was recommended by his orthopedist that he get an MRI (magnetic resonance imaging), which clearly showed the bulging discs as well as a couple of small, benign tumors on the left side of his spine near the area of the bulging discs. Gerald is generally a very athletic and active person and has found this debilitating condition catalyzing bouts of depression. Gerald's physician recommended that he begin taking an antidepressant. In addition, Gerald was put on some very strong pain and anti-inflammatory medications.

Before seriously discussing surgery for his discs and subsequent physical therapy, Gerald was referred by his orthopedist to a massage therapist and began receiving 30- to 45-minute treatments of deep tissue massage on the affected area. After the very first treatment, the shooting pain in his thighs diminished significantly. On the pain scale, he reported going from a 10, the highest and most painful, down to a 4. Although there was still some shooting pain left, it was an amazing experience for Gerald, one which began to instill a little hope that there was light at the end of the tunnel. After the next few treatments, the shooting pain fully disappeared. At that point, what remained was pain in the more localized area of the initial injury.

In addition to being a massage therapist, Gerald's practitioner was also a personal fitness trainer, and so Gerald began to do some light workouts with him. The big advantage here is that his massage professional was already very well versed on Gerald's specific problem and could design an exercise program that would be exactly fitted to his needs. Gerald continued his deep tissue treatments, alternating with full-body Swedish massage treatments.

After about eight weeks of treatment, Gerald is almost pain free, but must still be careful in his physical activities and work his way back up to working out at full intensity. Until Gerald gets another MRI it won't be possible to know if any or all of the protruding discs retreated back into their normal positions. More likely at this point the treatments, along with the exercise, helped to greatly relax and reduce the muscle spasms that were irritating nerves and aggravating the entire area, producing his pain. Gerald was also able to wean off of the antidepressants and anti-inflammatory medications and is overall a much happier individual.

Severe Lower Back Pain Due to Surgery on Left Knee Treated with Neuromuscular Therapy and Trigger Point Therapy

Susan is a 38-year-old school teacher who recently developed severe pain on the left side of her low back. After going through all of the standard medical tests and finding out from her orthopedist that medication and physical therapy were the least radical options available to her, she decided on an alternate route. Based on many of the positive stories she had heard Susan decided to seek out a massage therapy practitioner who specializes in **neuromuscular therapy**. She found one that came highly recommended and made her first appointment.

At the onset of that visit, Susan's neuromuscular therapist noticed that she had indicated on her intake form that she had recent surgery on her left knee. The therapist suspected she may have been compensating for the weakened knee by shifting her weight over to her right side. This would put a greater demand on the muscles in the left side of her low back. Susan stated that she hadn't had trouble with her knee since the surgery six months ago and had also resumed her exercise regimen, which included light weight training and walking a few miles at the beach a few times a week. As part of the initial intake, the therapist palpated Susan's back and saw a common cross-patterning of left low-back tightness, and right mid-back spasm resulting from the body's attempts to remain upright.

The therapist explained to Susan that he suspected she might still be suffering the consequences of the former knee problem. Her body may have learned a new way of compensating by positioning itself over her right leg in order to shift weight off the previously bad knee. He explained that walking on uneven surfaces such as on a sandy beach was not a good idea because it encourages further elevation of the hip in order to avoid having to lift the leg and bend the knee too much.

The therapist treated the areas using neuromuscular therapy techniques and specific trigger points, which reduced a lot of muscular tightness. This in turn encouraged the body to unwind and relax into a more balanced posture. However, recognizing that if Susan didn't begin to pay more attention to her posture and how she was walking and compensating for her left knee the treatments would only act as a temporary relief. The therapist decided that he would have to work with Susan in more detail on this issue.

The therapist taught Susan to stand more squarely over her hips and in front of a mirror he had her march in place without allowing her body to shift so extremely to her right side. Susan felt much better following her treatment. She reported noticing that she feels more balanced and agreed to practice at home. In a few more sessions the back pain had almost completely disappeared and after consistent practice on Susan's part, she was able to march in place more naturally without any pain. She was also able to walk without any perceptible shift to one side.

SUMMARY

The main purpose of this chapter was to present a detailed description of the Second Paradigm of practice and, in doing so, distinguish it from the First and Third Paradigms. During this chapter, it was explained how the scope of Second Paradigm massage therapy and bodywork practice is rooted in remediation, therapy, and pain relief. On the continuum of growth and development of a massage therapist, this level of practice reflects the middle ground between reducing stress and comprehensive holistic health care. Because of this, maturely evolved Second Paradigm therapists will naturally embrace qualities in their work of both the paradigm above and below, administering treatments that include relieving tension and stress, as well as stepping up into roles and responsibilities that are the primary work of Third Paradigm practitioners. This chapter also emphasized the importance of learning, developing, and adding new skills and abilities of the most useful adjunctive therapies that can be integrated into treatment within the scope of the Second Paradigm.

A number of brief case histories were also presented to help provide an understanding and appreciation for this paradigm of practice. They include histories of patients who were under the care of highly skilled Second Paradigm practitioners as they were treated for pain, physical ailments, and other issues that fall within the scope of the Second Paradigm. These histories also demonstrate how integrating various massage treatment techniques with other modalities broadens massage therapy practitioners' scope of care and begins opening the path into the Third Paradigm of practice.

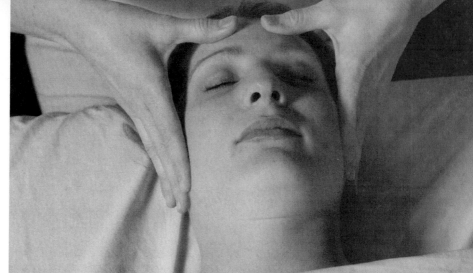

4

CHAPTER

Third Paradigm—Holistic Integration

CHAPTER GOALS

1. Develop an understanding of the Third Paradigm of practice.

2. Distinguish the First and Second Paradigms of practice from the Third Paradigm of practice.

3. Understand the Third Paradigm of practice as holistic and integrative in its approach to treatment.

4. Understand the importance of self-development as playing a significant role towards evolving into a Third Paradigm practitioner.

5. Recognize the important role Third Paradigm therapists must play intellectually and emotionally in order to appropriately engage their patients to take responsibility for their own health and well-being.

6. Understand the importance of the relationship between Third Paradigm-level massage therapy and bodywork practice and some of the most useful and most popular adjunctive therapies that can be integrated into treatment plans and treatment in order to greatly expand the scope of a therapist's practice, including but not limited to

   - Asian bodywork
   - Acupuncture
   - Chiropractic
   - Moxibustion

- Chinese herbalism
- Western herbalism
- Diet and nutrition
- Biofeedback
- Bach Flower Remedies
- Exercise
- Hypnotherapy
- Guided imagery
- Naturopathy
- Aromatherapy
- Homeopathy

7. Gain an appreciation for Third Paradigm practice through becoming familiar with some actual case histories that briefly illustrate how integrating massage therapy with various other modalities increases practitioners' ability to heal by expanding their practice into other dimensions of treating.

INTRODUCTION

Practitioners of the Third Paradigm are generally therapists who have a driving interest in helping others to heal, that is, to make them "whole." They practice from a holistic perspective that views humans as much more than their skeletal structure, muscles, tissues, and organs. They understand an individual to be a **mind-body-emotion-spirit complex**, where imbalances in this dynamic can lead to "dis-ease" and eventually to chronic and debilitating illnesses. Essentially, the role of Third Paradigm practitioners is to use whatever they have in their arsenals to help restore and maintain this balance. Generally speaking, the arsenals of First and Second Paradigm professionals are insufficient for this level of care because these practitioners do not have the knowledge and skills necessary to fulfill the roles and responsibilities of this level of practice.

For most practitioners of the Third Paradigm, evolving their understanding of the human condition goes hand-in-hand with expanding their education with more advanced or even new approaches to treating. At some point, these therapists recognize that their current knowledge and technique base is no longer adequate to accomplish this level of healing. They want to do more and find themselves hampered by their lack of knowledge and skills in assessing and treating, as well as in various other supportive modalities. They desire to evolve from technician into master practitioner and healer. Those that truly undertake this path recognize that to do so requires a great deal of study, persistence, commitment, and directed attention. They understand that such efforts will expand their consciousness and develop their palpatory and sensory awareness—ultimately transforming it into intuition. Some are born with this great gift of **intuition** already fully formed, but others can develop it through the practice of self-development while simultaneously expanding and honing their knowledge and skills.

THE WAY OF THE THIRD PARADIGM

In order to move into the Third Paradigm, whatever style or form of massage a person has learned must first be perfected. All too often students learn one form and then start learning other styles and mix and match what they have acquired. This then becomes a hodge-podge of techniques that does not produce healing and can even worsen a condition. For example, Asian body-work techniques meant to move and balance energy, or qi, are often used along with Swedish massage treatments, which are meant to move blood and lymph. Although this may relax and even improve some of the milder conditions, there is a clear loss of purpose and intention in the mix. Such treatments will usually not have a lasting effect and may often make the problem worse, for example, by catalyzing a headache or muscle spasm.

This is really not much different than beginners in one style of martial arts mixing in all kinds of techniques from other styles learned from a book or seminar. Although it may be more fun to practice this way, and may give one the impression of knowing a lot more, the true essence of the style cannot be effectively understood and therefore will not yield the most successful results when practicing it. It is not the way these modalities were taught and it is not the way they should be used—at least not until there is a much greater level of knowledge and experience on the part of the therapist. Intermingling techniques from different forms can only be accomplished properly with real purpose and understanding. This generally requires a teacher or master practitioner who can guide and give reasons for when and why it is or isn't appropriate. Third Paradigm practitioners always know and are aware of what they are doing and why. True aim and strong intention are the hallmarks of a Third Paradigm practitioner.

After Third Paradigm therapists learn a specific modality of massage therapy and bodywork, they must then perfect it, usually with the help of a teacher or mentor who is already considered a "master" or expert in that style. This is someone who can correct and guide his or her students into the world of higher palpation, sensitivity, and intuition. Even practitioners who have graduated from a certified program in massage are still only beginners in the field and need to work with someone who can help them perfect their knowledge, skills, and abilities in the particular form that they have chosen. In the world of karate, for example, attaining the coveted level of first degree black belt means that a student has graduated and attained the level of beginner. In the martial arts, "beginner" is considered the level where real serious study first starts. It is only when practitioners of the martial arts have achieved this level of black belt that they are truly prepared to begin the study and practice of advanced forms and techniques. Everything up until that point is considered preparatory and foundational.

In this same way, practitioners of massage must recognize that graduating from a program, even from the most comprehensive ones, means that they have only learned the basic techniques and now they must begin to learn, evolve, and practice in earnest. During the time that they are diligently at work they must also gradually begin to seek out and learn adjunctive therapies that will support, enhance and broaden their practices and treatments so that they can improve the results they get with their patients. This is the way of the Third Paradigm.

AN HOLISTIC/INTEGRATIVE APPROACH

A Third Paradigm or holistic approach to treatment is often best expressed, though not exclusively, by traditional Chinese medicine. As will be explained later in Chapter 9: The Bio-Energetic Layer of the Massage Therapy and Bodywork Continuum, the **energy system** is often attacked or impinged upon by a variety of external, as well as internal, factors. Although the causes of disease are often multiple and interrelated, it always results in some level of disturbance to the underlying balance of the energy system that then begins to manifest as illness in the physical body. Treating these energetic disturbances that have many causes most often requires a multipronged approach to achieve the best results.

One of the problems with western medicine is that it all too often takes a reductionist approach to the human body—always seeking to reduce the causes of disease down to the smallest possible common denominator. This approach assumes it will provide a better understanding of the cause of the problem, while often forgetting and neglecting the rest of the mind-body complex in the process. Holism provides a bigger perspective. It takes the position that to understand true health one must understand the whole person and must always approach healing with the awareness that the mind and the body are a unity. Practitioners must realize that any treatment of the body will affect the mind and any treatment of the mind will affect the body. The aim of Third Paradigm (holistic/integrative) treatment is not simply the absence of illness but also the creation of an ongoing positive state of well-being.

In **traditional Chinese medicine** (**TCM**) for example, there are five main branches: 1) massage and bodywork, 2) acupuncture, 3) herbalism, 4) diet and nutrition, and 5) exercise. Traditionally, a doctor of TCM had to be a master of all five branches in order to practice medicine successfully. Massage practitioners seeking to move into the Third Paradigm must follow a similar path. They have to recognize that their massage practices need to evolve well beyond technical mastery whatever the massage modality and that their work is enhanced by incorporating other adjunctive therapies such as diet, nutrition, supplementation, exercise, and relaxation techniques—all of which can improve the positive effects and benefits of their treatments. It is after years of concentrated and dedicated practice, constant self-correction, and earnest study that practitioners move into the realm of the Third Paradigm.

Third Paradigm practitioners seek to go beyond treating for relaxation and stress reduction (the realm of the First Paradigm) and must even go beyond remediation and pain relief, (the realm of the Second). Relaxation, remediation, and the reduction of pain are often the secondary or side benefits resulting from Third Paradigm treatment. Therapists at this level are not averse to taking on a larger and more primary role of responsibility in the overall care of their patients. They are also not averse to bringing their arsenal of massage modalities and **adjunctive therapies** to treat patients suffering from severe illnesses such as cancer, multiple sclerosis, Parkinson's disease, AIDS, diabetes, and so on. They see their treatments as helping to fortify and build the immune system, providing quality of life (and often longevity), and, in many cases, great improvement in the conditions being treated, including slower progression and even remission of some diseases. Often, along with the care of the patient's physician, Third Paradigm practitioners help their patients wean off of unnecessary medications, which in and of itself can help reduce many of the iatrogenic complications (illnesses that are unintentionally induced by medical treatment) and symptoms being experienced.

Third Paradigm practitioners often become patient advocates, work with other health care professionals, and act as liaisons between patient and doctor—helping to ensure that both parties gain a more complete and accurate understanding of their patient's current state of health, treatment results, and other treatment options that they may want to explore.

THE IMPORTANCE OF SELF-DEVELOPMENT

One of the most important aspects of evolving into the Third Paradigm is the practice and application to oneself of various self-development methods and techniques along the way. This may include, for example, different ways of increasing self-knowledge and emotional self-awareness through counseling, meditation, and stress management. Staying healthy and in shape through regular diet, cleansing/detoxification, and exercise regimens is also a very important part of the practitioner's development and growth. Through such practices, massage therapists become more balanced in mind, body, emotion, and spirit and also develop their level of consciousness. As a result they become much more capable of understanding the emotional and physical states of the patients that they work with. They can be more empathetic and compassionate, not only regarding a patient's present situation but also regarding the path of treatment and the expected reactions and experiences a patient may have during their practitioners' prescribed course of massage therapy treatment.

Massage therapists should try to become role models. They should try hard not to be like the doctor who tells his patients to stop smoking while a cigar hangs from his lips. When for example, practitioners talk about supplementation, diet, exercise, and herbs, it will always be more meaningful when it comes from their own experience of benefits gleaned and difficulties that they themselves have encountered.

Practitioners must also be educated about western drugs and their side effects so that they can properly assess their patient's symptoms and know when to refer the patient back to either their physician or to another health care practitioner. Massage therapists must continually read and expand their knowledge base about current research, disease patterns, new diseases, and treatments. At the same time they must study and learn how to promote wellness and incorporate age-old techniques and treatments when orthodox western treatments are inadequate and/or failing.

One of the hallmarks of Third Paradigm practice is that each patient is assessed individually and treatments are tailored to his or her own "pattern of disharmony." There is no "one way" to treat all patients. In addition, Third Paradigm therapists take responsibility for their patients that goes beyond the actual treatment itself. They regularly follow up by calling the patient to see how they are doing after treatment, check on and research their medications and side effects, speak with other health professionals when necessary, and strive to understand the patient's emotional and mental states without negativity, disdain, or judgment.

PATIENT RESPONSIBILITY

Third Paradigm therapists must also be able to intellectually and emotionally engage their patients to take responsibility for their own health and well-being. This means that the patient has to be educated on how to work with their therapist in their own healing process. Being under the care of a Third Paradigm **holistic practitioner** is very different from visiting a First or Second Paradigm practitioner. When patients leave a holistic practitioner's office they will usually be armed with an ongoing treatment plan, a lot of information, dietary guidelines, supplements, herbs, and exercises (although not necessarily all on the first visit) tailored to their specific needs. They must go home and begin to implement the changes discussed and practice what they have been taught in preparation for the next treatment. In this way, the practitioner and the therapist work hand-in-hand toward the same goal, and the chances for success are optimized.

First and Second Paradigm practitioners certainly provide useful information and make appropriate recommendations to their clients/patients as well when necessary. The primary distinction here has mostly to do with the extent of a practitioner's training and experience and the level of willingness and skill to take on, care for, work with, and follow through with more serious and complicated cases. Most practitioners in the First Paradigm will generally treat the same client only once or very infrequently, as, for example, in a resort spa setting. These clients come with no major complaints and with little expectation other than receiving a relaxing and stress-reducing treatment. Patients of Second Paradigm massage therapy practitioners will often be placing their health, at least in part, under their care and will usually require a level of involvement and responsibility beyond that of First Paradigm work. Over time First and Second Paradigm therapists, if they so desire, can work to evolve into Third Paradigm practitioners.

Generally speaking, holistic practitioners of the Third paradigm are therapists who understand and practice compassion to a very high degree. Two of the highest paths a person can take in life are healing and teaching. Practitioners of the Third Paradigm are persons who strive to embody both of these paths. When therapists have evolved to where they can understand the physical, mental, and emotional condition of their patients (because they themselves have worked through similar states of being) they become empathic. These therapists can then carefully and perceptively guide their patients to develop beneficial health practices while administering creative massage therapy treatments that help them to heal and become whole.

EFFECTIVE ADJUNCTIVE THERAPIES FOR THE THIRD PARADIGM PRACTITIONER

As already mentioned, part of what makes a massage therapist a Third Paradigm practitioner has as much to do with experience and self-development as it has to do with the arsenal of tools, techniques, and knowledge a practitioner brings to the table. The following section briefly details some of the most useful and most popular adjunctive therapies that can be integrated into treatment and can be used to broaden the scope of a therapist's practice. The list of therapies described below is by no means all inclusive but, rather, is meant to act as a guide for those practitioners interested to either seek them out for the benefits they provide, learning and adding them to their own arsenal of practice, or for practitioners to align themselves with other health professionals who are experts in these modalities for possible patient referral.

ASIAN BODYWORK

Asian bodywork is recommended and listed here first for practitioners of massage therapy who wish to evolve their perspective, knowledge, and skills beyond the limits of treating the physical body to include the energy body. While almost all massage treatment focuses on the soft tissue, that is, muscles, ligaments, and fascia, Asian bodywork modalities move things a step further by including the study and manipulation of the energy system—considered to be the underlying and enlivening layer of the human being complex. A working knowledge of the energy system, its principles of assessment, and skillful manipulation of the channels and points greatly broadens the scope of the kinds of conditions that a massage therapist can learn to treat. In Chapter 9, several of the major bioenergetic modalities of Asian bodywork are described. Although most massage and bodywork therapies, when mastered, can be used along with other adjunctive modalities listed in this section to treat many different and more serious conditions, training and practice in one of the bioenergetic modalities can provide a clearer path to Third Paradigm of practice. This is because of the potential expansion in scope of practice when the energetic system is included as part of one's training, overall perspective, and treatment.

ACUPUNCTURE

Acupuncture is one of the oldest documented health care modalities in history, dating back over 5,000 years. In China, physicians study not only western medical coursework but also acupuncture, bodywork, and herbs and then specialize in either eastern or western medicine. Acupuncture, once ridiculed in the West as quackery, now has become practically mainstream. Clinical trials using western research methods have demonstrated acupuncture's efficacy with regard to pain relief[1], addictions, nausea and vomiting, childbirth, infertility[2], and the treatment of many serious and chronic conditions. Many studies have shown the immune-boosting effects of acupuncture therapy.[3] Acupuncture is a wonderful adjunct to massage, especially in the treatment of musculoskeletal problems. Today, acupuncture schools across the USA are seeing certified and licensed massage therapists enrolled in their programs interested in broadening their knowledge, skills and abilities and scope of practice into the Third Paradigm. In acupuncture, very fine, sterile needles are inserted into the superficial layer of the skin and used to stimulate specific energy points that are chosen by the acupuncturist after an extensive process of assessment. The purpose of acupuncture treatment is to balance the energy system and assist the body in self-healing (Figure 4-1).

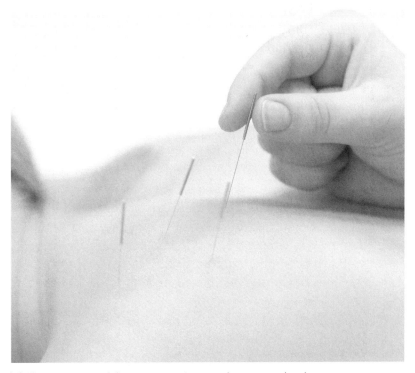

Figure 4-1 A woman receiving acupuncture on her upper back. *Image copyright 2009, Yuri Arcurs. Used under license from shutterstock.com.*

MOXIBUSTION

Moxibustion is the application of heat to acupuncture points generally utilizing a Chinese herb called *mugwort* in the West. There are many ways to apply moxibustion both directly to the skin or indirectly. The herb can be applied to the top of an inserted acupuncture needle and lit to transmit warmth through the needle directly down to the point. It can be molded into the shape of a small cone or rice grain that can be placed directly on prepared skin to prevent burning. Other mediums such as sliced ginger root or salt can be heated and used over an acupuncture point and removed as soon as the person feels the heat. Moxibustion can also be utilized through the use of a moxa stick, which resembles a thin cigar. The stick is lit and, without touching the skin, is held over an acupuncture point or used by waving it above and along the channel pathway to warm the area, stimulate the flow of blocked energies and relieve pain. Moxa is a wonderful adjunct to massage therapy and very helpful for stimulating energy in persons who suffer from cold, damp, and deficient conditions as are found in common forms of arthritis and many autoimmune diseases. It is also very beneficial in the treatment of sprains, strains, and muscle spasms. (Figure 4-2) Many workshops and

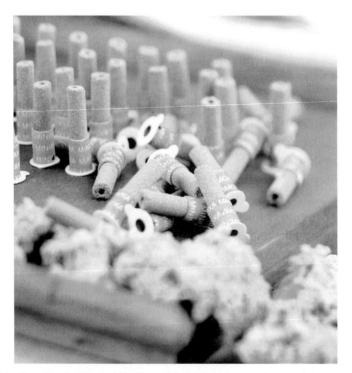

Figure 4-2 Moxibustion is the application of heat to acupuncture points generally utilizing a Chinese herb called mugwort. *Image copyright 2009, WizData, inc. Used under license from shutterstock.com.*

seminars are offered throughout the year that are open to professional massage therapists interested in learning this useful treatment modality.

CHIROPRACTIC

Chiropractic treatment is a wonderful complement to massage therapy treatment and massage therapy treatment is a wonderful complement to chiropractic adjustment. In other words, they work very well together, particularly in the treatment of conditions of the musculoskeletal and the nervous systems. Chiropractors often find that after a patient has a massage therapy session they are able to adjust and maintain the spine's alignment with greater ease and effectiveness. Massage therapists find that their patients who regularly see chiropractors for adjustment maintain better states of heath and wellbeing overall. They also find that while treating patients for specific musculoskeletal conditions, those who are also receiving chiropractic adjustment generally experience a speedier recovery.

Although many think that chiropractors only treat back problems, skilled chiropractors can provide adjunctive therapy for a wider range of physical disorders. Chiropractors generally recommend specific exercises to their patients and often recommend massage therapy as well. If a massage therapist is also not a doctor of chiropractic (there are a few in the industry), it is very helpful for a massage practitioner to network with several chiropractors, to be able to communicate with them about patient care, and, when appropriate, co-manage particular cases. When referring patients for chiropractic, it is important that the massage therapist experience a chiropractic adjustment from the chiropractor he or she intends to recommend. The therapist should feel confident with the chiropractor's level of skill, gentleness, and efficacy (Figure 4-3).

CHINESE HERBALISM

Chinese herbalism is one of the five limbs of Chinese medicine and its use is thousands of years old. It follows the same underlying principle of all the limbs, that the body is capable of healing itself once the proper conditions are provided. Whereas the Asian bodywork therapist assesses the patient and then treats the energy (qi) by manipulating the soft tissue to balance the energy system, and the acupuncturist diagnoses according to the principles of Chinese medicine and then inserts fine, sterilized needles into acupuncture points to achieve balanced energy, the herbalist employs natural substances such as leaves, bark, roots, and flowers to move the energy system towards the same goal of achieving balance in order to produce an optimum state of health.

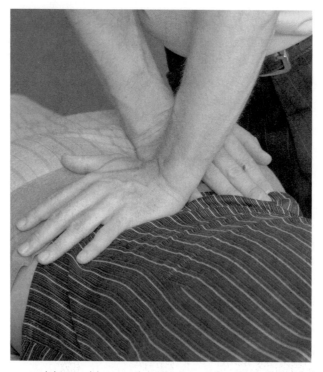

Figure 4-3 A man receiving a chiropractic adjustment for chronic lower-back pain.
Image copyright 2009, Garry Wolsey. Used under license from shutterstock.com.

Herbs are chosen not only for their specific symptom-controlling properties but also for the particular quality of energy they provide. Most western drugs have side effects and some of them are dangerous or addictive. Herbal therapy may be used as a means of avoiding western drugs, replacing them where possible or using them as an adjunct to minimize their unpleasant side effects. Practitioners skilled in Chinese herbalism generally have graduated from a school of Oriental Medicine that includes extensive training in Chinese herbs and they should be certified by a national examination in order to practice. Chinese herbalism is a wonderful adjunct for practitioners who advance themselves in the practice of Asian bodywork and massage therapies (Figure 4-4).

WESTERN HERBALISM

According to the World Health Organization, herbs are the primary choice of 80% of the world's population (that's approximately 4 billion people) for the treatment of disease.[4] The use of herbal medicine has been found to be a significant part of all indigenous peoples' traditional medicine and is common in naturopathic

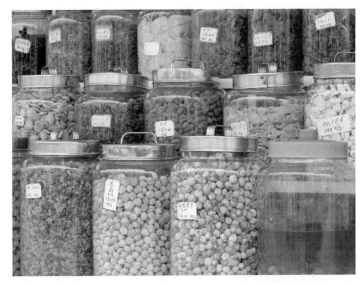

Figure 4-4 Jars of Chinese herbs, containing natural substances such as leaves, bark, roots, and flowers can be combined into various formulas to help achieve balance for an optimum state of health. *Image copyright 2009, Charles Taylor. Used under license from shutterstock.com.*

medicine, Native American Indian medicine, Ayurvedic medicine, homeopathy and traditional Chinese medicine. The ancient Greeks, Romans, Egyptians—all of the great cultures of the ancient world covering every continent—evolved the knowledge and use of herbs in their medicines. Europe had a strong herbal history that predates the discovery of America. In the United States, much herbal knowledge was learned from the Native American Indians, who have a long oral tradition regarding herbal treatments. Herbs were the primary source of medicine in America until the introduction of antibiotics, which were heralded as the cure-all for everyone's ailments. Doctors formed alliances with the pharmaceutical industry and shunned herbal medicine. In the past 40 years, however, herbal medicine has had a resurgence as people search for less harmful ways to treat themselves. Herbal remedies can be in the form of teas, powders, capsules, pills, liniments, and so on. There are numerous schools of **herbalism** where practitioners can earn certificates or diplomas of completion of the required coursework. Herbalism is a wonderful adjunct to the massage therapist's career.

DIET AND NUTRITION

Proper nutrition is essential in the prevention and treatment of disease, yet most people are not educated about correct eating and have poor nutritional habits. Obesity is on the rise, and with it, chronic, degenerative diseases.

Educating patients about what foods can help their specific conditions is a natural fit with massage therapy since food can act as medicine and produce a therapeutic effect. There are many different philosophies regarding nutrition; however, what a person eats should contain the nutrients their body needs to be healthy. Some medical systems include dietary therapy as part of their treatment programs, such as traditional Chinese medicine and **Ayurveda**. These systems are concerned with the energetics of food. Western nutrition deals with the scientific knowledge of the nutritional function of foods and the daily requirements for optimal health. Nutritionists work with the client to avoid processed and chemically treated foods and to choose proper food combinations for a healthier lifestyle. Massage therapists interested in diet and nutrition can become credentialed in one of a number of ways including online degree and non-degree programs, as well as more traditional training in colleges and universities across the country. Nutritionists are also skilled in recommending the proper vitamins, minerals, and **nutraceuticals** that accompany dietary change and help build the body's own defenses (Figure 4-5).

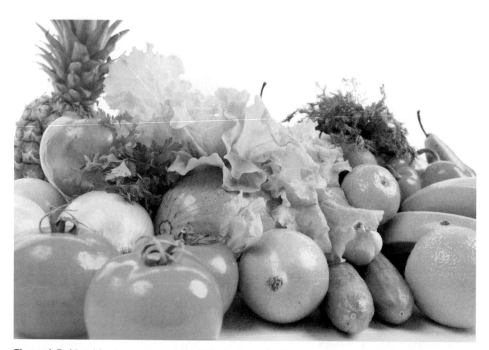

Figure 4-5 Nutritionists recommend fresh organic fruits and vegetables to help avoid processed and chemically treated foods for a healthier lifestyle. *Image copyright 2009, Kiselev Andrey Valerevic. Used under license from shutterstock.com.*

BIOFEEDBACK

Biofeedback is a noninvasive technique that helps patients learn to control or manage the body's response to stress. The biofeedback therapist teaches the patient relaxation exercises and uses sensitive computerized instruments to measure response. This information is then "fed back" to patients using light, sound, or metered feedback, so that patients increase their self-awareness and learn to make subtle adjustments, helping them to move towards a more balanced emotional and physiological state. This new awareness of the mind-body connection helps patients to control their muscle tension, skin temperature, anxiety, heart rate, and brainwave activity. Health concerns such as headaches, high blood pressure, anxiety, attention deficit hyperactivity disorder (ADHD), and many other problems that are triggered or exacerbated by stress can be reduced or eliminated. Biofeedback is an excellent adjunct for massage therapists seeking to expand the reach of their knowledge and practice (Figure 4-6). Biofeedback training courses are available throughout the USA which lead a national certification exam offered by the Biofeedback Certification Institute of America (BCIA), recognized as the standard in the field.

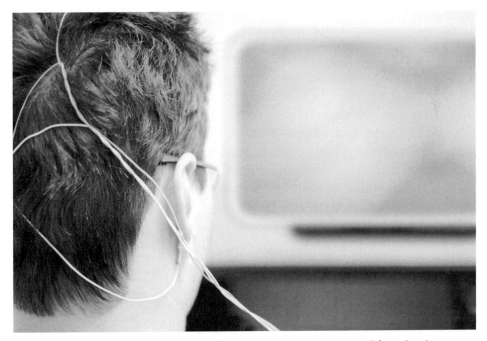

Figure 4-6 A young boy during a biofeedback session being treated for migraine headaches. *Image copyright 2009, Stephen Strathdee. Used under license from shutterstock.com.*

BACH FLOWER REMEDIES

Bach Flower Remedies were created and founded by Dr. Edward Bach, a British-trained physician who believed that natural healing, non-invasive therapies, were the way to improve people's health. He was trained as a bacteriologist and a homeopath, and after much study and investigation concluded that most diseases resulted from negative emotions, which he classified into seven categories. Dr. Bach discovered that the essences of certain flowers contained specific energies that could help to balance emotional and physical symptoms. Remedies are chosen based on personality types that are determined by the therapist through specific questioning during a consultation. Bach remedies are very safe and do not interfere with other treatments. They are good not only for adults but for children and pets as well. The Bach remedies are a good adjunct for the massage therapist's practice. There is no licensing for Bach Flower Remedy therapists; however, the Bach Center in England offers professional training leading to certification. There are also a number of certified therapists who offer courses in the United States.

EXERCISE

It is now common knowledge that exercise is a vital component for maintaining health and vitality, starting in early childhood and extending all the way to our senior years. Practitioners who regularly exercise and who have studied specific types of exercise to the point of mastery are ones who can effectively enhance not only their own health but those of their patients as well. They can instruct their patients on specific exercises that will help their particular conditions or help them to maintain a healthy lifestyle. Although there are many different forms of exercise, some stand out as being more beneficial to treating the whole body and are more complementary with a massage therapy practice. For example: Yoga, tai chi chuan, qi gong, and body building through personal training.

Yoga

Yoga is a profound spiritual philosophy and consists of eight branches of study. Most people are familiar with Hatha Yoga, the branch that consists of an exercise system that can positively affect the body, mind, and emotions through breathing exercises, specific postures (called *asanas* in Sanskrit), and meditative techniques. Yoga helps to improve energy circulation through the mind-body complex, resulting in increasing levels of vitality and health. Yoga is not a competitive sport and can be adjusted to people's specific body limitations. Becoming a qualified yoga instructor, for example, can help to expand the massage therapist's practice in a number of ways, including running classes for patients with specific problems

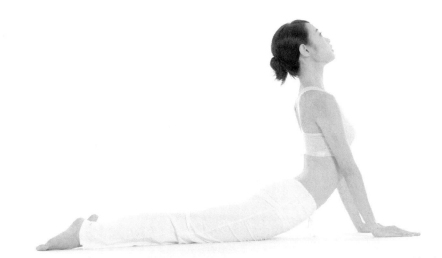

Figure 4-7 A woman practicing Hatha Yoga, a system of exercise that can positively affect the body, mind, and emotions. *Image copyright 2009, Apollofoto. Used under license from shutterstock.com.*

or interested in maintaining wellness and recommending specific exercises for home practice directed towards resolving a particular condition that the massage practitioner is treating (Figure 4-7).

Tai Chi Chuan

Tai Chi Chuan is an ancient Chinese exercise system (one of the inner schools of the martial arts) that is sometimes referred to as a "moving meditation" or the "Grand Dance for Health." Many research studies have shown the benefits of Tai Chi Chuan (commonly known as Tai Chi) for improving balance, postural alignment, increasing focus and concentration, and improving circulation and overall vitality. Tai chi helps to bring harmony to the mind, body, and emotions while seeking to balance the body's energy system. Tai chi also increases flexibility and strength through a set series of slow, continuous, relaxed movements that are done with great detail and attention. Practitioners who study Tai Chi not only improve their own health but also increase their energy levels and stamina, allowing them to provide more effective treatments. In addition, those that go on to master Tai Chi and to teach it will be able to offer an extremely valuable service to their patients (Figure 4-8).

Qi Gong

Qi Gong is another ancient Chinese martial art that can also be practiced and utilized for cultivating and maintaining health, as well as for the treatment of various diseases. Qi Gong is focused on the art of energy generation

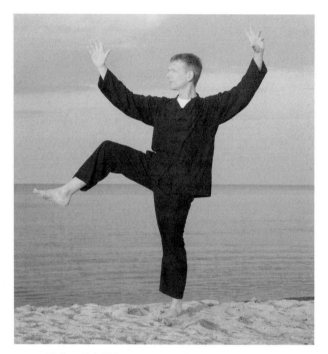

Figure 4-8 A man practicing Tai Chi, a system of exercise that helps to bring harmony to the mind, body, and emotions while seeking to balance the body's energy system. *Image copyright 2009, Riekephotos. Used under license from shutterstock.com.*

and balance through a series of simple yet profound exercises. With regular practice, practitioners can strengthen the mind-body connection, develop an internal state of peace, and provide more effective treatments to their patients. In addition, very specific exercises can be learned and taught to patients for the treatment of different illnesses.

Personal Training

The personal training industry has grown very rapidly in the last decade. Personal training complements massage therapy very well and the two make a potent combination for leading patients towards wellness. Massage therapists who seek some form of training and certification in this growing field study the physiological principles and hands-on skills needed to design and implement safe and effective exercise and fitness programs for their clients and patients. These programs can focus on strength training, flexibility, weight control or weight reduction, or training for a specific sport. More focused exercise programs may be designed for healthy adults interested in improving and maintaining their fitness levels or for clients with special needs, including those with orthopedic injuries, diabetes, or hypertension. They can also be easily customized to be

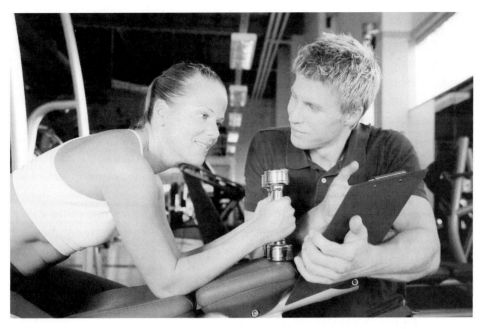

Figure 4-9 A woman working out with her massage therapist/personal trainer.
Image copyright 2009, Arne Trautmann. Used under license from shutterstock.com.

done with clients at their local gym or in the home before or after a massage or on other regularly scheduled days. Some programs prepare massage therapists to take personal trainer certification examinations. (Figure 4-9).

HYPNOTHERAPY

Hypnotherapy is a wonderful adjunctive therapy that helps to reinforce the benefits of massage, as well as other treatments. While most people think of hypnosis as something performed on a stage for fun, it is actually a state of being in focused concentration where suggestions for change can be more easily accepted. Modern hypnotherapists use basic techniques to put the patient into a light trance during which they can suggest ideas that the patient can use to change certain beliefs or behaviors such as stopping smoking or overeating. Self-hypnosis can also be taught to help people deal with stress, pain, or self-defeating habits. Hypnosis is a very well-researched modality that is used to help relieve patients of pain and anxieties and effectively demonstrates the mind-body connection. Hypnotherapy can only be successful if the patient is seeking change and is willing to work with the therapist. A patient cannot be hypnotized to do something against their belief or will. In the United States, the National Board for Certified Clinical Hypnotherapists and the American Council of Hypnotist Examiners certify professionals in the field of hypnotherapy.

GUIDED IMAGERY

The connection between mind and body has been scientifically proven by the emerging field of **psychoneuroimmunology.** Research has demonstrated that a person's thoughts and expectations about surgery, treatments, or medications can have significant impact on the outcome.[5] In addition, numerous scientific studies have shown that imagery is a very effective tool for eliciting the relaxation response. In a therapy session with a trained health care provider, the patient can learn cognitive-behavioral restructuring to "reframe" fears and negative thoughts into positive ones. Visualization therapies harness the mind to create positive images that are used for healing. For example, cancer patients can be taught to imagine that their medication (or some other entity) is destroying cancer cells or dissolving tumors. Imagery therapy can be used for inducing states of relaxation and helping to resolve stress or helping people to cope with and overcome difficulties or illnesses through positive thinking. Massage therapists can seek post-graduate training for health professionals in guided imagery that supports their efforts to integrate other means into their practices for helping their patients.

NATUROPATHY

Naturopathy is the use of natural therapies for the treatment of illness. In some states naturopaths are licensed as doctors and are trained in some western medical techniques such as taking blood pressure, reading X-rays, tending to wounds, drawing blood, and so on. They may also be skilled in acupuncture, hydrotherapy, nutrition, herbs, and supplements. Naturopaths believe that if the body is given the proper tools this will stimulate the vital energy of the body to fight disease and restore the body to energetic balance. Some naturopaths also are skilled in counseling. Several schools of naturopathy have four- and five-year programs leading to degrees that are recognized by many states.

AROMATHERAPY

The use of essential oils in the treatment of disease is centuries old, dating back to the time of the ancient Greeks, Romans, and Egyptians. While essential oils are currently common in massage therapy treatments, their benefit extends way beyond being massaged into the skin. Today, the uses of essential oils as

aromatherapy extends into hospitals for cancer patients, women in labor, and even cardiac patients. In Asia, some forward-thinking engineers are utilizing different scents and aroma systems in new buildings. Some essential oils are known to be antiseptic and antiviral, while others are analgesic and stress relieving and can also improve one's mood. Essential oils can be applied directly to the skin through massage to promote relaxation and stress reduction. They can also be utilized in baths, as compresses, to treat burns, or used in diffusers or vaporizers through which their aromas can be inhaled to relieve headaches, sinus problems, coughs, and colds. Aromatherapy is also a wonderful adjunct for massage therapists to incorporate into their practices because many massage therapists already employ the use of essential oils in their treatments. Many continuing education training courses exist in aromatherapy for massage therapists who want to become proficient in its many uses and applications. (Figure 4-10).

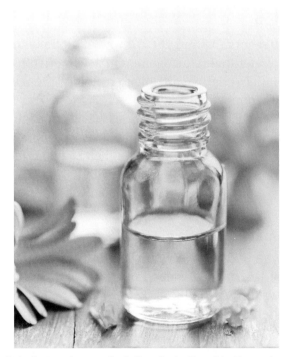

Figure 4-10 Essential oils can be applied directly to the skin through massage to promote relaxation and stress reduction. Essential oils also have many other therapeutic uses and applications in massage. *Image copyright 2009, Liv Friis-larsen. Used under license from shutterstock.com.*

HOMEOPATHY

Homeopathy is very popular in England and throughout Europe, where homeopathic physicians have equal status with traditional allopathic physicians. Homeopathy was discovered by a German doctor, Samuel Hahnemann, in the nineteenth century but its principles actually date back to the time of Hippocrates. One of the major principles of homeopathy is the principle that "like cures like." That is, a substance given in a large quantity that can cause specific symptoms in a healthy person can treat those same symptoms when given in tiny dosages. Homeopaths conduct extensive case histories, which include questions on diet and lifestyle. Once the practitioner has arrived at each person's pattern of disharmony, a specific remedy that matches their symptom picture is recommended. Because they are so diluted, homeopathic remedies are considered to be extremely safe. Training programs in the U.S. and Europe, online and in class, exist for interested practitioners.

CASE HISTORIES

The more practitioners expand their knowledge base and repertoire of techniques, the greater their effectiveness in accomplishing their main goal as health professionals—helping people to restore, cultivate, and maintain a healthy mind-body connection.

Below are some brief, actual case histories that illustrate the Third Paradigm of practice by demonstrating how integrating massage therapy with other modalities enhances a practitioner's ability to heal by expanding their practice into other dimensions of treating.

Severe Rheumatoid Arthritis

June is a 50-year-old female who was suffering from severe rheumatoid arthritis of the hands, knees, and feet. A health care practitioner herself, June was concerned that if she was unable to use her hands or stand for long periods of time, she would be unable to make a living. Even though she was on western drugs for this disease, she was still experiencing debilitating pain and mental anguish over her increasingly deteriorating condition. She began treatments with Amma therapeutic massage, a form of Asian bodywork therapy, and gradually expanded her treatments to include acupuncture so that she was receiving one Amma and two acupuncture treatments per week. These treatments focused on moving energy

CASE HISTORY

blockages, strengthening weak areas, and relieving pain, stiffness, and discomfort. Herbal liniments were applied and moxibustion was used intermittently, especially on cold and rainy days. In addition, June made numerous dietary changes to help strengthen her digestion and absorption of nutrients and to decrease inflammation caused by sugars, additives, and toxic chemicals in foods. Supplements and Chinese herbs were incorporated into her daily routines to optimize her healing potential and she began taking weekly classes in Qi Gong to increase her joint mobility, balance, and internal well-being. She has a home practice of Qi Gong, breathing exercises, liniment application, and she makes efforts to conserve her energy by not overworking. Amma massage treatments are also an opportunity for her to dialogue about things that upset her and to ask questions about her diet, Qi Gong practice, and lifestyle changes. As a result, after two years, her arthritis has not progressed, her pain level has significantly decreased, and she has decreased her treatments to alternating one Amma and one acupuncture treatment per week. She is still able to work and function normally and her mental outlook is good.

Emotional Disturbance

Greg is a 23-year-old male who was born with a cleft palate and suffered numerous surgeries as a small child that left him with a very poor self-image and poor social skills. His parents tried to help by sending him away to special schools, but these had the opposite effect of causing him to retreat further into himself to the point where he had not left his home to venture out into the world in over two years. His mother, already an experienced Asian bodywork patient, finally convinced him to go for "just one treatment," which he reluctantly did. After the initial intake process, the practitioner explained his problems to him using the principles of traditional Chinese medicine (TCM) and he said that this was the first time that anyone was able to explain his condition exactly as he felt it. From a TCM perspective, Greg suffered from Heart Heat and Kidney Deficiency, which were brought into balance relatively quickly with regular shiatsu treatments and an occasional acupuncture tune-up. He said that for the first time he understood his condition in a way that not only made sense to him but also gave him the hope of having a normal existence. He continued to come for regular treatments and used his therapists as sounding boards for ideas and concerns and for navigating his way through college and his social life.

He was recommended supplements and herbs, which he preferred to take over drugs, and he is very impressed with how he can stave off a cold and recover quickly from injuries by diligently taking herbs when he starts to feel ill. He is doing very well, and his parents consider his progress miraculous. Now in his third year of college, he plans to become a lawyer.

Tourette's Syndrome

Theresa is a 5-year-old female child who suddenly began manifesting twitches and spasms, and throwing her head back. She said that she did this voluntarily because she had headaches, but it was clear through observation that it was happening involuntarily as well. Soon after Theresa was diagnosed with Tourette's syndrome by her neurologist. She presented with very tight shoulders, which she didn't like rubbed, a fidgety nature, and a weak constitution. She also worried a lot and complained about pains in her legs, especially at night. She was treated with craniosacral therapy, as well as vitamin and herbal therapies, including Bach flower remedies. She did very well and the symptoms subsided greatly. Her therapists spoke with her about Shoni Shin, which is a Japanese system of pediatric noninsertion acupuncture. Theresa loved this because she got to pick out her own tools and, as stimulating as the process seemed, she responded by lying quietly, relaxing, and enjoying the whole experience. Today she is calmer, has no pain in her legs, and has not had any Tourette's episodes in almost eight months. Shoni Shin is a wonderful modality that massage therapists can easily be trained in and is very useful to add to their skills, especially for pediatric patients.

Disease Prevention and Maintenance of Well-Being

Jack is an 82-year-old male who still plays tennis and is actively working at several businesses. He has a history of heart disease that includes bypass surgery and several stent implants. He is taking medication for high cholesterol and a blood thinner to prevent clotting at the stents. He was treated for prostate cancer by having radioactive seed implants, and has had a successful knee replacement surgery. He goes for regular massage therapy treatments and also takes vitamins and nutraceuticals for the specific purpose of maintaining his positive state of well-being and healthy lifestyle. About 6 months ago, Jack had been complaining about pains in his leg. His therapist, who has made it a point to study western pharmacology, advised him that it might be a side effect of his medication. As a result, Jack brought this to the attention of his doctor who decided to take him off the medication responsible for this and placed him on a different one.

Recently, Jack was complaining of a strange rushing sensation in his head, especially when he lay down. Being concerned about his heart, Jack's therapist referred him to his cardiologist, who determined that the problem was not his heart but again the medication that he was taking for high cholesterol. Jack considers his massage treatments not only necessary for maintaining his health and well-being but also important for educating him about his medications and providing him with important questions to ask his doctors.

Breast Cancer

Ann is a 50-year-old female with stage IV breast cancer who had been told she had only two months to live. Now still vibrant and active six years later, she receives Amma therapeutic massage once a week in combination with acupuncture treatments twice a week and occasional moxibustion treatments. She takes vitamins, nutraceuticals, western and eastern herbs, has radically changed her diet, and has regular personal training sessions. She looks good, feels wonderful, and continues to amaze her oncologist. This is an example of the importance of supporting the immune system when undergoing chemotherapy and/or radiation therapy in traditional cancer treatment. Often these medications achieve the intended effect of shrinking tumors and regulating blood levels but they do so at the expense of the patient, who can become so ill from the treatment that it results in death. Here, massage and other holistic therapies work to support the immune system, relieve the symptoms associated with the side effects of drugs, and lift the spirits of patients so that they can continue healing on many levels.

Sleep Apnea

Tara is a 4-year-old, overweight female child suffering from sleep apnea. She was under a doctors care for this condition but was not making any progress. Unusual for a child, she was unable to sleep more than three or four hours a night with her anxious mother constantly checking her to make sure she was breathing. With only four massage therapy treatments, some herbal therapy, and strict dietary changes, she was able to avoid invasive surgery and now sleeps seven to nine hours per night with minimal snoring. While massage therapy should not be considered stand-alone treatment for sleep apnea, with all its physiological benefits it certainly is complementary to a multipronged approach including herbs, dietary changes, exercise and weight loss.

Malignant Melanoma

Sandy is a 40-year-old female suffering from a malignant melanoma who was given a grim prognosis of nine months to live. After resigning herself to her inevitable demise, her sister's massage therapist recommended she investigate Cancer Care of America. With a bit of prodding from her sister, Sandy eventually sought the help of Cancer Care and is currently seeing a naturopathic physician who is providing nutritional counseling and prescribing herbs alongside having chemotherapy. She is also receiving regular massage therapy from a practitioner trained in guided imagery therapy. This multipronged approach has sent her cancer into remission and her current prognosis is good.

As you can see from the above examples of Third Paradigm practice, integrating massage therapies with additional modalities that enhance the constitution and improve the immune system while treating the symptoms as well greatly improves the patient's health and well-being. It also improves quality of life and rewards practitioners with the knowledge that they have helped to heal another human being and alleviated suffering in the world.

SUMMARY

The main purpose of this chapter was to present a detailed description of the Third Paradigm of practice and, in doing so, better distinguish it from the First and Second Paradigms. During this chapter, it was explained how the Third Paradigm of massage therapy and bodywork practice is also very holistic and integrative in its approach to treatment. In order to further demonstrate this point, the importance of the relationship between Third Paradigm level of practice and some of the most useful adjunctive therapies that can be integrated into treatment were briefly discussed. These included but are not limited to Asian bodywork, acupuncture, chiropractic, moxibustion, Chinese herbalism, western herbalism, diet and nutrition, biofeedback, Bach Flower Remedies, exercise, hypnotherapy, guided imagery, naturopathy, aromatherapy, and homeopathy.

The importance of self-development as playing a significant role towards developing into a Third Paradigm practitioner was also greatly emphasized. It was explained how Third Paradigm therapists must step up and intellectually and emotionally give of themselves in order to appropriately engage their patients to take responsibility for their own health and well-being. A number of brief case histories were presented to help provide an understanding and appreciation of Third Paradigm practice. These case histories illustrate how integrating different modalities of massage therapy with various other modalities increases a massage therapist's ability to heal by expanding their practice into other dimensions of treating.

CHAPTER REFERENCES

1. National Cancer Institute, US National Institutes of Health. Retrieved April 18, 2009, from http://www.cancer.gov/cancertopics/pdq/cam/acupuncture/patient/Page2
2. Paulus, W. E., Zhang, M., Strehler, E., El-Danasouri, I., & Sterzik, K. (2002). Influence of acupuncture on the pregnancy rate in patients who undergo assisted reproduction therapy. *Fertility & Sterility, 77*(4), 721–724.
3. National Cancer Institute, US National Institutes of Health. Retrieved April 18, 2009, from http://www.cancer.gov/cancertopics/pdq/cam/acupuncture/patient/Page2
4. Farnsworth, N. R., Akerele, O., Bingel, A. S., Soejarto, D. D., & Guo, Z. (1985). Medicinal plants in therapy. *Bulletin the WHO, 63*, 965–81.
5. Johnston, M., & Vogele, C. (1993). Benefits of psychological preparation for surgery: A meta analysis. *Annals of Behavioral Medicine, 15*(4), 245–256.

5
CHAPTER

History and Evolution of Massage Therapy and Bodywork

CHAPTER GOALS

1. Develop an understanding and appreciation for the history and evolution of massage therapy and bodywork, including its prehistoric origins in Babylonia and Assyria; its development in Egypt, India, China, Japan, The Philippines, Russia and the Ukraine, the ancient Americas, North America, Hawaii, Central and South America, Europe and the evolution of modern medicine, Greece, Rome, the Middle Ages, the Renaissance, the seventeenth, eighteenth, and nineteenth centuries; and massage today.

INTRODUCTION

The evolution of massage was not a linear path; it was a natural and organic process. Evidence of the field of massage exists throughout history, suggesting that humanity and massage evolved together in some form from the very beginning of the human race. Today, the field of massage therapy is enormous and diverse. Due to its independent and sometimes parallel evolution in many different cultures, its history is complex. Many of the myriad forms of massage, some of which are interrelated, have their own unique and independent history and lineage and have come into existence at different times throughout world history. Many are thousands of years old and have been carefully passed down, remaining essentially the same pure art form over time. Newer approaches, some based on their ancestral forms, have evolved into effective, complex systems of massage and bodywork therapy. In addition, more recent times have given rise to yet other modalities that have become popular and are presently included in the greater framework of practice within the profession.

This text does not engage in a deep and detailed explanation of the history of massage. A brief overview highlighting the beginnings of massage during major historical time periods in different countries or regions of the world will provide a proper sense of the roots of massage therapy and bodywork being practiced today. Those interested in researching more of the history can begin with some of the suggested resources from the bibliography provided in Appendix I.

PREHISTORIC ORIGINS

Massage has been an integral aspect of nearly every ancient civilization with an understanding and usage that has widely varied. In its earliest stages it was an instinctive reaction to relieve the hurts and pains of one another by the simple yet powerful act of human touch.[1] Massage then became a method of anointing people for protection or to enhance a sense of well-being. It also came to be used to improve physical appearance. Even in prehistoric times, it was a natural action for the suffering, sick, and wounded to reach out for the compassionate touch that only a human hand can offer.

Ancient systems of massage were almost always tied to spiritual endeavors and continued to be practiced in a shroud of magic and mysticism for thousands of years before **rite** and ritual gave way to logic and reason.

European cave paintings (dating to as early as 15,000 BCE) reveal evidence of healing touch in the prehistoric world.[2] This was an untempered age where spirits and demons roamed freely, evil deeds invoked the wrath of gods, and sickness and death were punishment for a life lived sinfully. In this mystical time, the noble shaman stood between humans and the gods to serve as a guide and protector of the human race. Shamans were the first priests and spiritual leaders of the civilized world.

As leaders, the shamans played many vital roles. They were civilization's first historians—keepers of knowledge and traditions, especially of the healing arts. It is from their ritualized healing practices that many of our modern healing procedures are derived. Evidence of these holy healers has been found throughout the continents of Asia, Australia, and Africa—sites coinciding with the birth of mankind.

Disease, commonly believed to be the result of invasion by a malevolent demon, was warded off with magic potions, charms, and talismans. Ritual dances, chants, and incantations were performed to free the body of the possession. For early humans, the act of massage was part of a holy ritual designed to purify the body. Sometimes the shaman would gingerly brush the body with herbs, leaves, and plasters to usher the spirit out. At other times he would vigorously knead the abdomen and purge the invading demon out through the top of the head.[3] Not uncommonly, more extreme measures were taken; for example, the patient would be fed noxious potions that caused violent vomiting or a hole would be cut into the patient's skull to allow the spirit a route to escape.[4]

THE FIRST CIVILIZATIONS

Babylonia and Assyria

Babylon, the world's first metropolis, assumed its greatness under the judicious rule of King Hammurabi, whose most impressive feat was his capacity to provide law, order, and direction for his people. It was his code of laws and edicts that made famous the expression "An eye for an eye." Within the Code of Hammurabi, the oldest legal text known to humanity, scholars have discovered inferential evidence of massage as part of ancient Babylonian culture: "If a physician heals the broken bone or the diseased soft part of man, the patient shall pay the physician five shekels." Scholars believe that manual manipulation was utilized to heal the "diseased soft part of man."

In Herman Kamenetz's (1980) chapter entitled "History of Massage" in the book *Manipulation, Traction and Massage,* M. Jastrow, a massage historian, describes the medical practice of ancient Babylonia-Assyria: *"If a man has cramps...place his head downwards and his feet under him, manipulate his back with the thumb, saying 'be good,' manipulate his arms 14 times, manipulate his head 14 times, rolling him on the ground."*[5] Here, massage was not necessarily performed on the patient, but on the offending demon that either had to be coaxed or forced out.

Egypt

Pictographs discovered in the tomb of Akhamor, known as the physician's tomb, depict evidence of massage dating back to an ancient Egyptian culture that existed over 4,000 years ago. The translation of their earliest medical papyri (medical records written on papyrus) has unearthed the statement "rubbed with vinegar." Some scholars say that this refers to the application of a potion or a vinegar-based poultice that was rubbed or massaged onto the body as part of a ritual practice.[6] This may be the earliest written record of massage in history.

Dating around 4,000 BCE, Isis, Divine Mother and daughter of Earth and Sky, is said to have played a central role in the healing arts. Elisabeth Brooke, author of *Medicine Woman*, writes:

> Her priestesses, consecrated to purity, had to bathe daily, wore linen robes free from animal fiber, and were strict vegetarians... [They] were also physicians. They used "rational" medicine, herbs, massages, baths, and so on, and combined them with the "irrational medicine" of prayer, incantations and ritual.[7]

It is commonly accepted that Hippocrates is the "father" of medicine. According to Sir William Osler, Hippocrates was the *"first figure of a physician to stand out clearly from the mists of antiquity"*.[8] However, Egyptian historians claim that another man deserves the crown of medicine's originator, Imhotep. Imhotep, who lived in the reign of King Djoser (2650–2631 BCE) of the third dynasty and about 2,200 years before Hippocrates, was more than just a physician. He was the architect of the first pyramid, vizier (a high government official) to the Pharaoh, and high priest of the sun god Ra.

Osler also reveals that *"Imhotep diagnosed and treated over 200 diseases, fifteen diseases of the abdomen, eleven of the bladder, ten of the rectum, twenty-nine of the eyes, and eighteen of the skin, hair, nails and tongue. Imhotep treated tuberculosis, gallstones, appendicitis, gout and arthritis. He also performed surgery and practiced some dentistry. Imhotep extracted medicine from plants. He also knew the position and function of the vital organs and circulation of the blood system."*[9]

Imhotep is considered to be the author of the Edwin Smith Papyrus, in which he describes 48 injuries and over 90 anatomical terms. He is also believed to have founded a medical school called Asklepion.[10] His contributions were instrumental in shaping the course of medicine for the next 1,500 years. He was renowned by the Egyptians as the world's first genius, and his brilliance so captivated the ancient world that 2,500 years after his death he was deified by modern Egyptians as the god of healing.

Egypt was a "superpower" of the ancient world, with a highly developed system of commerce and a rich culture of education that was devoted to the advancement of medical knowledge. Their physicians spent rigorous years training in the arts of inspection, examination, and palpation.[11] They had specialists for the head, the eyes, the intestines, etc. Therefore, scholars believe they had specialists in massage as well. Egyptian medicine was so well respected that scholars and physicians traveled from distant empires to study at their institutions. Egyptian physicians themselves traveled widely to research new progress while sharing their own knowledge of medicine.

India

Ayurveda, literally the *science of life*, is the supreme mystic discipline that forms the core of Indian medicine. While originally mentioned in only a small, but significant part of the Vedas (the primary documents outlining Hindu wisdom and spirituality), the Rig Veda, Ayurvedic medicine extended into its own field because it dealt with the healing aspect of spirituality. Scholars believe that the system is one that has existed for over 8,000 years through the oral tradition but did not take written form until the second millennium BCE.

Early Indian medical science was married so intimately with spirituality that no delineation was between humanity and the powers above. Hindu culture is based upon the belief in this sacred union, between man and God, which provides the meaning of life, form, and existence. The origins of this belief system began when the great rishis (seers of truth) of the Himalayas gathered in prayer and meditation to request compassion from the heavens for the human suffering below. It is believed that through means of their perseverance and devotion they saw existence through the eyes of God and thus attained a direct link to the truths of the higher realms and accessed the secrets of healing and longevity. With this came the understanding of the workings of the world, which included greater understanding of herbs, foods, aromas, gems, colors, yoga, mantras, lifestyle, and surgery.[12]

Because of this supernatural origin, Ayurveda later came under the criticism of scientific minds that demanded empirical validation. Although this brought about scrupulous investigations into the theory and practice of Ayurveda, this rigorous process of scientific testing actually served to forge the system into a substantiated medical system, with theories that hold true to this day.

There are three main texts of Ayurveda: the *Charak Samhita* (compilation), the *Sushrut Samhita,* and the *Ashtanga Hridaya Samhita* (a concise version of Charak and Sushrut). While other systems have lost bits and pieces over the years, these texts have been preserved in their original form. Written over 1200 years ago, they form the most complete medical system in existence today.[13]

In approximately 1,500 BCE, Ayurveda was organized into eight main courses of study. The two main branches were the Atreya School of physicians led by Charak and the Dhanvantari School of surgeons headed by Sushrut. Charak discoursed lengthily on the subjects of physiology, anatomy, etiology, pathogenesis, diagnosis, prevention, and longevity. He detailed and prescribed the medicinal use of herbs and offered treatments for the reversal of the aging process. His body of work even included month-by-month descriptions of a developing fetus that has been verified with recent technology.

Sushrut's contribution to Ayurveda was his sophisticated understanding of the human anatomy and a mastery of knowledge of various surgical procedures. His text presents detailed discussions of surgical equipment, plastic surgery, amputations, fractures, burns, and so on. He also reveals extensive knowledge of the skeletal system, joint functions, the nervous system, and the circulatory system that has been validated by modern science as well. It is in Sushrut's work that marma points (vital points) are described. **Marma points** lie on the body and can be found where muscles, veins, arteries, nerves, tendons, bones, and joints meet. Many of these points coincide with acupuncture points and may have also influenced the Chinese meridian system used in acupuncture.

Even with the relentless advancement of modern science, the people of India never forgot or discarded their origins. Ayurveda is a system of medicine that embraces all aspects of human existence—the body, mind, and spirit. The revelations of the great rishis revealed the singular nature of the universe and described how health, wisdom, and life flow down in a continuous chain from the One-Absolute. Health is not merely the absence of disease. It is defined as the experience of bliss of the soul.[14]

In this sacred system, the foremost cause of human suffering is an interruption of the Divine union. All forms of illness, be they mental, physical, or spiritual, are considered to be a direct consequence of the severance of humanity from their higher self. The job of the Vaidyas, or Ayurvedic physicians, was to reestablish that vital link to God.[15]

Ayurveda's main mode of treatment is through food and nutrition, herbs, and massage with aromatic oils (Figure 5-1). The taking of life is discouraged altogether, so fruits and vegetables are recommended as opposed to the consumption of animals. Yoga will often be prescribed along with treatment. Although Ayurveda and Yoga developed separately, they share the same principles and blend well together. The system in its complete form also incorporates Vedic astrologers, who may prescribe the use of certain gems befitting the patient's condition since minerals possess energetic healing qualities.[16]

Ayurvedic treatment is based on the balance of the three **doshas** (natures): vata, pitta, and kapha. These three fundamental energies are found throughout nature and, as all things in the universe, are reflected in humanity, in this case

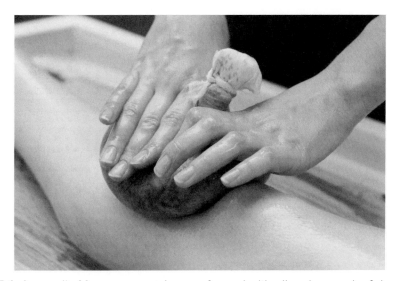

Figure 5-1 Ayurvedic Massage procedure performed with oil and a pouch of rice, herbs, and spices. *Image copyright 2009, Niderlander. Used under license from shutterstock.com.*

in the doshas. They describe the different emotional, physical, and intellectual faculties of different types of people. Figure 5-2 summarizes the characteristics found within the three doshas. While a modern western doctor may ask, "What kind of disease is this person suffering from?", an Ayurvedic physician would ask, "What kind of person is suffering from this disease?" Massage for each type varies according to an individual's principle nature.

Evidence suggests that medical theories born in India pollinated much of the known world. It is believed that through the veins of the Persian Empire, Indian medicine and philosophy was transmitted to the European nations. Principles at the core of the Vedas, such as self-knowledge, sprang into the forefront of Greek minds. The theory of the tri-dosha, the idea of viewing people as a combination of elements that radiate certain characteristics, is mimicked in Greek medical theories with their four basic substances of the body that they called the four **humours** (Figure 5-3). This theory held that when these four essential substances were in harmony the human being was in a healthy state. Conversely, disease was the result of an imbalance due to an excess or deficiency of one or more of these four substances. The four humours were black bile, yellow bile, phlegm, and blood. This idea, introduced by Hippocrates, became deeply embedded into European medical sciences and was not displaced until the nineteenth century CE.

Three Doshas of the Ayurvedic System:

DOSHA	Vata	Pitta	Kapha
Representation	Movement	Metabolism	Structure
Elements	Air and Space	Fire and Water	Earth and Water
Governs	Breathing, muscle movement, beating of the heart	Digestion, assimilation, nutrition, absorption, regulation of body temperature	Forms tendons, muscle, bone; nourishes joint and skin; immune system vitality
In Balance	Promotion of flexibility and creativity	Intelligence and understanding	Calm, loving, forgiving
Out of Balance	Produces fear and anxiety	Jealousy, anger, hatred	Greed, envy, attachment
Weather Association	Cold, dry, and windy as in Autumn and early winter	Heat and humidity as in late spring and summer	Cold and damp as in winter and early spring
Personal Traits	Thin narrow bodies, don't typically gain weight easily, restless	Well proportioned bodies, average build, active minds, impatient, good sense of humor, warm	Sturdily built, have weight problems, naturally athletic, need motivation, sensitive, need understanding, turn to food for emotional support
Massage	Gets the most benefit from massage, should be gentle, with soothing relaxing strokes, use of warm and sweet scented oils	Blend of both the gentle massage with oils and the vigorous massage with very little oil	Vigorous massage, use of little or no oil

Figure 5-2 Ayurvedic treatment is based on the three doshas (natures): Vata, Pitta, and Kapha. They describe the different emotional, physical, and intellectual faculties of different types of people.

The Four Humours:

Blood	Yellow Bile	Phlegm	Black Bile
Sturdy, confident, optimistic, happy	Angry, irritable, bitter, distasteful	Slow, cool, impassive	Depressed, sad

Figure 5-3 The ancient Greek's four basic substances of the body called the four humours. It was believed that when these essential substances were in harmony, good health was the natural result.

In the Chinese medical systems there are obvious parallels between their Five Element theory and acupuncture points to Ayurveda's system of the three elements and its marma points (vital points). Today, we also see the knowledge of ancient India expressed through western modalities such as polarity therapy, an energy-based form of bodywork therapy (See Chapter 10).

China

One of the fundamental principles that pulses through the entire culture of China is that of the primary duality of complementary yet opposing energetic forces, yin and yang (Figure 5-4). The Chinese view is that all things created are the result of the dynamic interplay of these two primary energies. **Yin and yang**, in all their myriad combinations, permeate everything from the clouds in the heavens to a single blade of grass. Through the interplay of these polar opposites, the world is born, dies, and is born again. This principle is the foundation of Taoist philosophy, out of which eventually arose the traditional Chinese medical system.

The origin of Chinese bodywork is often credited to the legendary Chinese yellow emperor, Huang Ti, who is believed to have lived over 5000 years ago.

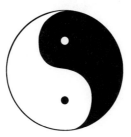

Figure 5-4 The yin yang symbol expresses a primary underlying principle of Chinese Taoist philosophy and represents the dynamic interplay of these two forces, or energies, responsible for the creation of the Universe—everything in it and the balance between all things.

Huang Ti is the author of the oldest written Chinese medical text, entitled *The Yellow Emperor's Classic of Internal Medicine.* The first written descriptions of massage therapy are found in this book (Figure 5-5).[17]

Over 3000 years ago, priests of the Shang Dynasty, through years of intensive meditation, penetrated higher spiritual realms. After piercing through the thick veil of the physical world, they experienced a spirit world underlying all of existence. In this formless, boundless dimension, all things were interconnected. They realized that humanity was not a segregated entity but was an integral part of a greater cosmic universe. The preserved works of these Shang priests have provided a legacy of some of the most ancient texts and philosophies of mankind, such as the I Ching, or the Book of Changes.[18] These contained the seeds that would later sprout to form the basis of traditional Chinese medicine (TCM).[19]

As the empire changed hands, the Shang priests were adopted as favored sons of the new Chou Dynasty and they rose in stature to the level of scholarly sages. Their studies continued to evolve and they developed the concepts of the **five elements**. Similar to the ancient Greeks and Indians, the Chinese sought to describe the different universal forces that interact with each other externally in the world and that are also reflected within the human being.

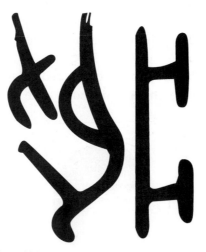

Figure 5-5 This is an ancient Chinese ideogram (a written symbol that represents an idea or object) for massage, which depicts a body lying on a table, perhaps a pregnant woman, with a hand hovering above, about to begin treatment. (Easier viewed when rotated 90 degrees to the right.)

In traditional Chinese medicine the five elements, represent the five energies that correspond to the climates, organs, emotions, tissues, seasons, colors, sounds, and so on. The principle of five elements is used as one of a number of important diagnostic tools by Asian medical practitioners such as acupuncturists, herbalists, and Asian bodywork therapists in the assessment and treatment of their patients (Figure 5-6).

Chinese knowledge of anatomy was limited to conjecture and speculation because it was considered inconceivable to disrespect their ancestors by dissecting what was once the residence of their venerable soul. This bred a system of medicine that honed its tools of diagnosis by physicians who were masters of energy development and movement and who carefully studied the patterns of disharmony that a patient exhibited. Signs and symptoms were considered against the landscape of the patient's home environment,

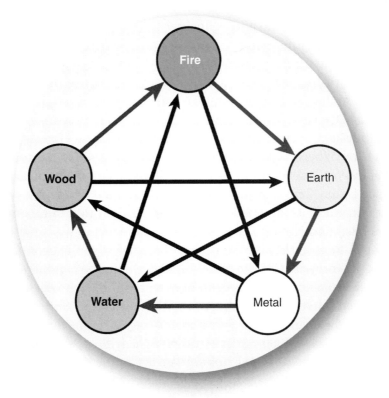

Figure 5-6 The five elements of traditional Chinese medicine is used as one of a number of important diagnostic tools in the assessment and treatment of patients.

while taking into consideration the patient's normal personal state in order to test for abnormal fluctuations. The physicians' diagnostic process, including examination of the tongue and pulses, evolved to such a high level of sensitivity that they became capable of sensing and distinguishing the subtlest fluctuations in the internal system of the body. Because these nuances could only be detected by subtle palpation, it was required that practitioners of acupuncture and oriental medicine have mastery over bodywork as well.[20] Physicians were also trained in the martial arts, usually in several styles, so that they could master and develop the physical body and sensitivity to the energy system that is the basis of TCM. As mentioned in Chapter one, according to TCM, the vital force, or Qi (pronounced chee), of the universe infuses the human body and flows through it in a complex system of energy channels, some of which can be accessed through palpation and pressure in massage and through needling of specific points in acupuncture (Figure 5-7). The mind, the body, and the emotions are all a part of and a manifestation of this energy system. It is the disturbance of this energy system that creates disease or "dis-ease" and its balancing that is the hallmark of health and wellbeing.

Amma (also known as ammo, anma or anmo), Chinese massage, is considered by many to be the grandparent of all other manual and energetic therapies.[21] The word *amma*, the oldest known word for massage, dates back to the period of the Yellow Emperor, Hwang Ti, and is translated as "push and pull." After the Han Dynasty of China (206 BCE–220 CE), Asian bodywork was known as *anmo*, translated as "press and rub." Then during the Ming Dynasty of China (1368–1644 CE) it became known as *tuina*, meaning to "lift and press." As this form of bodywork spread throughout the Orient, the original term amma was maintained by the Koreans, while anma was used by the Japanese.

It was during the Han Dynasty (206 BCE–220 CE) that medicine began to evolve based on Huang Ti's written treatise. During the Tang Dynasty (618–907 CE), bodywork achieved such a high level of sophistication and respect that the Imperial College of Medicine in Xian, the capital of the Tang Dynasty, offered a doctoral degree in bodywork.[22] This land, rich in knowledge, attracted thirsty minds from around the world.

Perhaps to distinguish themselves from the ways of the previous ruling social ranks, the Sung dynasty (960–1279 CE) turned a "high brow" to the manual therapies, and touching became an inappropriate act for the rich and powerful upper class. Popularity of massage rose and fell in the dynasties that followed.

During the period of 1911 to 1949, China's republic was experiencing hardship. To begin with, in 1911 there was the start of the Communist Revolution, and then the Chinese, with help from America, had to fight off Japan.

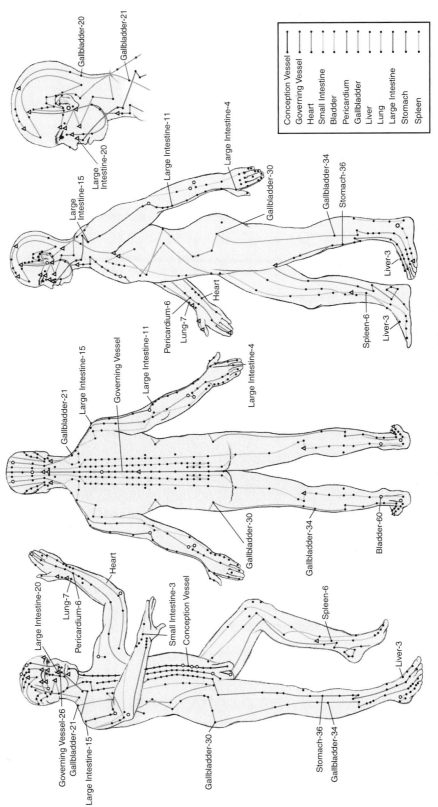

Figure 5-7 The twelve organ channels of acupuncture and their points are located bilaterally on the body.

This continued into World War II until the Japanese finally surrendered. Then the Civil War (1945–1949) began in China and was one of the most violent acts in Chinese history.

During this period, Chinese doctors studying abroad reported home that they had seen the way of the future. They were dazzled by the complexity of western medicine and came to believe that their traditional ways were weak and archaic. In order to thrust the nation into the twentieth century, they relied heavily on everything western and adopted the use of surgery and potent drugs while purging their traditional ways.[23] But their medical system, alive and incubating within the fertile Chinese culture for thousands of years, was rooted too deeply, especially in the countryside among the common folk, who did not have access to expensive western medicine and so it remained alive and well. Although the pulse of the old ways remained constant and vital in the middle and lower classes, it wasn't until the war between the Nationalist troops and the Communists that traditional medicine again attained a proper seat of respect.

During China's brutal civil war, following World War II, Communist troops, driven hard into the mountains, were cut off from western medicine with only the traditional ways to heal their sick and wounded. Traditional medicine, having proven its value even in times of war, was reinfused into the medical system. Since there were only a handful of western trained doctors available to service a nation of hundreds of millions, traditional practitioners were called upon to satisfy the everyday medical needs of the abundant population. These "barefoot doctors," in many cases the only physicians for miles around, enjoyed a lasting reputation throughout the countryside of China.[24]

Today the profound ancient system of traditional medicine of China intermingles freely with the modern technology of the West, and hospitals exist side by side that are devoted exclusively to either system. Therapeutic massage receives recognition as a distinct specialty with schools and hospitals dedicated to its practice and advancement. Today, modern massage techniques are still called **tuina** in China, in Japan anma and shiatsu, and in Korea, the ancient name of amma has been retained.

Japan

Envoys from China established commercial trade routes to Japan in the sixth century BCE, opening a dynamic interaction between the two countries. Buddhist priests, traveling with the Trade Embassy of China, brought with them extensive knowledge of spirituality and the medicine of Imperial China.

These seeds sown by the Buddhist priests bloomed and peaked during the Edo period (1603–1867 BCE). The Japanese temperament was drawn to the manual element of Chinese medicine, which resulted in the extensive development of shiatsu (their own interpretation of Chinese massage), acupuncture, moxabustion, and **palpatory diagnosis**.

In the fashion of China in the millennium prior, doctors were required to master bodywork before being allowed to diagnose or handle needles. The major force behind this movement was Waichi Sugiyama (1610–1694 BCE). Blind since an early age, Sugiyama left his home in Kyoto as a teenager in hopes of studying anma massage and acupuncture in Edo (now called Tokyo). He worked under the tutelage of two of the most prominent sighted masters of oriental medicine of his time. Fatefully, after a total of about five years with his first teacher and three years with his second teacher, Sugiyama was found lacking in the competence of a serious pupil necessary to be able to practice on others and was dismissed back to Kyoto.

Before returning home, Sugiyama made a pilgrimage to the isle of Enoshida to implore of the Goddess Benten (the Hindu Goddess Saraswati) for an answer to his failed life's quest. Benten is one of the seven Japanese deities of good fortune and the only female goddess of that group. After several weeks of fasting and prayer, Sugiyama left his cave after a fast. There he stumbled and fell, and as the story goes a pine tree needle stuck deeply into his leg. He removed it and noted that it was sticking out from within a bamboo shoot. There he had a vision and a deep inspiration. Sugiyama felt that the Goddess Benten had blessed him and instructed him to return to Edo with the needle-insertion guide-tube (Figure 5-8) that revolutionized Japanese acupuncture. Eventually, Sugiyama came to be known as the "Father of Japanese Acupuncture," surpassing the fame of even his once greatly admired teachers.[25]

Later in his life, Sugiyama was called upon to treat a famous Shogun, Lord Tsunayoshi, who suffered a painful abdominal illness that none of the court physicians had been able to remedy. Under Sugiyama's expert care, the Shogun's health rapidly improved. The Shogun expressed his profound gratitude by making acupuncture and anma massage a special province of the blind. By the time of his death in 1694, Sugiyama had established over 45 medical schools for the blind throughout Japan.

During the Meiji period (1867–1911 CE), European traders brought to China the wonders of western medicine. Enchanted by the glitter of technology, the aristocrats hailed the new medicine as superior to their own and banned the teaching of their native therapies. As a result, anma, once a

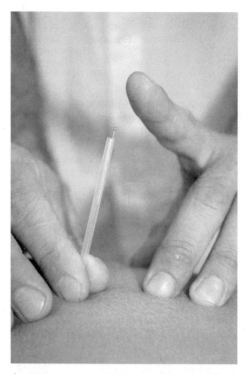

Figure 5-8 The modern Japanese acupuncture needle and guide tube. The guide tube helps to minimize the sting of an acupuncture needle being inserted and in the accuracy of accessing points. *Image copyright 2009, Paul Prescott. Used under license from shutterstock.com.*

powerful form of massage therapy with a sophisticated system of diagnosis, degenerated to such a low level that it became nothing more than a pleasurable indulgence for the rich.

The ancient ways were fading rapidly until 1919 when Shiatsu developed. Its originator, Tamai Tempaku, published the revolutionary treatise *Shiatsu Ho* (finger-pressure method). The book was a combination of anma, a form of abdominal massage called *ampuku,* Do-In (therapeutic exercises), and a modern knowledge of western anatomy and physiology. This produced an effective method of treating a variety of western ailments. With Shiatsu Ho, Tempaku effectively revived the ancient ways and brought them to the forefront of the twentieth century. Many practitioners eagerly followed his works, and in 1925 the Shiatsu Therapists Association was formed in order to distinguish professionally trained practitioners from the generic anma "body-rubbers."[26] Students of Tempaku went on to further the field of Japanese bodywork, including three whose lineages still exert a major influence on the study and practice of shiatsu/anma today: 1) Katsusuke Serizawa, 2) Shizuto Masunaga's mother (Shizuto Masunaga became the founder of Zen Shiatsu), and 3) Tokujiro Namikoshi.

After studying with Tempaku, Serizawa went on to study physical therapy. In 1951 at Tokyo University he began doing physiological research and in 1955 became a research fellow at the Tokyo University School of Medicine. Serizawa received his doctorate degree in 1961 for his well-known research into the **tsubo** (the points that lie along the 14 traditional acupuncture meridians) system. Previous skepticism of any therapy that works by stimulating or sedating these vital points along the body, was eliminated with the advent of the electrometric measuring device that was used to prove beyond doubt the physical existence of the tsubo vital points. As a result, Katsusuke Serizawa created tsubo therapy, an Asian bodywork therapy based on his landmark research and codified in his 1976 book *Tsubo: Vital Points for Oriental Therapy.*[27] The style of shiatsu, also known as acupressure, is a western derivative of tsubo therapy.

Shizuto Masunaga brought shiatsu back to its Asian foundations, resulting in a style of shiatsu that reintegrated its original core of spirituality and energy. With his special interest in exploring the mental, emotional, and spiritual components of the human entity, Masunaga crafted a system, known as Zen shiatsu, that merged theories from western psychology, traditional Chinese medicine, modern understanding of the body, and Zen Buddhism. He developed his system around the treatment of the meridian extensions, which go beyond those energy pathways recognized in the traditional Chinese view. He also introduced the assessment principle of *kyo/jitsu*, which, dependent on the therapist's palpation skills and sensitivity, reveals energy imbalances in the meridians, according to deficiencies (kyo) and excesses (jitsu). Masunaga is also known for the development of a particular form of abdominal diagnosis known as **hara diagnosis**. His work continues to gain widespread popularity in Japan, Europe, and the United States.[28]

The most famous of Tempaku's students, credited with being the single most influential man in spreading shiatsu across the globe was Tokujiro Namikoshi. To distinguish the new modes of shiatsu therapy from that of the anma body-rubbers, Namikoshi petitioned to have shiatsu recognized separately as a distinct medical specialty. To further distance his new field of scientific massage from its roots, Namikoshi removed all theories connected to traditional energy based concepts and displaced them with modern, scientific terms to create a version of shiatsu that was neuromuscularly based (Figure 5-9).

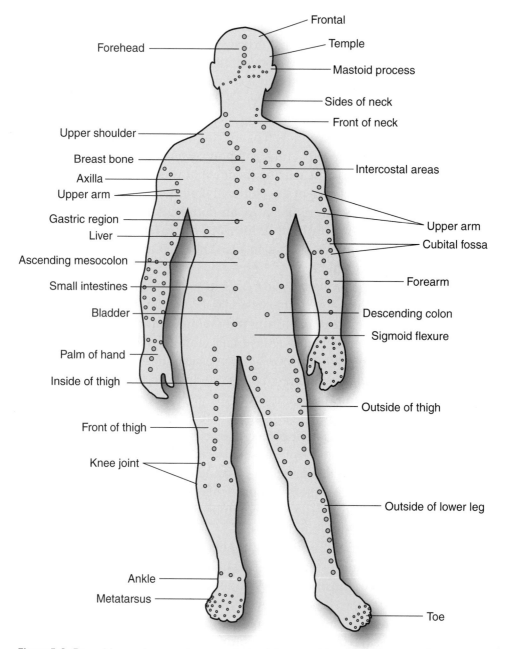

Forehead

Frontal

Temple

Mastoid process

Sides of neck

Front of neck

Upper shoulder

Breast bone

Axilla

Upper arm

Intercostal areas

Gastric region

Liver

Upper arm

Cubital fossa

Ascending mesocolon

Small intestines

Forearm

Bladder

Descending colon

Sigmoid flexure

Palm of hand

Inside of thigh

Outside of thigh

Front of thigh

Knee joint

Outside of lower leg

Ankle

Metatarsus

Toe

Figure 5-9 Based in modern anatomy and physiology and located on or over the muscles, nerves, blood vessels, lymph vessels, bones and endocrine glands Namikoshi's pressure point system directly affects the nervous system, which in turn affects the internal physiological organ systems of the body. (Posterior view)

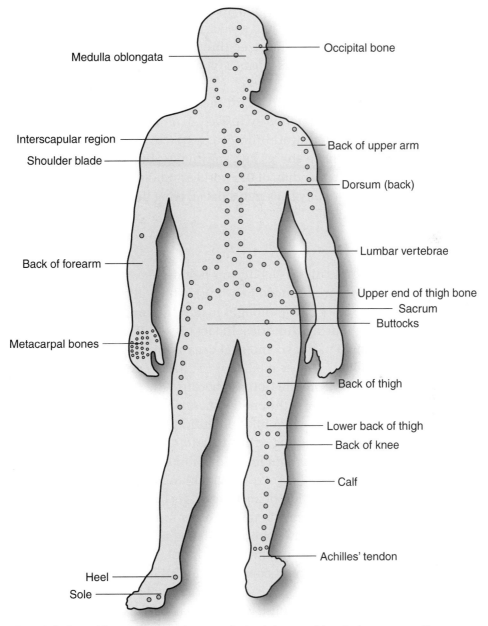

Figure 5-9 Based in modern anatomy and physiology and located on or over the muscles, nerves, blood vessels, lymph vessels, bones and endocrine glands Namikoshi's pressure point system directly affects the nervous system, which in turn affects the internal physiological organ systems of the body. (Posterior view)

Establishing the legitimacy of shiatsu even more firmly, Namikoshi was called in to treat a honeymooning Marilyn Monroe, the famous actress, who had become deathly ill and unresponsive to western medical treatment. Namikoshi treated her every day and a week later she made a remarkable recovery. The story was widely publicized throughout Japan, and in 1954, shiatsu was finally recognized by the Japanese government as a legitimate form of treatment.

When shiatsu instructors arrived in the United States, they taught the Namikoshi neuromuscular method exclusively in order to present a legitimate, scientific face to the western world. This was a system that had been stripped clean of any connections to energy and spirituality, but American students, starved for deeper understanding of the world around them, reinstated theories of energy and spirituality back into shiatsu, tying the new system back to its ancient roots.[29]

The Philippines

Often called "oriental rubbers," Filipino healers developed a system of massage called **hilot** (pronounced hee-lote), which also included the use of herbs and magic. Hilot is also thought to have ties to and may have been imported from neighboring countries. In fact, the hilot system of treatment includes the principle of the six internal organs, an important part of the teachings of traditional Chinese medicine, (TCM). Its underlying principles seem to have stemmed from the Chinese because they also approached the body with an understanding of the energy channels. Hilot may be considered a form of deep tissue massage. A hilot practitioner prepares the patient for this deeper work by first working lightly to soften the muscles and increase the overall circulation throughout the body. And like any good practitioner, the hilot therapist will vary the pressure depending upon the patient's tolerance and the specific condition being treated. Its techniques include many similar strokes common to deep tissue and other forms of bodywork, including those that are performed away from the heart and cross-fiber techniques. Before the actual massage begins, the patient is put through a series of range-of-motion exercises, an element commonly found in Thai and other Asian systems.[30]

Today, this traditional Filipino massage has become a major trend in spas. In fact, in 2005, hilot was nominated as the "Spa Treatment of the Year" during the Baccarat Inaugural Awards in Hong Kong. Posh resorts and spas all over the world have now begun adding hilot to their menu of offerings.

In the Philippines, all the spas accredited by the Department of Tourism are now required to incorporate hilot in their massage therapy and bodywork offerings.[31]

Russia and the Ukraine

Russia and the Ukraine enjoy a rich and long history of massage. Since there is little written documentation on the origins of this subject in that region, it is assumed that, as in most other regions of the world, massage evolved here first as part of the various folk remedies of the culture practiced by the religious groups of its time. Eventually, massage evolved to the point where it became recognized by the medical establishment.

Until the 1980s, Russian massage was virtually unknown in the United States, even though in Russia patients received massage treatment as part of their physical rehabilitation, whether outpatient or inpatient. According to Zheny Kurashova Wine, a well-known Russian massage teacher now living in the United States, massage in Russia and other Soviet countries gained widespread popularity and use because it was heavily researched in Russia for more than 130 years. Manual therapies were used as a part of folk medicine for centuries, but were not studied or used scientifically in Russia until 1860. Up until the 1990s, when Russian society opened up with the advent of Perestroika, the program of economic and political reform in the Soviet Union initiated by Mikhail Gorbachev in 1986, the teaching and receiving of massage was limited. Massage was taught only in medical and athletic institutions and a physician's prescription was necessary to receive treatment as a rehab patient. If you were a valued member of a sports team, treatment went without saying. Also, the very privileged had easy access to massage therapy treatment.[32]

The ancient Slovaks would perform a treatment called "twigging" with the softened leaves of a birch tree. They were the first to provide a written record of their work in massage. According to Zheny Wine, a therapist in the sauna *"would hit the body...and follow by rubbing the body with the branches. After this the masseur would pour water (hot first, followed by cold) on the body... That process was repeated several times during the bathing, and was finished with a bather going for a dip in the snow. This severe amount of friction prevented the body from serious over-cooling and helped the bather to better adapt to the cold temperatures of Winter Russia."*[33]

By the end of the nineteenth century, centers for the study and teaching of massage could be found all over Russia and the Ukraine in their medical schools, military academies, and in their sport and athletic institutions. To this day, massage continues to play an important role in the treatment of a broad range of conditions, including musculoskeletal, neurological, cardiovascular, and other dysfunctions.[34]

THE ANCIENT AMERICAS

North America

The original Native Americans had no written language, so the historical evidence of massage in this culture has only been documented since the arrival of the European colonies. With entire tribes wiped out, little of their culture and tradition has survived. Without a documented history, traces of their medical past can only be found in living practitioners.

In Native American medicine, the root of all imbalance is found in the world of spirits. Native Americans had great respect for the sick, and their preferences were always honored. It would be impossible to establish harmony if the treatment was disagreeable to the patient or forced.[35]

Native American healers revered the uniqueness of each individual's case so much that there was no set payment plan. Instead, patients evaluated the severity and importance of their own disease and made an offer to the healer. Negotiations were never done face-to-face. Instead, the patient left the offering at the healer's door. If it was gone the next morning, it signified that the offering was accepted and treatment could begin. If it was still there, the patient could make another offer, or find someone else to treat him or her.

Once the price was established and the offering accepted, the medicine man would consider many factors, including the patients' own valuation of the healing process, their readiness for treatment, and their willingness to be healed. Often the patient would be given a task to strengthen resolve, such as ending a dispute with a family member, performing an act of selflessness, or climbing a sacred mountain. The healer would recommend that the patient engage in self-study to identify what patterns were causing the illness. Treatment included lifestyle modification, prayer, herbs, and massage and could include various rituals and ceremonies such as sweat lodges and vision quests.[36]

Reports from colonial settlers of the New World describe massages given by the Native American Indians as ritualistic ceremonies that would sometimes span a number of days. The medicine man would rub the hides and horns of animals on a patient's limbs, chest, and back while hooting and chanting words of purification and power. Sometimes they would channel the spirit into their own bodies and either purge it themselves or transfer it to another medicine man who would then expel it back into the heavens.

Today massage lives on only in a handful of Indian nations where it is used mostly during childbirth and the treatment of abdominal pain.[37]

Hawaii

In the Pacific Islands, **lomi-lomi** (Hawaiian massage) was an integral part of the traditionial healing arts. This style, distinguished by its long, flowing strokes, rhythmic patterns, and use of forearms, resembles the Esalen massage of California. The kahuna, or spiritual leader, who played a similar role as the shaman, was often secretly taught by his grandmother or grandfather until he either proved his worth or exhibited true sincerity in the desire to become a kahuna healer.[38]

Lomi means "to rub," "to knead," "to work in and out," or "to weave."[39] The kahuna united love and spirit while unraveling stagnant and unhealthy belief patterns. Old blockages were removed and restrictions were unbound in order to create a space within the patient to receive visions of healing and transformation. The process was to enlighten the receiver's inner being and awaken them to their true calling.

In the temples of ancient Hawaii, a powerful and unique lineage of lomi-lomi was practiced called Ke Ala Hoku, or "Pathway to the Stars." Entrance into this spiritual tradition required divine ordinance received in the fervor of holy ceremony. Surrounded by blazing fires, tribal chanting, drum beats, and shamanic dancing, the kahunas would call upon the wisdom of their ancestors to request a vision that would foretell who was to be initiated as a kahuna healer. The initiate, once chosen, would receive lomi-lomi treatment for 10 hours or up to 15 days nonstop by multiple practitioners.[40]

Traditionally, lomi-lomi was performed on the king and queen after eating so that they could continue their royal consumption of food without being limited by the constraints of a full stomach. Apparently, lomi-lomi was believed to aid in the digestive process.

It was also customary to offer massage to an honored guest.[41] Captain Cook, allegedly the first European to visit Hawaii, had been suffering from severe rheumatism until a somewhat fateful visit to Tahiti. To help the captain, the local chief called upon his women relatives and practitioners and had them pummel, squeeze, elbow, knee, and stand on Captain Cook's sprawled-out body. After only a few minutes, the captain stood up, amazed to find his pain alleviated. They asked if the captain wanted more, to which he hastily replied, "Indeed!" He jumped back down onto the ground, whereupon no less than 12 large women pounced on him again. In only three more sessions, his pains were fully resolved.[42]

It was often said that the lomi-lomi practitioners of old had the power, knowledge, and ability to communicate deep to the bones of those they treated, palpating for blocked areas and then by moving their palms, thumbs, knuckles, and forearms in rhythmic, dance-like motions, dispersing them. From generation to generation, lomi-lomi has continued to thrive and be practiced within Hawaiian communities and has expanded to other regions of the United States.[43]

Central and South America

When Hernando Cortes and his Spanish Conquistadors marched on the capital of the Aztec nation, they marveled at a civilization surpassing anything they had previously experienced—even in all of Europe. The Aztec nation's streets were paved with bricks of mud and their buildings were expertly engineered with stones cut to fit so snugly that they didn't need cement to bind them together. Their statues were precisely carved out of massive stones imported from inland volcanoes. An advanced sanitation system collected garbage regularly, they had clean public toilets, and they had pharmacies that sold plasters, ointments, and ready-to-drink remedies. Their medical world was already well developed, with formulas available to treat a wide range of disorders from sore muscles, post-pregnancy pain, exhaustion, rheumatism, to neuralgia. Although the Aztec physicians were learned enough to incorporate medicinal plants and herbs into their system of healing arts, they still lived in a world where disease was seen as the consequence of a displeased deity. Unique to this region, the price for regaining the favor of the gods was paid for with human sacrifice.

Although the Spanish didn't invade the Aztec nation until the 1500s, it was clear that Aztec practices had been developing for thousands of years. The Aztecs built tremendous steam baths called Temazcalli, which housed a large exercise area along with hot and cold rooms where slaves administered daily massages to the slaveowners. These treatments were sometimes applied with ointments brewed from herbs, animal fats, oils, and special leaves. [44]

EUROPE AND MODERN MEDICINE

Greece

The third century BCE marked a turning point in the history of mankind as Greek influence spread in the wake of Alexander's conquering legions. The Hellenistic period ushered in a bold new breed of thought born from the fertile union of insight, intellect, opportunity, and experimentation.

As the new science fermented among the Greeks, they produced a way of medicine that broke free from previous superstitions. Hippocrates, the father of medicine, pioneered the exploration of human anatomy with a piercing lens that saw clear through the holy shroud of magic, mysticism, and ritual. According to Robert Calvert, massage historian, Hippocrates was the *"first to separate physicians from the historical roots of cosmological speculator and philosopher of nature."* Hippocrates single-handedly revolutionized the previously mystical world of medical diagnosis and treatment (Figure 5-10).

His predecessor and teacher Herodicus was also an avid proponent of massage who helped establish its place in Greece's ancient medical culture. Herodicus's methods were so effective in healing the infirm that he was reproached by Plato for causing them greater suffering by extending their lives.[45]

Up until this time, disease was perceived to be either an invasion by an evil spirit or as suffering caused by the punishment of an angry god. Although the Greek physicians were trained in a system of medicine that was based on mystical and religious causes of disease, these theories fell apart and gave way to the new logic led by Hippocrates. This shift in thinking and science was the

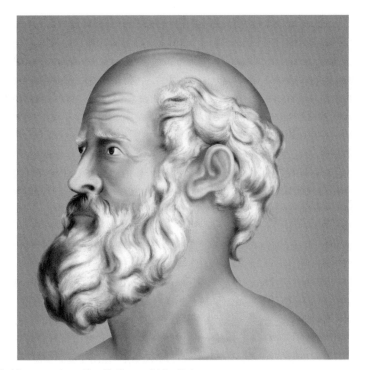

Figure 5-10 Hippocrates, the Father of Medicine.

discovery and exercise of human reason. Through Hippocrates, a new science was born.

To this day, Hippocrates is the most written-about medical practitioner in history. He developed a system of medicine that was based on keen, scientific observations of the patient's signs and symptoms with a thorough diagnosis that factored in the patient's internal and external conditions. *Anatripsis,* the Greek word for massage, played a small but vital role in his new medicine. He wrote, *"The physician must be experienced in many things, but assuredly also in rubbing."* He goes on to say, *"Rubbing can bind a joint which is too loose, and loosen a joint which is too hard."* [46]

The word *anatripsis* means "the process of rubbing up." This is significant because it marks the shift away from superstitious beliefs that were common in previous eras. In every form of ancient massage, the technique was always from the core out. The process would start at the abdomen and the stroking, pulling, scraping, and brushing would be directed out to the extremities. This process of "rubbing down" was utilized to move the evil spirit out from the core of the body to be extracted through the head or limbs. The new method was completely opposite. The strokes started at the extremities and were directed toward the center. [47] Today this method is known to benefit the body, increasing the circulation of blood and lymph by pushing toxins to the center of the body where they can be better processed and eliminated.

The ancient Greeks realized the close association of physical well-being and the mind and emotions. Everyone, from the wealthy patrician to the impoverished slaves, desired massage treatment—some for mere pleasure, and others to hasten recovery from illness and injury. For the ancient gladiators it was used to heal their broken and battered bodies after battle. [48] But the most common association of ancient Greek life with massage was made in their baths and gymnasiums. Gymnasiums were beautiful centers dedicated to the advancement of the intellectual, spiritual, and physical components of humanity. It was an open arena available to all free-born citizens where the low-born could learn, discourse, and compete freely with the noble class.

The *alliptae* (slave masseurs, or "rubbers" as they were often referred to) anointed the youthful wrestlers before their matches to invigorate their bodies and again afterwards to alleviate any strains or pains. [49] In addition to massage, skin scraping, and anointing with oil, the alliptae regulated the diet of the wrestlers by prescribing the exact quantity, quality, and time of every meal. [50]

In other areas of Greek society massage was still tied to magic and religion. It was used in the ritual of preparing a person for "temple sleep." Here the ailing patient would be prepared to sleep in a temple where Aesclepius (the god of health and medicine) and his daughters, Hygeia and Panacea, would visit in a dream to wash away the disease.[51]

Rome

With the conquest of Greece, medicine arrived in Rome. The practice of medicine was unregulated in ancient Rome and was practiced by almost anyone, even those with no previous experience or training. Many were mere charlatans hawking ineffective cures to diseases about which they had no understanding. The early Roman physicians would employ all manner of perverse methods to obtain patients, including following them home from the local taverns.[52] Often, it was the common household slave who practiced bleeding and surgery while the masseur dabbled in medicine and healing cures.[53] Because of the distrust that was bred from the abysmal success rate of treatments and the unethical behavior of those who dispensed them, doctors were scorned and the profession was relegated to that of foreigners of no status.[54]

War had ravaged the lands of the once-proud Greeks and the country became poverty stricken. Physicians sold themselves as slaves to be able to practice their art in Rome, where many were able to buy their freedom.[55] This educated class of Greek physicians eventually took control of the field of medicine. Once Julius Caesar granted their freedom they were able to attain a level of professionalism worthy of society's trust and confidence.[56] Through this new wave of competent physicians, the Hippocratic model (with a special niche for massage) was carried on. Then, in the early third century BCE, knowledge of human anatomy took an evolutionary leap forward.

Under the piercing scrutiny of the rapidly developing rational sciences, the mysticism of the ancient cultures began to evaporate and the laws that bound the hands of physicians for thousands of years were slowly pried loose. Human dissection, once seen as an atrocious act of treason against the souls of one's ancestors, was partially legalized.[57] Physicians were limited to the bodies of select, condemned criminals, but even with these constraints, they finally had the freedom to view the inner mechanisms of the human body.

Heir to these exciting times, Asclepiades, favored son of both Rome and Greece, made solid advancements in the budding field of massage therapy. He was one of the Greek physicians practicing in Rome, where he founded a school of medicine called the Methodists. The Methodists subscribed to a simplistic way of healing that mostly utilized massage, diet, and bathing.[58] Asclepiades hypothesized that the optimum functioning of the body necessitated the rebalancing of its "nutritive fluids" to allow for their free flow. Although he was educated in all the modern medicines, he eventually abandoned conventional methods to rely exclusively on massage to cure disease.[59] He championed the humane treatment of the mentally ill and treated many with natural therapies, including diet and massage.[60] It was even rumored that he brought a dead man back to life with physical manipulation.[61]

Massage continued to advance into the flourishing age of ancient Rome. Cicero remarked that he owed his health equally to his masseuse and his physician. Caesar, suffering from neuralgia, had himself pinched daily to alleviate his pains. Pliny, writer, encyclopedist, and the foremost authority on science in his time, wrote to the emperor about how his life had been saved by a physician who employed rubbing and anointing.[62]

Although there were many followers of Hippocrates, none have come closer than Galen (129–99 CE). Considered by many to be the greatest physician of antiquity after Hippocrates, his first professional appointment was surgeon to the gladiators. In Rome, he achieved a brilliant career as a physician.[63] His fame became widespread, and soon he rose to the ranks of court physician to the emperor Marcus Aurelius.[64]

He took five centuries of Greco-Roman theory and practice of massage therapy and produced volumes of texts in the field of medicine and philosophy. Although many of his theories were later proven to be wrong, he is still recognized for his enormous contributions to anatomy, especially in the area of muscles, tendons, and ligaments. He was also one of the first people to connect anatomy to physiology.

As an impassioned disciple of Hippocrates, he held massage in the highest regard and expressed obvious contempt for those who would reduce it to mere sexual favors.[65] He expanded on the specific use of massage for both athletes and nonathletes. He outlined preparatory massage for before exercising and described treatments for afterward. He expounded on Hippocrates's theory of the necessity of applying strokes in every direction to achieve the greatest release of bound muscle fibers and developed nine different forms of massage, each for different applications and problems.[66]

By the second century CE, caring for the sick had become a province of the church. Some early Christians were powerful healers who ministered remediation through the laying-on of hands and the anointing with oil.[67]

Middle Ages

With the fall of the Roman Empire in the fifth century, medicine in Europe descended into a thick fog of religious dogma and did not resurface for almost a thousand years. There was a return to obscure and theurgic medicine, with Saints and their relics believed to harbor miraculous healing powers.[68] With a zealous faith in God, the people came to believe that all manifestation was an act of the higher powers. Illness happened because God willed it for a greater good; therefore, it was wrong to attempt interference upon his divine plan.[69]

This dark Christian era of the Middle Ages bred an increasing intolerance for pleasures of the body that resulted in the outlawing of the bath houses and the closing of the Olympic Games. It also marked an end to an important period of time where both massage and exercise were highly valued. Even the great concern for the hygiene and care of the physical body steadily declined under the oppressive weight of religious influence. Yet, it was the women of the very same church who were responsible for keeping the tradition of massage alive. Whereas in prior eras massage was almost the exclusive domain of the men, particularly in the athletic and medical specialties, it was the women of the church who undertook the task of healing the sick through natural means and helping to keep the art of massage alive. Abandoned temples were converted into hospitals and hospices and new healing centers were founded and funded by wealthy citizens, staffed by volunteers, and led by the sisters of various religious groups.[70]

By the late Middle Ages (twelfth to fourteenth centuries), however, claims of possessing healing powers were considered heresy and punishable by death.[71]

> "Many a poor woman was burned at the stake in northern Europe during the Middle Ages because she knew a little more than another person and cured suffering men by massage, a magic which was looked upon as a power of Satan."[72]

While Europe turned its back on the classical sciences, the rest of the world sustained its steady march forward toward the advancement of medicine and massage. The quest for empirical medical knowledge first undertaken by Hippocrates was continued by the Arab world. Medical knowledge was kept alive in large part and spread by translating the classics into Arabic and other **Semitic** languages.[73]

The Renaissance

It wasn't until the Renaissance that a fresh breeze blew through Europe, invigorating the stiff and stagnant minds with the crisp logic of rational science. With the increased tolerance of human dissection, studies in the old concepts of anatomy and physiology were resuscitated and universities again made it a central theme of their medical studies. By the sixteenth century, a number of significant works concerning "mechanical treatments" were produced from all over Europe.

Paracelsus (1493–541) of Switzerland, the man who is recognized as being the first to realize the necessity of keeping wounds clean, also developed theories on the connection between the emotions and the physical body. He wrote:

> A man who is angry is not only angry in his heart or in his fist, but all over... all the organs of the body, and the body itself, are only form-manifestations of previously and universally existing mental states.

Andrea Vesalius (1514–1564) of Brussels made significant contributions toward the study of human anatomy. In order to attain the bodies necessary to satisfy his curiosity of the inner workings of his fellow humans, he would cut down the bodies of hanged criminals—an act that earned the disdain and reproach of church authorities. Later, he performed public autopsies and lectured to the large crowds that gathered around him. His discoveries unleashed a vast body of knowledge and charted new courses in the dimension of medicine.

Studies in massage during this time coincided heavily with the groundwork laid out by Galen and Hippocrates. The threads of previous research were rediscovered and woven into new theories of health and healing. These new modes of therapy often included movement exercises, and many of these hybrid styles emphasized the use of massage for joint mobilization, fluid circulation, and muscle conditioning. This new wave of movement therapy developed for centuries and eventually infused the western minds of the 1800s.[74]

THE SEVENTEENTH, EIGHTEENTH, AND NINETEENTH CENTURIES

The power of healing, once attributed to the gods and goddesses of the ancient world, was naturally passed down to kings and queens, who claimed divine rights to their throne. It was believed that a person could merely be touched and cured by a royal hand. However, the practice of the laying-on of hands was not confined to royalty. Healers from many lands claimed such powers, but none so effectively as Valentine Greatrakes (1628–1683), also known as "The Stroker," a soldier of Ireland who enjoyed an enormous reputation as a powerful healer.[75]

As time went on massage continued to gain momentum, with greater and greater bodies of work being developed concerning its efficacy in treating disease. There was such strong support for massage that some reported that almost all diseases could be cured through it, including syphilis. There were even reports of a woman who had lost her vision through a trauma but regained it with massage.[76]

The idea of achieving a healthy state of both mind and body through exercise had already been recognized for thousands of years. New autopsies of the body revealed its likeness to a powerful machine capable of self-regulation. A divide began to emerge between naturalists and conventionalists. The naturalists stood solidly in their beliefs and empowered the individual to recognize their body's innate ability to heal itself through natural means without the interjection of harsh substances into the body's delicate ecosystem and without the invasive, dangerous, and often unnecessary practice of surgery. The conventionalist position, rooted in allopathic medicine, relied upon emerging science, technology, and pharmaceuticals to treat the body. This fostered a reductionist approach to the treatment of disease that became the dominant viewpoint of western medicine moving into the nineteenth, twentieth, and twenty-first centuries.

Although others actually developed medical gymnastics (systems of exercise and movement applied to the treatment of disease), it is Peter Henry Ling, a Swedish military officer, medical gymnast, and fencing master (1776–1839) who is most closely associated with these ideas. He is widely considered to be the father of Swedish massage and physical therapy. Ling studied massage early in his life after being cured of a debilitating form of rheumatoid arthritis that he had unsuccessfully tried to heal himself for many years. Undeterred by his failures to resolve his painful condition, he traveled to France, Germany, and then the Far East to find a cure. There he learned the principles of Chinese medicine and studied kung fu with Taoist priests. He also acquired great proficiency in fencing and gymnastics.

While previous forms of movement therapy already existed among his contemporaries, it wasn't yet an exact science. Ling was the first to formulate a specific series of exercises in order to achieve health benefits. When he perceived the human body, he envisioned the interplay of dynamic forces found within both humanity and the universe. Although not a doctor, his keen intuition understood that there was a hierarchy of existence in the Universe in which people play a fractional but vibrant role.

His form of gymnastics included active exercises, which the patient performed unassisted and passive movements, in which the patient was moved and manipulated by the therapist. These passive movements, which included stroking, kneading, **friction**, and stripping, eventually evolved into what is now popularly known as Swedish massage. Although Ling did much to systemize therapeutic massage, he documented little on the subject. His work, however, was carried on by his pupils (who wrote as if they were the creators of massage).[77]

Ling's system was first introduced exclusively to the military academies, but soon knowledge of its value became known and was adopted by almost every medical school, college, and university throughout the country. His work was praised for its effectiveness in treating chronic illnesses and his system was hailed by the medical community as a landmark achievement. Ling's work was embraced throughout Europe, and eventually made its way to America.

In 1880, George H. Taylor, M.D., a forefather in the fight for the acceptance of natural medicine, including movement and massage, boldly exclaimed in his book *Health by Exercise:*

> In glancing at the history of movements, the reader will wonder why an art so easily practiced...should not in modern times have come more generally into popular favor. The answer to this inquiry will be found in the fact of the maze of obscurity that has prevailed in the general mind in regard to the true curative value of drugs. But while all possible things have been both asserted and denied in regard to drugs, the value of movements has never been denied or questioned, but only at times neglected.[78]

John Harvey Kellog (1852–1943), was one of the leading proponents of massage on the new frontier of American soil. In fact, some consider him to be the father of massage in America. He was a writer, inventor (the cornflake breakfast cereal was his creation), physician, and entrepreneur. He was an advocate of vegetarianism and ran a famous sanitarium at Battlecreek, Michigan, using holistic modalities that included nutrition, hydrotherapy, massage, and enemas. One of his most famous books, *The Art of Massage: A Practical Manual for the Nurse, the Student and the Practitioner* published in 1929, is still being used in some massage schools across the country. His main contribution to the profession of massage therapy is that he was able to help it become mainstream, particularly in the medical spa environment.

> Fifty years ago there were in this country few if any persons who were really skilled in massage. It was only by visiting Stockholm, Sweden, and Germany and France that it was found possible to obtain a practical knowledge of the subject.[79]

In 1878, S. Weir Mitchell of Philadelphia, the leading neurologist of the time, published *Fat and Blood, and How to Make Them,* which helped to establish the credibility of manual therapies. The book had a separate chapter on massage, and throughout the rest of the text one could find numerous references to the use of massage as an important part of recommended treatment for many different conditions.[80] But in the late 1800s, publications appeared around the world announcing the abuses and misuses of massage, including quackery and prostitution. The field came under attack after increases in scandals concerning massage; but Mitchell, whose credibility by now far exceeded the limits of Philadelphia and even the United States, joined with others in an effort to promote the struggling field and reestablish it as a respectable medical practice.

Since Hippocrates little had been written about the appropriate amount of pressure to be used in treatment. Some believed in the gentle approach while others subscribed to theories that say "great violence" is necessary for effective results. Still others adopted the flexible middle path, where some cases required the gentle techniques while other situations called for stronger methods.

In the mid 1800s, Johan Georg Mezger brought Amsterdam to the center of the massage world. He was renowned for not only his effectiveness, but for his forceful and painful methods. He actually described his work as the tearing of subcutaneous vessels. Despite the acceleration of the rate of international scientific research, massage was still a somewhat questionable field. But Metzger, being a physician, was able to penetrate the medical field much more deeply than Ling ever was, and he was able to improve the field to such a degree that it developed into its own special branch in the art of medicine. He influenced the field so much that the French terminology he used to describe the strokes of Swedish massage (**effleruage**, **petrissage**, and **tapotement**) are still used today.[81] Prior to this, the process of massage went by many names, including friction, rubbing, masseing, passive movement, passes, atouchements, and more.

The medical world continued to pour research into the dynamic field of massage therapy. Russia's Supreme Medical Board appointed members of their Medical Council to research the effects of movement and manipulation. New studies developed that sought to understand the physiology of massage. Many different conditions were experimentally treated with massage, including fractures, prostate enlargement, gynecological issues, pregnancy complications, neuralgia and more.

By the start of the twentieth century, massage came to be used through-out the West. The First World War provided ample opportunity for the practice and continued development of the manual therapies, or mechano-therapies, as they were often called. Demand for bodywork increased as societies and organizations formed to organize and advance the field of massage therapy. The qualities that they outlined included not only soundness of mind and body, but strength in moral fiber as well.[82]

In 1894, the Society of Trained Masseuses formed in Great Britain to pro-vide structure and guidance for the quickly developing field. They worked not only to train emerging therapists but also to provide guidelines for them to operate under. They established a solid massage curriculum and a board-certification program. They were responsible for the accreditation and regular inspections of massage schools and they worked to improve the quality of edu-cation by requiring specific qualifications of their teachers. By the end of WWI, the society was 5000 members strong. By 1939, that number had more than doubled, to over 11,000.

In 1943, graduates of the College of Swedish Massage in Chicago gathered to form the American Association of Masseurs and Masseuses (AAMM). In 1958, they changed their name to the **American Massage Therapy Association** (AMTA).[83] Today the AMTA, the largest and oldest professional association in the United States representing massage therapists, is about 58,000 members strong.

MASSAGE TODAY

Today, because of small groups of individuals throughout the United States who resurrected the principles of holistic health in the 1970s, myriad styles of massage and bodywork are once again flourishing in this country. Dozens of different methods or modalities of massage have been developed, mostly in the United States, since the 1960s.[84] **Holistic, alternative, integrative** and **comple-mentary health care** has become one of the fastest growing industries in the country. More and more people are realizing the efficacy of treating the ailments of the modern world with natural and noninvasive therapies. **Integrative med-icine** is evolving and becoming a regular part of the everyday man or woman's health care in order to lead a healthy and happy life. People are seeing the limi-tations of **allopathic medicine** in the treatment of chronic disease and have be-come disenchanted with the dehumanization of the modern health care world. In this aversion toward the cold sterility of modern medicine, massage and other holistic practices are beginning to enjoy a fervent renaissance. Science is again realizing the fundamental truth that human touch is integral to human health and that the human body responds most favorably to human touch.

SUMMARY

This chapter discusses the history and evolution of touch and presents an overview of the roots of massage during major historical time periods in different countries and regions of the world. By highlighting the growth and development of touch through time, it can be seen that its evolution through history until today has not been linear, but instead a very organic, yet complex, progression due to its independent and sometimes parallel development in many different cultures. The chapter also looks at, and briefly discusses, diverse forms of touch including those that have evolved in prehistoric times, Babylonia and Assyria, Egypt, India, China, Japan, The Philippines, Russia, and Ukraine, The Ancient Americas, North America, Hawaii, Central and South America, Europe, Greece, Rome, Middle Ages, the Renaissance, the 17th, 18th, and the 19th centuries, and massage as it exists today. The chapter discusses how some of these hands-on healing arts are thousands of years old and have been carefully passed down, remaining essentially the same pure arts through time and how other newer approaches, some based on their ancestral forms, have evolved into effective, complex systems of massage and bodywork therapy. It also points out how the more recent times have independently given rise to yet other modalities that have become popular and are included in the greater framework of practice within the profession.

CHAPTER REFERENCES

1. Beck, M. (2006). *Theory and practice of therapeutic massage* (4th ed.). Albany, NY: Cengage Learning.
2. Salvo, S. (2003). *Massage therapy—Principles and practice* (2nd ed.). St. Louis: Saunders/Elsevier.
3. Calvert, R. (2002). *The history of massage.* Rochester, VT: Healing Arts Press.
4. *Medicine.* Retrieved March 6, 2008, from http://encarta.msn.com/encyclopedia_761567832_2/Medicine.html#p76
5. Kamenetz, H. (1980) "History of Massage" in *Manipulation, Traction and Massage.* Baltimore, MD: William and Wilkins.
6. Calvert, R. (2002). *The history of massage.* Rochester, VT: Healing Arts Press.
7. Brooke, E. (1997). *Medicine women.* Illinois: Quest Books.

8. *Imhotep*. Retrieved March 6, 2008, from http://en.wikipedia.org/wiki/Imhotep

9. Dunn, J. Imhotep, doctor, architect, high priest, scribe and vizier to King Djoser. Retrieved March 6, 2008, from *http://www.touregypt.net/featurestories/imhotep.htm*

10. Dunn, J. Imhotep, doctor, architect, high priest, scribe and vizier to King Djoser. Retrieved March 6, 2008, from *http://www.touregypt.net/featurestories/imhotep.htm*

11. *Medicine*. Retrieved March 6, 2008, from http://encarta.msn.com/encyclopedia_761567832_2/Medicine.html#p76

12. Douillard, J. (2004). *Encyclopedia of ayurvedic massage*. Berkeley, CA: North Atlantic Books.

13. *Ayurveda-history and philosophy*. Retrieved February 26, 2008, from http://www.healthandhealingny.org/tradition_healing/ayurveda-history.html

14. *Ayurveda-history and philosophy*. Retrieved February 26, 2008, from http://www.healthandhealingny.org/tradition_healing/ayurveda-history.html

15. Gerson, S. *Basic principles of ayurveda*. Retrieved February 26, 2008, from http://niam.com/corp-web/basicstoc.html

16. Morningstar, S. *The new life library: Ayurveda*. United Kingdom: Lorenz Books.

17. Sohn, R., & Sohn, T. (1996). *Amma therapy*. Rochester, VT: Healing Arts Press.

18. Calvert, R. (2002). *The history of massage*. Rochester, VT: Healing Arts Press.

19. Calvert, R. (2002). *The history of massage*. Rochester, VT: Healing Arts Press.

20. Dubitsky, C. (1997). *Bodywork shiatsu*. Rochester, VT: Healing Arts Press.

21. Salvo, S. (2003). *Massage therapy—Principles and practice* (2nd ed.). St. Louis: Saunders/Elsevier.

22. Dubitsky, C. (1997). *Bodywork shiatsu*. Rochester, VT: Healing Arts Press.

23. Sohn, R., & Sohn, T. (1996). *Amma therapy*. Rochester, VT: Healing Arts Press.

24. Sohn, R., & Sohn, T. (1996). *Amma therapy*. Rochester, VT: Healing Arts Press.

25. Dharmananda, S. R. Retrieved December, 13, 2008, from http://www.itmonline.org/arts/japacu.htm

26. Dubitsky, C. (1997). *Bodywork shiatsu*. Rochester, VT: Healing Arts Press.

27. Dubitsky, C. (1997). *Bodywork shiatsu*. Rochester, VT: Healing Arts Press.

28. Dharmananda, S. R. Retrieved December 13, 2008, from http://www.itmonline.org/arts/shiatsu.htm

29. Dubitsky, C. (1997). *Bodywork shiatsu*. Rochester, VT: Healing Arts Press.

30. Calvert, R. (2002). *The history of massage*. Rochester, VT: Healing Arts Press.

31. Juvida, S. F. Retrieved December 13, 2008, from http://www.workspresso.com/20070601%20edition/archives/2006/may16-31-06/current/features_current/feature2.html

32. Wine, Z. K. (April, 2008). A history of Russian medical massage. *Massage Today, 08*(4).

33. Calvert, R. (2002). *The history of massage*. Rochester, VT: Healing Arts Press.

34. Wine, Z. K. (April, 2008). A history of Russian medical massage. *Massage Today, 08*(4).

35. *Native American history and philosophy*. Retrieved March 5, 2008, from http://www.healthandhealingny.org/tradition_healing/native-history.html

36. *Native American treatment approaches*. Retrieved March 5, 2008, from http://www.healthandhealingny.org/tradition_healing/native-treat.html

37. Calvert, R. (2002). *The history of massage.* Rochester, VT: Healing Arts Press.
38. Calvert, R. (2002). *The history of massage.* Rochester, VT: Healing Arts Press.
39. *Hawaiian temple bodywork—Out of the temples, into our hearts.* Retrieved March 6, 2008, from http://www.hawaiiantemplebodywork.com/Introductionlomilomi1.html
40. *Hawaiian temple bodywork—Out of the temples, into our hearts.* Retrieved March 6, 2008, from http://www.hawaiiantemplebodywork.com/Introductionlomilomi1.html
41. Mitchell, S. (2000). *The complete illustrated guide to massage: A step-by-step approach to the healing art of touch.* Shaftesbury, Dorset, UK:Element Books Ltd.
42. Calvert, R. (2002). *The history of massage.* Rochester, VT: Healing Arts Press.
43. Mondragon, T. (2000, July). History of lomilomi. *Massage Magazine.*
44. Calvert, R. (2002). *The history of massage.* Rochester, VT: Healing Arts Press.
45. Kamenetz, H. (1980). History of Massage. In *Manipulation, traction and massage.* Baltimore, MD: William and Wilkins.
46. Kamenetz, H. (1980). History of Massage. In *Manipulation, traction and massage.* Baltimore, MD: William and Wilkins.
47. Calvert, R. (2002). *The history of massage.* Rochester, VT: Healing Arts Press.
48. Kamenetz, H. (1980). History of Massage. In *Manipulation, traction and massage.* Baltimore, MD: William and Wilkins.
49. Kamenetz, H. (1980). History of Massage. In *Manipulation, traction and massage.* Baltimore, MD: William and Wilkins.
50. Calvert, R. (2002). *The history of massage.* Rochester, VT: Healing Arts Press.
51. Calvert, R. (2002). *The history of massage.* Rochester, VT: Healing Arts Press.
52. *Ancient Roman medicine.* Retrieved March 6, 2008, from http://www.crystalinks.com/romemedicine.html
53. Calvert, R. (2002). *The history of massage.* Rochester, VT: Healing Arts Press.
54. Fiorin, L. *Hellenistic-Roman medicine. Arab medicine. Medieval times.* Retrieved March 6, 2008, from http://pacs.unica.it/biblio/lesson2.htm
55. Fiorin, L. *Hellenistic-Roman medicine. Arab medicine. Medieval times.* Retrieved March 6, 2008, from http://pacs.unica.it/biblio/lesson2.htm
56. Calvert, R. (2002). *The history of massage.* Rochester, VT: Healing Arts Press.
57. Calvert, R. (2002). *The history of massage.* Rochester, VT: Healing Arts Press.
58. Salvo, S. (2003). *Massage therapy—Principles and practice* (2nd ed.). St. Louis: Saunders/Elsevier.
59. Calvert, R. (2002). *The history of massage.* Rochester, VT: Healing Arts Press.
60. *Asclepiades c.129–40 BC Greek Physician.* Retrieved March 6, 2008, from http://www.hyperhistory.com/online_n2/people_n2/persons2_n2/asclepiades.html
61. Calvert, R. (2002). *The history of massage.* Rochester, VT: Healing Arts Press.
62. Kamenetz, H. (1980). History of Massage. In *Manipulation, traction and massage.* Baltimore, MD: William and Wilkins.
63. *Galen.* Retrieved March 6, 2008, from http://www.med.virginia.edu/hs-library/historical/antiqua/galen.htm
64. *Galen.* Retrieved March 6, 2008, from http://en.wikipedia.org/wiki/Galen
65. Calvert, R. (2002). *The history of massage.* Rochester, VT: Healing Arts Press.

66. Kamenetz, H. (1980). History of Massage. In *Manipulation, traction and massage.* Baltimore, MD: William and Wilkins.

67. Mumford, S. (1998). *The healing massage: A practical guide to relaxation and well-being.* USA: Plume.

68. Fiorin, L. *Hellenistic-Roman medicine. Arab medicine. Medieval times.* Retrieved March 6, 2008, from http://pacs.unica.it/biblio/lesson2.htm

69. *Medicine and religion in the middle ages—"The cure comes from god."* Retrieved March 6, 2008, from http://intermaggie.com/med/religion.php

70. Calvert, R. (2002). *The history of massage.* Rochester, VT: Healing Arts Press.

71. Salvo, S. (2003). *Massage therapy—Principles and practice* (2nd ed.). St. Louis: Saunders/Elsevier.

72. Nissen, H. (1923). *Practical massage.* Philadelphia: F. A. Davis.

73. Kamenetz, H. (1980). History of Massage. In *Manipulation, traction and massage.* Baltimore, MD: William and Wilkins.

74. Calvert, R. (2002). *The history of massage.* Rochester, VT: Healing Arts Press.

75. Kamenetz, H. (1980). History of Massage. In *Manipulation, traction and massage.* Baltimore, MD: William and Wilkins.

76. Kamenetz, H. (1980). History of Massage. In *Manipulation, traction and massage.* Baltimore, MD: William and Wilkins.

77. Kamenetz, H. (1980). History of Massage. In *Manipulation, traction and massage.* Baltimore, MD: William and Wilkins.

78. Taylor, G. H. (1883). *Health by exercise: What exercises to take and how to take them, to remove special physical weakness. Embracing an account of the Swedish methods, and a summary of the principles of hygiene.* New York: American Book Exchange, John B. Alden.

79. Kellogg, J. H. (1929). *The art of massage: A practical manual for the nurse, the student and the practitioner.* Whitefish, MT: Re-published by Kessinger Publishing, 2004.

80. Mitchell, S. W. (1882). *Fat and blood: And how to make them.* Lanham, MD: Re-published by Rowman Altamira, 2004.

81. Salvo, S. (2003). *Massage therapy—Principles and practice* (2nd ed.). St. Louis: Saunders/Elsevier.

82. Mitchell, S. (2000). *The complete illustrated guide to massage: A step-by-step approach to the healing art of touch.* Shaftesbury, Dorset, UK:Element Books Ltd.

83. Salvo, S. (2003). *Massage therapy—Principles and practice* (2nd ed.). St. Louis: Saunders/Elsevier.

84. Salvo, S. (2003). *Massage therapy—Principles and practice* (2nd ed.). St. Louis: Saunders/Elsevier.

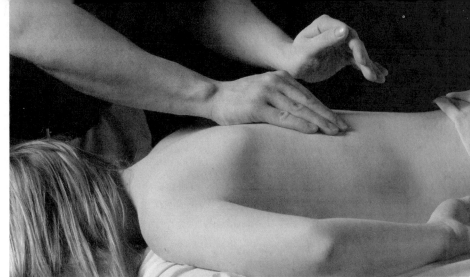

6
CHAPTER

The Continuum of the Four Massage Therapy and Bodywork Levels

CHAPTER GOALS

1. Develop an understanding of the origin of the concept of the continuum of the four massage therapy and bodywork levels.

2. Discuss the fable of the Four Blind Men and the Elephant to demonstrate that depending upon one's perspective, truth may be relative and exist on many levels.

3. Discuss the fable of the Four Blind Men and the Elephant and its relationship to viewing and understanding the notion that the essential difference between each of the many diverse forms of touch lies primarily in its intention to treat and effect a specific layer or level of the human being.

4. Develop an understanding of the importance of a practitioner's underlying intention in the practice of any modality within the continuum of the four massage therapy and bodywork levels.

INTRODUCTION

In 1990, I (author of this text) had the good fortune to be part of a small group of professional massage therapy and bodywork organization leaders brought together by the American Massage Therapy Association (AMTA) to form the Job Analysis Advisory Committee (JAAC) of the National Certification Program. The Committee was composed of practitioners representing various massage therapy and bodywork disciplines. At that time, I was also serving as the first president of the American Organization of Bodywork Therapies of Asia (AOBTA) and was asked to participate in this ground-breaking project to represent the voice, interests, and perspectives of the Asian bodywork community in the United States.

The JAAC's mandate was to begin the process of developing a Job Analysis Survey for the massage therapy and bodywork profession. In December of 1990, the results were published in a document called "A National Study of the Profession of Massage Therapy/Bodywork." It would be the first time that the field took a really good look at itself in order to ascertain from the broadest cross-section of practicing professionals what massage and bodywork therapists actually do. It was an attempt to distill from all the information gathered what skills, knowledge, and abilities were considered necessary for entering into the practice of massage therapy and more accurately define its scope of practice. Armed with this information, a statistically valid and legally defensible national certification examination program was developed and the JAAC evolved into the first National Certification Board for Therapeutic Massage and Bodywork (NCBTMB). Today, 43 states regulate the profession of massage therapy, and of those, 33 states plus the District of Columbia currently require passing the NCBTMB examination for licensure and/or certification for practice.

The information gathered from the survey gradually became the basis for massage therapy school program curricula that more accurately reflected the field of practice, its latest trends, and where the profession was headed. With a new blueprint for practice, state regulators, associations, and educators developing new or revamping old standards or school programs could now use the new research information to better reflect the present state of the profession. As a result of the development of the NCBTMB, the education and training of massage therapy and bodywork professionals across the country was greatly benefited.

THE CONTINUUM OF THE FOUR MASSAGE THERAPY AND BODYWORK LEVELS

For me, the most profound and influential ideas emerged from the first set of grassroots discussions we had as we attempted to wrap our minds around all of the diverse techniques being practiced under the umbrella of massage therapy and bodywork and how we were going to address all of those in one examination. To this day I can clearly recall our efforts at listing every modality and discipline that we could think of. After a few hours and much debate, we were left with a room full of easel paper covering the walls from floor to ceiling containing lists of more than one hundred different forms of massage. Those lists led to some very long and deep discussions over several days, out of which eventually came the ideas we named the Three Paradigms and the Five Approaches. Ultimately, our insights were published in a brief article entitled, "Three Paradigms, Five Approaches" in the *Massage Therapy Journal,* Summer 1991, and was co-authored by Carl Dubitsky, ABT, LMT, Patricia Benjamin, PhD, Raymond Castellino, DC, RPP, Jeffery Maitland, PhD, and me, Steven Schenkman.

The Three Paradigms describe the continuum of levels that form the scope of possible practice of massage therapy and bodywork. They describe the depth and extent of knowledge and technical training that form the context from which massage therapists practice. They are covered fully in Chapters 1 through 4, and have been expanded to include several new ideas.

The **Five Approaches** resulted from an in-depth analysis of all the modalities that were listed during the JAAC meetings and judged to be part of the profession of massage therapy and bodywork. Discussion led to grouping modalities with common philosophies, principles, and cores of knowledge into five categories, which included at that time 1) traditional massage; 2) contemporary western massage and bodywork; 3) structural/functional/movement/integration modalities; 4) Asian bodywork; and 5) energetic bodywork (Figure 6-1). This was an interesting way to look at and order the field; however, the more I lectured and thought about this over the years and the more I engaged in lengthy dialogues with some of my advanced students about this idea, a new way of looking at touch began to emerge.

Through years of intense training rooted in the Asian traditions, I was very used to looking at things in terms of levels and layers. As I viewed the various components of a human being in this way, a new view of all the modalities evolved. I realized that although these many forms of massage and bodywork may have originated at different times and from different places on the earth, the thing that really distinguished one from the other was the specific *layer* of the body it was intended to target and treat as its primary objective. Some forms were intended to treat and heal from a physical standpoint by addressing muscles, tissues, nerves, bones, and the movement of lymph and blood. Some sought to treat and heal and bring about positive change by delving deeply into the structures of the body to make important physical adjustments and corrections, as well as affect a person's overall psychology. Some sought

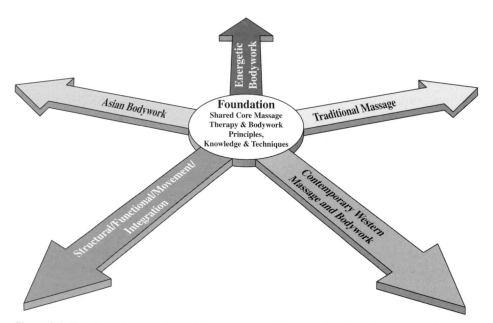

Figure 6-1 The Five Approaches of Massage and Bodywork: The original classification of massage therapy and bodywork modalities grouped into five categories according to common philosophy, principles, and core of knowledge.

to treat and heal from an energetic perspective by focusing on the channels, points, and flow of energy (Qi) through the manipulation of the soft tissues of the body. And still other forms sought to treat the body's radiance or aura, by holding and moving the hands over key areas without touching the body. The aura is the energy field that emanates from and surrounds living creatures. It is the extension beyond the body of the same energy system of acupuncture meridians and points described in traditional Chinese medicine.

The Five Approaches, which essentially placed everything on the same plateau within a common base of core information, evolved into its new form—the Continuum of the Four Massage Therapy and Bodywork Levels. These Four Levels describe a continuum of touch along which each modality is categorized according to its intention and specific focus on primarily targeting, treating, and affecting one of the four layers of the body-mind-energy complex. The four levels of massage are 1) somatic, 2) somato-psychic, 3) bioenergetic, and 4) energetic (Figure 6-2).

The **somatic layer** has to do with modalities that deal primarily with the treatment of the physical body. Practitioners of these forms seek to affect changes purely on a physiological level. These include but are not limited to Swedish

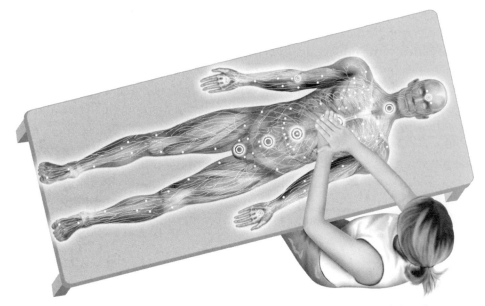

Figure 6-2 The Continuum of the Four Massage Therapy and Bodywork Levels: Classifies each modality according to what level or specific layer of the body-mind-energy complex it is intended to target and treat as its primary objective.

massage, neuromuscular therapy, myofascial release, manual lymphatic drainage, trigger point therapy, sports massage, and orthopedic massage.

The next layer deals with modalities that also primarily seek to treat the physical body, but at the same time deal with related issues of psychology. What does it mean that a certain muscle or area of the body is constricted and as a result restricted? What are the psychological implications and significance that the body is postured in a certain way? What is the impact of the emotions on the body and how can a person's psychology be impacted through deep and intense structured touch? These treatments are specifically intended to impact the body-mind connection to affect changes at the psychological level as well as the physical, hence the name **somato-psychic**. These include but are not limited to Rolfing®, Soma Neuromuscular Integration, Hellerwork, Alexander Technique, Feldenkrais®, and craniosacral therapy.

In the **bioenergetic level** of bodywork we explore the invisible world of energy. These modalities seek to treat an underlying layer of the body commonly referred to as the "energy body." Although this is accomplished through a rigorous manipulation of the physical body, the specific intention and focus is to create changes at the energetic level, including the meridians and acupuncture points, in order to balance and heal the overall system. These forms include but are not limited to several forms of shiatsu, tuina, acupressure, amma therapeutic massage, Jin Shin Do®, and Thai massage.

And finally, the **energetic level** includes modalities whose intent is to affect changes in the underlying energy body by directly accessing and affecting the energy body's extension, the aura, with little or even no direct physical contact. These include but are not limited to Reiki, therapeutic touch, and polarity therapy.

There are often very positive side effects of treatment with these modalities that have carryover benefits on one or more of the other levels of the body-mind-energy complex not directly targeted as the primary intention. When practiced properly, these far reaching and positive repercussions greatly contribute to the overall healing effects of any massage therapy and bodywork approach.

THE FABLE OF THE BLIND MEN AND THE ELEPHANT

When I think back to those initial meetings of the JAAC and the diverse and often very strong views of how the total field of the Massage Therapy and Bodywork profession could, or even should, be organized, I am reminded of an old fable known as "The Four Blind Men and the Elephant." Though there are many renditions of the story that have been told and even some questions about its origin, they all seek to teach the same lesson. The story goes something like this:

Four blind men approached an elephant. The first blind man approached the elephant's rear and grabbed its tail. After a few moments of examination, he declared, "An elephant is like a rope!" The second blind man encountered the elephant from the side and felt one of its legs. He then stated with great authority that "an elephant is like a tree." The third blind man approached the elephant from the front and took hold of its trunk and with much certainty declared, "An elephant is like a snake." Finally, the fourth blind man touched the elephant's side with both hands and exclaimed, "An elephant is like a great wall!" And so learning that they were in complete disagreement, each of the blind men, asserting their position, began to argue with the other over who was right. A sighted man observing their quarreling knew each was right from their position, but wrong and incomplete from an overall perspective or view.

The parable of The Four Blind Men is often told to demonstrate that depending upon one's perspective, reality may be viewed very differently, pointing out how truth may be relative and exist on many different levels all at once. It also points to the existence of a higher truth, one that encompasses and reconciles the lower truths. In the case of the four blind men, it is the elephant in its entirety that encompasses and reconciles the lesser or part-truths that result from each of the men's limited perception (Figure 6-3). Generally speaking, the higher the truth, the more inclusive it is even of viewpoints that may at first appear divergent.

Viewing and understanding the myriad massage therapy and bodywork modalities within a continuum of four levels, each modality able to be practiced from Three Paradigms, provide a profound and encompassing insight into the notion that the Universe and practice of massage and bodywork is multidimensional (Figure 6-4). In addition it demonstrates that the essential difference between each of the many diverse forms of touch included within the profession lies primarily in each one's specific intention to treat and effect a particular layer or level of the human being, thus bringing positive and healthful benefits, balance, and harmony to the whole person.

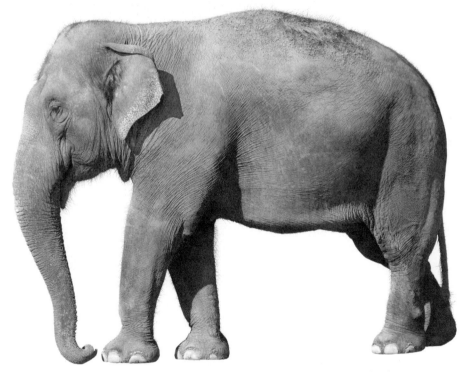

Figure 6-3 The elephant in its entirety encompasses and reconciles the lesser or part-truths that result from each of the blind men's limited perception. *Image copyright 2009, Rey Kamensky. Used under license from shutterstock.com.*

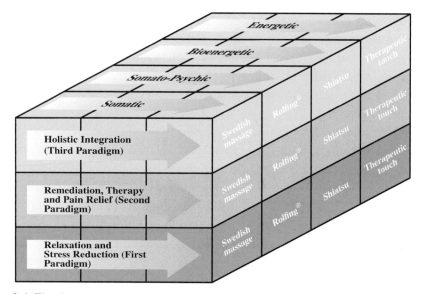

Figure 6-4 The "universe" of massage therapy & bodywork composed of The Three Paradigms and the Continuum of Four Massage & Bodywork Therapy Levels can be represented as a solid made of three dimensional cubes. Each vertical column of 3 cubes (3 high) represents a specific modality (i.e., Swedish massage of the Somatic level or Therapeutic Touch of the Energetic level) and its' level of practice at either the First, Second or Third Paradigm.

THE IMPORTANCE OF INTENTION

This powerful notion that intention to treat and affect one of the Four Levels of the human body-mind-energy complex is at the root of what distinguishes one modality from another demonstrates the real role the mind plays in the profession of touch therapy. How strong, focused, and directed a practitioner's intention is while applying the hands to a client's or patient's body will directly affect the outcome of the treatment whatever the particular modality being used. Even the best massage technicians, those who are great with their hands, will fall far short of becoming a true master of their craft if they do not learn to direct and concentrate their attention and develop a deep and powerful intention for their particular modality.

To the untrained eye, massage and bodywork therapists practicing any form of touch from any level of expertise can look almost identical. Yet depending on the therapist's intention and degree of focused attention, there can be a great difference. Take for example a therapist appearing to treat the soft tissue of the upper arm of a client. A practitioner trained in sports massage, a modality of the somatic group, may apply a compression technique on the biceps muscle of the upper arm with the intent of alleviating muscle soreness, increasing blood circulation, and improving nerve conduction. A practitioner trained in a modality from the bioenergetic group, such as shiatsu, who outwardly appears to be treating the exact same area with the exact same stroke, may have an entirely different intention and purpose. In this case, the shiatsu practitioner is treating the Lung Energy Channel and specific acupuncture points that lie along the same muscle area of the upper arm in order to affect the lung organ to help alleviate a chest cold.

A somato-psychic practitioner, for example a Rolfer, may be focused intently on the treatment of a client's back pain and postural misalignments while another Rolfer, from the same school, is completely distracted. Although the second practitioner may be applying the exact same techniques as the first, his attention is absorbed on the argument he had with his spouse earlier that day. It all looks the same, but the two practitioners are worlds apart in terms of the level of attention and intention underlying what their minds and therefore their hands are doing and accomplishing.

In order for massage therapy students to evolve into professional practitioners they must absorb and then integrate their training and practical experiences into a kind of blueprint of understanding. With the right attention and efforts, this understanding can grow into a comprehensive framework commensurate with their efforts to embrace their education and hone their technical skills. Ultimately, the level of framework developed becomes expressed as a powerful intention through the hands of these practitioners. In the end, it is the client that becomes the fortunate recipient of such a practice that emanates as pure intention through the massage therapist's hands. And, essentially, when you boil things right down, that is a reflection of what a massage therapist brings to the table.

MODALITIES OF THE CONTINUUM OF THE FOUR MASSAGE THERAPY AND BODYWORK LEVELS

The next four chapters take a serious look into 26 of the most commonly practiced massage therapy and bodywork modalities. Each modality discussed within each of the four levels includes a brief description of its founder and history, the significance of the modalities within the same level, how they differ, and how they are similar to each other. Also provided is a basic detailing of the underlying theory and principles, along with a description of the process of assessment and the specific hand techniques used in each modality. In addition, there is a discussion of a general treatment session using each of the modalities, which will enable the reader to become somewhat acquainted with what it might be like to experience a treatment. Discussions also include who should seek this form of treatment, contraindications and precautions, and what conditions are most benefited by each of these modalities. Information including training, licensing, certifications, and requirements necessary to practice each of the modalities is also briefly presented.

SUMMARY

This chapter begins with a brief history of the development of the first National Certification exam in Massage Therapy and Bodywork, a discussion of the author's role in that process and how out of that experience came the origin of the concept of "The Continuum of the Four Massage and Bodywork Therapy Levels." The four levels describe a continuum of touch within which each massage modality is categorized according to its intention and specific focus on primarily targeting, treating, and affecting one of the four layers of the body/mind/energy complex. The layers are 1) Somatic, 2) Somato-Psychic, 3) Bioenergetic, and 4) Energetic. The chapter includes a discussion of the well known "Fable of the Four Blind Men and the Elephant" in order to illustrate that there is rarely ever a single way of seeing things, that Truth is relative, it exists on many levels, and that larger or higher truths are more encompassing and inclusive. An understanding of this principle makes it easier to comprehend how the real essential difference between each of the many diverse forms of massage therapy and bodywork lies primarily in its intention to treat and affect a specific layer or level of the human being. The chapter also points out how to an outside observer, a practitioner may appear to be treating the soft tissue, but in fact he or she is treating the energy. The other major point made in this chapter is how a strong, focused, and directed intention, independent of massage modality, will directly and positively affect the outcome of treatment, while a weak and scattered intention will reap weak or no results.

The Somatic Level of the Massage Therapy and Bodywork Continuum

CHAPTER GOALS

1. Develop an understanding of how the modalities of Swedish massage, deep tissue massage, neuromuscular therapy, trigger point therapy, orthopedic massage, myofascial release, manual lymphatic drainage, and sports massage fit into the somatic approach of massage.

2. Recognize the significance of these modalities, how they differ, and how they are similar to each other.

3. Develop a basic understanding of the theory and principles of each of the modalities.

4. Develop a basic understanding of the process of assessment used in each of the modalities.

5. Develop a basic understanding of the techniques involved in each of the modalities.

6. Become acquainted with the general experience of a session in each of the modalities.

7. Identify who should seek this form of treatment and what conditions are most benefited by each of the modalities.

8. Become aware of contraindications and precautions related to each of the modalities.

9. Become knowledgeable about the training, licensing, certifications, and requirements that one needs in order to practice within each of the modalities.

INTRODUCTION TO THE SOMATIC LEVEL OF MASSAGE THERAPY AND BODYWORK

Although the techniques of each modality in the somatic level of massage therapy and bodywork touch the various layers of a human being, their focus, intent, and effects reside mainly in the physical level and are primarily meant to induce positive changes in the body. Even though each modality within this level has found its own special niche, they are not far removed from one another. When reduced to their greatest common denominator, it can be seen that many of these modalities are a direct offspring of Per Henrik Ling's groundbreaking developments in massage therapy and bodywork that later came to be known as Swedish massage.

Since Ling's death in 1839, new generations of bodywork modalities have promoted the growing field of massage. Scientific developments have altered the way we look at the body, and the theories and practices of massage therapy and bodywork have come to reflect these changes. As bodywork explorers experimented with depth, pressure, timing, and sequence, they discovered that they could access different layers of the body. With deep, penetrating pressure they found that they could release chronic tensions that had been building for years. When they softened the strokes to such a degree that they moved just the skin, they found that they could start a chain reaction of fluids pumping throughout the entire body to diminish swelling while boosting the immune system. When they held a stroke 10 to 20 times longer than normal, they found that certain tissues would literally melt beneath their hands. When they quickened the pace of other strokes, they found that they could charge the muscles with nutrients and oxygen to prepare the body for an all-out athletic performance.

As each system evolved, it fed and nourished the other systems. Works like deep tissue, sports massage, orthopedic massage, neuromuscular therapy, and trigger point therapy build directly upon the foundations of their parent Swedish system. Neuromuscular, sports massage, and orthopedic massage can be seen as deep tissue work taken to the next level, while deep tissue can be viewed as the natural advancement of Swedish massage. Modalities like manual lymph drainage and Myofascial Release may seem unrelated at first glance, but when inspected more thoroughly, it is revealed that their theories and practices draw from the same foundational and understanding of the body. The guiding principle that bred these systems of massage therapy and bodywork were the same. While their techniques may appear vastly different, they are still reading from the same map and navigating with the same compass.

An interesting aspect of this level of massage is that a therapist versed in one somatic modality is often likely to be skilled in several of the other somatic modalities as well. Most therapists don't only practice Swedish massage, even if this was the main core of their training. They will usually apply deep tissue techniques while naturally borrowing at least some theories and principles from Neuromuscular and Orthopedic Massage. This is because each modality in the Somatic Layer of Massage Therapy and Bodywork is complementary to the others. Although each of these styles has gelled into its own specialized form, they all follow the same universal theories and principles of this level of bodywork and can be practiced side by side, even within the same treatment. Most treatments will in fact require a mixture of many of the techniques of these therapies to achieve maximum results. For advanced and experienced practitioners, the modalities represented in the somatic family of massage therapy and bodywork can function as one complete system when they are knowledgeably and skillfully brought side by side to work together.

SWEDISH MASSAGE

Swedish massage is *the* most common form of massage therapy and bodywork practiced in the United States today. It is considered a classic system and often serves as the foundation for many of today's styles. Although therapeutic in nature, its unique pampering qualities have made it highly prized in the spa industry, and it is sought out time and again by men and women who need a helping hand to wind down and help reduce stress (Figure 7-1).

This form of massage carries an innate gentleness that makes it optimal for times when a tender touch is necessary. Because of this, a wide range of clients from infants to the elderly can benefit enormously from this soft, caressive modality. Its simple, elegant qualities are especially appealing to newcomers of massage, and this style often serves as the gateway for them to try other forms of bodywork.

History

As stated earlier, Swedish massage was developed over the last two centuries in Europe and the United States. It was founded by Per Henrik Ling (1776–1839) of Sweden, whose interest in medicine, like many great healers, stemmed from the drive to cure his own ailments. Early in his life, Ling suffered from a debilitating form of rheumatoid arthritis for which he could find no cure. Undeterred by his early failures of a resolution to his painful condition, he traveled to France, Germany, and then the Far East to find a cure. There he

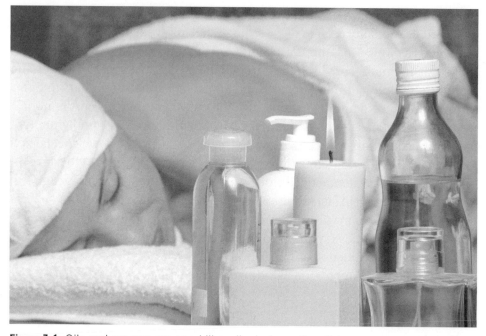

Figure 7-1 Oils and creams are used liberally during a Swedish massage session. Also, these sessions are most commonly done at spas all around the world. *Image copyright 2009, Leah-Anne Thompson. Used under license from shutterstock.com.*

learned the principles of Chinese medicine and studied Kung Fu with Taoist priests. He also acquired great proficiency in fencing and gymnastics.

Ling integrated his understanding of gymnastic exercises, ancient methods harnessed from the Orient, and emerging western medical knowledge to formulate a scientific system of treatment and exercise. Eventually he perfected his work, and in doing so was able to utilize his own methods to restore his health completely. His form of gymnastics included active exercises, which the patient performed unassisted, and passive movements (the treatment), in which the patient was moved and manipulated by the therapist.

Excited by his results, Ling eagerly sought to share his new system with the rest of world. At first, the traditional medical establishment denounced it as nothing but quackery, but over time Ling's persistence allowed his method's undeniable effectiveness to be revealed. Soon afterwards, Ling's system received widespread popularity and was even used by the Swedish cavalry. The Swedish government further promoted Ling's system via the Royal Swedish Central Institute in Stockholm, to which students traveled from all over Europe and from overseas to learn his new techniques of healing. By the time of his death in 1839 Ling's method had received worldwide recognition and his system eventually evolved into the Swedish massage as it is known today.

Theory and Principles

Of the sizable research conducted on the effectiveness of massage, one of the most important scientific explanations as to why it feels good to the body is that massage promotes the body's relaxation response by stimulating the release of endorphins. These neurochemicals are commonly known as the body's natural painkillers and are instrumental in fighting the negative effects of stress. Many experts believe that as much as 80 percent of today's illnesses are caused by stress because it inhibits the body's immune system, slows its rate of repair, and accelerates the aging process.

One of the chief features of Swedish massage is its ability to improve the circulation of blood and lymph. The circulation of both of these fluids is vital to every cell and tissue in the body. Blood brings oxygen, water, and nutrients to nourish the body's terrain and soothes tired, achy muscles and joints by bathing it in healing chemicals. Lymph plays a huge role in the body's immune system. The circulation of lymph is *the* major method of defense against dangerous, microbial intruders. When the immune system is engaged, the **lymphatic system** releases hordes of guardian cells that ward off invasions of germs and bacteria.[1]

The Technique

The basic techniques that compose this system of massage are akin to the palette of colors that an artist may use. Depending upon the style, composition, pace, and intensity of application, entirely different effects can be produced. And just as a painting reflects the artist's level of mastery over his or her medium, so too will the massage reflect the therapist's skills and abilities. There are five characteristic strokes that make up the Swedish system: effleurage, petrissage, friction, tapotement, and vibration.

Effleurage, or "touching lightly," has an inherent softness that lends itself well to being utilized as an introduction to touch. These are long, sweeping strokes conducted with the broad, flat, palmar surface of the hands which convey a sense of warmth, caring, and connectedness. With this embracing stroke the client gets a sense that the body is being heard and recognized. The therapist will utilize this time to lay down a foundation of oil, cream, or lotion while familiarizing himself or herself with the textures, contours, and condition of the client's body beneath the hands. Using effleurage, an expert therapist will be able to feel knots, tightness, areas of inflammation, and muscular imbalances. This stroke is especially soothing for people experiencing tension, nervousness, irritation, or restlessness.

In addition to being used as an introductory movement, effleurage is also applied as an intermediary stroke to smooth the transition as the treatment progresses from one part of the body to another. It is also an excellent finishing stroke to end a treatment session. Following deeper work, it is often used to flush out toxins and bring in a fresh supply of blood to warm and nourish the muscles. Like all the strokes in this system, it is applied in the direction of the heart to encourage the return of venous blood for cleansing and recirculation.[2]

A heavy effleurage has the effect of stretching and broadening the muscles while enhancing the body's circulation. This is an effective way to warm the muscles and lay the foundation for deeper work to take place. A lighter version of this technique is the "nerve," or "feather" stroke. Applied with the hands or fingertips, it is intended to either stimulate or sedate, depending on the number of passes. By lightly triggering nerve activity, a few passes will produce a mild and refreshing sensation while continued application will act to sedate. This stroke is popularly used as a finishing touch to smoothly close the session.

Petrissage, or "kneading," is the second layer of touch in the Swedish system. Following the initial phase of effleurage, the pace and pressure of the strokes become deeper and more enthusiastic. Here the muscles are squeezed, rolled, and kneaded to further relax and soften the tissue. As opposed to the global application of effleurage, petrissage targets specific muscles using the hands, thumbs, and fingers to lift, pull, and squeeze the musculature into pliancy. This action milks toxins and fluids out of the muscles to make room for a fresh supply of nutrients. Although this stroke can be applied anywhere, it is most effective on the thicker tissues of the body, including the shoulders, upper arms, legs, and calves, where the muscle tissue is dense and abundant.

Friction, or "rubbing," refers to the deepest work of Swedish massage. It is a slow, circular, or transverse stroke that is applied with the fingers, thumbs, or elbows to a concentrated area. This is the therapist's most powerful tool in softening adhesions (internal scar tissue) and providing mobility to areas that have been locked or limited, especially after injury. This can be a somewhat intensive procedure and the heat and pressure generated by friction may cause the overlying skin to redden. This is a positive indicator that the highly beneficial process of hyperemia, the increased circulation of blood, is taking place.

Tapotement, or "tapping," is a percussive stroke that can be utilized to either stimulate or relax, depending upon the length of application. When utilized for less than 10 seconds it excites and stimulates the nerves and is beneficial for when muscles have become weak and have lost their tone. When performed for longer periods (up to 60 seconds), the nerves become exhausted and the musculature relaxes. Because of its ability to subdue and "dampen" nerve reactivity, it is an effective technique for when areas are highly sensitive or ticklish.

The action of tapotement is performed with the fists, cupped hands, or fingers in "karate chop" fashion. The amount of force and pace can vary depending upon the outcome desired. A short burst will cause the nerves to become stimulated and will increase muscle tonicity, while a longer application will overtire nerves and produce a numbing effect.

Vibration, or "shaking," is done by placing the hands or fingers on an area and rapidly shaking them. This action either stimulates for cases of decreased muscle tonicity or desensitizes when a nerve is hyperactive.

Light pressure is used over sensitive or thin tissue. Heavier movements are reserved for thicker and deeper areas. Slow, gentle movements are applied to soothe and relax while quicker, more vigorous movements are designed to stimulate.

The Session

Since practitioners of Swedish massage liberally utilize oils, lotions, and creams, the recipient is unclothed but modestly draped at all times with either a sheet and/or a towel. The only area that is exposed is the area being addressed. The recipient is lying on a table face down for the first half, then face up for the second half, or vice versa. The session can be as short as 30 minutes, but in order to experience the full benefits of this treatment it is recommended that the session last from 1 to 1½ hours.

The session will begin with light, sweeping strokes (effleurage) meant to familiarize the therapist's hands to the client's body. Since the therapist's hands are often their most accurate organs of "sight," they will utilize this phase to conduct an assessment of the body to find out if specific areas will require more focused attention.

As the hands pass over the body they mold to the contours of the skin, soaking up valuable clues as to the underlying condition of the patient. By noting the patient's muscle tone, body temperature, skeletal alignment, and overall condition, the therapist forms a mental game plan that outlines the parameters for the treatment's pace and pressure. This is a continuous process that accompanies the length of the entire treatment. Each aspect of the body may be different, and it is imperative that the therapist always be focused and listening to messages that the body may be sending.

As the session progresses, the tempo will gradually crescendo and the therapist's work will become more specific, depending upon the client's needs. Each stroke should blend into the next, creating a soothing composition that flows effortlessly from one part of the body to the next. An expert therapist will never depart his or her hands from the body abruptly or noticeably. Even the resting moments are smoothly transitioned into the next, whether it is to pause for draping purposes or for another application of oil, lotion, or cream.

As the session builds the pace quickens and the pressure becomes more concentrated. The broad, expansive strokes of effleurage give way to the kneading, rhythmic strokes of petrissage. As muscles are pulled, pushed, lifted, and squeezed into pliancy, a fresh supply of blood rushes in to replace the tired, depleted fluids. Once the tissue is sufficiently warmed, the penetrating strokes of friction are applied to access the deepest layers of the muscles. This slow, methodical pressure is applied only to the patient's level of tolerance. Beyond this threshold the hands of the therapist are felt by the body as an intrusion, triggering a defensive response where the muscles clench and the body locks, making it almost impossible for any effective treatment to continue. At this level, real damage can occur to not only the body but also to the trust between patient and therapist. Following the fine detailed work of friction, another layer of effleurage is applied to sweep through the area and smooth out the work. This allows toxins that may have been released to be flushed out and brings in a fresh supply of blood and fluids.

Methodically, the treatment progresses from one section of the body to the next as each issue is addressed in turn. The time allotted to each section depends upon the severity of the problem. While other forms of therapy may spend most or even all of the treatment time on just a few areas, Swedish massage treatment seeks to encompass the entire body. This global approach allows other forms of massage to use the Swedish system for laying a treatment foundation into which other techniques and modalities are integrated.

The Swedish system is perhaps the most well known for its smooth transitions and its soft, wavelike maneuvers where the end of one stroke becomes the beginning of the next. Although the pace may vary, the movement never stops and the edges of each stroke blend together so that the hard line distinguishing one technique from another disappears. Although the hands and elbows are the only parts that are in contact with the patient, the practitioner commits his entire body to each movement. The whole body moves in sync with the hands—crouching, bending, twisting, and turning as the need arises. Because of the rhythm and style, therapists often describe the experience of giving this treatment as a dance.

The treatment will end as gently as it started and contact is disengaged in a manner that is more akin to melting away than breaking off. The end of the treatment usually occurs at the natural and obvious locations such as the head or feet. The finishing touch is often a short sequence of light sweeping gestures that connect and seal the entire treatment. This can be accompanied by lightly cradling the head, gently holding the feet, or simply placing the hands on the patient's chest in a symbolic gesture representing the peace and quiescence of stillness. This is a moment taken to provide closure not only for the patient, but for the therapist as well.

Benefits

- Enhanced feeling of well-being
- Reduction of stress
- Decreased muscle tension and soreness
- Improved elimination of toxins
- Lower blood pressure
- Improve blood and lymph circulation
- Decrease anxiety and depression
- Increased flexibility and range of motion

Contraindications and Precautions

- Fever, vomiting, nausea, diarrhea, jaundice, arthritis in one joint, or pain due to unknown cause: These are signs of infection and Swedish massage should be avoided due to risk of spreading the infection.
- Cancer and some skin disorders: The patient should have these conditions checked by a doctor before receiving Swedish massage.
- Phlebitis, thrombosis, varicose veins: Swedish massage directly over the affected areas may transport blood clots, which can result in a stroke or heart failure. Swedish massage above or below the affected areas, however, is beneficial.
- High blood pressure/heart problems: Abdominal massage should not be done as it can increase stress to the heart.

- Fractures, bruises, bleeding, keloid scars: These areas should be avoided.
- Pregnancy: Women should not receive Swedish massage in the first trimester. As a general rule, pregnant clients should not lie on their stomachs nor should they lie on their right side (especially during the later months of the pregnancy) because the extra weight may put too much pressure on the liver.

If there are any unknown or uncertain symptoms it is always advisable to check with a physician before providing or receiving any type of massage.

Training of a Therapist

The education and training requirements for becoming a massage therapist vary widely from state to state. Some states have no regulations; others require credentials issued by separate cities, towns, townships, villages, and other locales within their states, such as in California, to practice legally. Some states require only a few hundred hours of training, while others require a minimum of 1000 hours of schooling in addition to passing a state or national examination for state licensure. To become a professional member of the American Massage Therapy Association (AMTA), the largest professional massage therapy organization in the country, practitioners must either meet one or more of the following qualifications: graduate from a 500-hour in-class program; hold a current license from a state that regulates the profession; or hold current certification offered by the National Certification Board for Therapeutic Massage & Bodywork.[3]

Most schools and programs that meet the minimum 500 hours of schooling have basic curricula that include anatomy and physiology, kinesiology, pathology, hands-on training, clinical internships and externships, and courses in professional development, business, and ethics. Programs with more hours are naturally able to offer more extensive hands-on training in the basics, as well as advanced training in other specialty modalities like deep tissue, neuromuscular therapy, trigger point therapy, shiatsu, sports massage, and even spa therapy techniques.

DEEP TISSUE MASSAGE, NEUROMUSCULAR THERAPY, AND ORTHOPEDIC MASSAGE

Although deep tissue massage is one of the most highly sought-after forms of massage today, it is actually not a specific modality, but rather an integration of other modalities. The term "deep tissue" is more of a colloquial term used to describe a type of massage with the specific intent of targeting deep-seated aches and pains. It achieves this by utilizing the classic Swedish system as its platform, while employing theories and techniques from other modalities, including neuromuscular therapy and orthopedic massage.

A deep tissue session would not be complete or even half as effective if it did not liberally employ the work of these other modalities. Stripped of these accompaniments, there would be a very thin frame left. In fact, the relationship of these modalities is so symbiotic that it can be said that they are the same treatments with a slightly different face and focus. Another way to look at this relationship is that deep tissue is a fledgling form of orthopedic and neuromuscular therapy. Just as deep tissue builds upon the foundation of Swedish massage, neuromuscular and orthopedic build upon the foundation of deep tissue. In other sources, these approaches may be defined and described as separate modalities, but because they are often integrated, here, in this section, they will be discussed together.

Deep Tissue Massage

The main focus of a **deep tissue-style massage** is to restore chronically shortened muscles to their original supple form. Normal muscles are soft and elastic and have a uniform consistency. They are not tender to the touch and the underlying structures including bones, joints, and viscera can easily be palpated. When healthy muscles contract, they return to normal shape, length, and pliancy after the contraction.

Dysfunctional muscles, on the other hand, contract, but do not return to their proper form. They often become locked in a shortened position, blocking blood flow, limiting range of motion and causing pain. Over time the tissues harden and become permanently contracted. As the muscle tissue loses its suppleness and elasticity, its ability to perform diminishes. These contracted muscles create patterns that can commonly be seen in people with elevated shoulders, rounded backs, and craning necks. When these conditions become chronic, other things begin to deteriorate. The flow of blood and fluids become constricted—further hardening the area. The strength of the muscle diminishes as does its mobility, and nerve conduction becomes impeded as well (Figure 7-2).

Muscular Imbalance

Muscles in the body are naturally paired like two ends of a seesaw. If one end goes up, the other must go down and vice versa. In similar fashion, muscles are paired so that some pull the body forward while others pull the body backwards. Some muscles lift the arm, others help to bring it back down. Some allow you to turn to the right and others allow you to turn to the left.

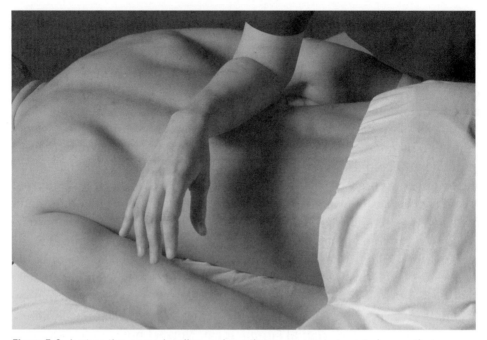

Figure 7-2 Just as the name implies, a deep tissue massage targets issues that are often deep-seated in the soft tissues of the body. Because of this, knuckles and elbows are often used for their penetrating effects.

The muscles perform these functions by contracting and releasing. Nerves engage the muscles, muscles pull the bones, and the whole structure moves accordingly. After their job is done, the muscles should release so the body can return to its normal and healthy state of balance. However, when the muscles contract but do not release, they disrupt the symmetrical forces that keep the body balanced. After a while, the short, contracted muscles take a toll on the body's structural equilibrium.

In this state, the structure of the body is compromised because the contracted muscles are pulling bones out of their natural, resting alignment. This creates a state of constant tension that leads to wear and tear. Imagine if you were trying to stand still and someone was constantly trying to push you over. Think about how tired you would become from constantly having to fight with this kind of persistent force. This same pattern can be seen in automobiles with wheels that are not aligned. Not only do the tires wear out much faster, it adds a great deal of stress to the whole vehicle due to the excess friction that has to be absorbed.

But it doesn't end there. The uneven, haphazard pulls on the body create stress points that the body must reinforce by building extra tissue around them. This provides support for the destabilized structure, but at the expense of making the body more rigid. Muscles in this chronic state of "stuckness" are far more prone to injury because they lack the ability to adapt to strain or stress.

Accidents and Illnesses

A similar condition arises when the body has been subject to trauma. In the case of automobile accidents, the muscles lock to brace themselves from the shock of impact. Ideally, following the impact the muscles should let go, but often this is not the case. A muscle can sometimes become semi-permanently locked and result in conditions such as "frozen shoulder," where the arm is unable to move freely.

One of the primary ways the body defends itself from infectious diseases is by producing an inflammatory response. When someone is running a fever, his or her body is basically at war, and like in any war, there are often civilian casualties. The body drives up its temperature to make it uninhabitable to foreign invaders, but if the heat is too long-standing it can damage the body's own tissues. In cases like this, even after the battle the damage done may long persist.

Toxic Buildup

In order for muscles to function properly, they rely on a steady influx of oxygen and nutrients. Like all things in nature, whatever consumes must in turn eliminate. What results is a byproduct of metabolic waste that is released from the muscles into the bloodstream. Normally this waste is carted away, but if this cycle is disrupted, the waste accumulates and the area becomes toxic. This internal toxicity not only irritates muscle and nerve fibers, it also causes the muscles to harden. This weakens the muscle and often causes pain. This buildup of toxins also taxes the immune system and makes the body more prone to disease. Common causes of this type of condition are over-exercise, poor diet, and living an unhealthy lifestyle.

Unfortunately, people with these kinds of conditions often do not seek out treatment until the problem has long been ingrained. Often these conditions have been quietly building in the body, sometimes for years, without any notice. It's not uncommon for someone to seek treatment for a recent pain that was actually initiated by some long-forgotten injury or illness. Because the condition has had such a long time to incubate, it often requires intensive and ongoing treatment to alleviate.

Neuromuscular Therapy (NMT)

Neuromuscular therapy (NMT) is a specialized form of soft tissue manipulation that utilizes static pressure on specific points, often trigger points, to help relieve pain. NMT techniques are also used to treat the soft tissue of the body, which includes the muscles, tendons, and connective tissue, to help create an overall balance between the central nervous system, (comprised of the brain, spinal column, and nerves) and the musculoskeletal system.

When the human being is balanced in this way, nerve impulses are freely and slowly transmitted throughout the body. This allows for pain-free movement of the body. Traumatic injuries and accidents, chronic stress, and postural habits and distortions create interference that often severely impairs nerve transmission by unnaturally speeding it up. This can result in various debilitating, painful patterns and syndromes, which if not treated, can lead to dysfunction and disability.

> NMT seeks to effect balance and harmony in the body by treating the following five major causes of pain:
>
> 1. Trigger points
> 2. Nerve compression or entrapment
> 3. Postural distortion
> 4. **Ischemia**
> 5. Biomechanical dysfunction

Trigger Points

One of the highlights of NMT is the intensive work that has been done with a condition that often arises in the muscles called "trigger points" (commonly known as knots). Simply put, **trigger points** are the most dysfunctional area of a muscle and they can affect a person by radiating pain, limiting mobility, and hindering normal, everyday activities like walking, writing, eating, and even sitting down. Trigger points often occur due to some form of trauma, which catalyzes a rapid transmission of nerve impulses into other areas of the body often far from the actual site of the pain. This process causes stagnation and imbalance in the surrounding and affected areas often greatly reducing proper blood flow. Prolonged, reduced blood flow can eventually cause ischemia, a lack of blood supply to the tissues, which in turn causes increased pain and discomfort.

Finding a trigger point is often fairly easy since they are the hardest and most tender part of the muscle. These little lumps can feel like marbles that have been imbedded underneath the skin. Take a quick trip to your upper trapezius muscles (shoulders) with your hands and you'll more than likely feel a few of these hard nodes in the muscle's belly. This is a common area for trigger points to develop as is between the shoulder blades, down in the lower back, and deep in the hips. Although they are highly treatable, once they form, they are not very likely to go away on their own.

By far the most famous name attached to trigger point work is Dr. Janet Travell. She has done more extensive research on trigger points and their treatment than probably anyone else and she developed a two volume series *Myofascial Pain and Dysfunction*, and the *Trigger Point Manual*, which have basically become the "bible" of this branch of study. In addition to being a highly regarded pioneer in the field of bodywork, Dr. Travell was the first woman to be appointed White House physician and served under Presidents Kennedy and Johnson. According to Senator Goldwater, Kennedy's greatest gift to the American people has been bringing Travell's work to the public's attention.[4]

There are two types of trigger points—latent and active. Both are similar in construction and design and wreak similar damage, but **latent trigger points** must be pressed to radiate pain whereas **active trigger points** can do this all by themselves. A latent trigger point can be seen as a lesser form of the active version, but can become active if left untreated. Some trigger points not only produce pain but also induce visual disturbances, nausea, changes in skin temperature, and tearing of the eyes.[5]

As medical doctors, chiropractors, and other health care professionals studied trigger points, they noticed the emergence of a distinct pattern. They discovered that certain trigger points always radiate pain to specific areas of the body. This came to be known as a referral pattern because they *refer* pain to another location. Trigger points in the large muscles of the upper trapezius will often refer pain up around the side of the head and around the ears. Pain directly above the eyes may mean trigger points in the neck, and a trigger point deep in the muscles of the hips will send pain down the back of the leg, mimicking sciatica pain. This pattern of referral has been thoroughly mapped and is commonly available in NMT or trigger point textbooks. Incidentally, nearly 75 percent of trigger points are identical to the location of acupuncture points[6] (Figure 7-3).

Techniques of Neuromuscular Therapy

Although there are many techniques for alleviating trigger points, the most common method utilized by massage therapists is the application of a steady

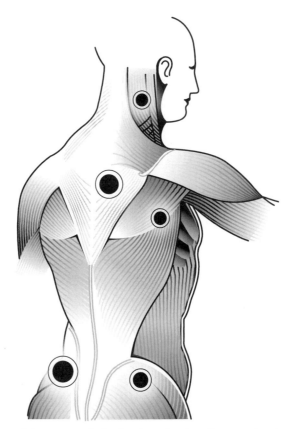

Figure 7-3 Trigger point maps and charts show the locations and pain patterns of the most common trigger points in the body. These make great tools for new therapists beginning in this field of study.

pressure straight into the core of the trigger point. Done with just the right touch, this can illicit that "good pain" for which people often seek massage. Done with too heavy a hand, however, this can result in a lot of pain and discomfort. Areas that have developed trigger points often have poor circulation and this means that there is likely a buildup of metabolic waste, which can cause the area to become hypersensitive. As well as being painful, techniques that are too hard and too fast can also be damaging because the muscle may respond by tensing further in order to protect itself. In those cases, instead of working with the body, the therapist is fighting with it—dramatically increasing the chances that the tissue will be injured.

Normally, pressure is held for 10 to 20 seconds or until the muscle gives. This rule, however, is not hard and fast and pressure can be applied longer or in 10- to 20-second intervals if necessary. Trigger points that have been lodged in the body for years will often take considerably more time to release than one that has been more recently formed. The proficient therapist will be able to discriminate just how much time and pressure are necessary for each specific case. Even in the same client, this timing can greatly vary. This method can be coupled with a deep, slow friction and then a stretch afterwards to keep the disbanded trigger point from reemerging.

When the trigger point releases, there will be a dramatic difference in the quality of the muscle. The area will be palpably softer, pain will diminish, and movement will be much easier. Once the muscle has been returned to its natural, supple state, it is important to analyze and correct other factors that may have initially contributed to the dysfunction. Postural distortions, improper use of the body, and poorly designed work-stations are some of the most common culprits for creating dysfunctions in the body. For President Kennedy, Travell had to redesign all his seats, including those in his boat, his helicopter, and his plane, Air Force One. In addition because JFK had one leg that was slightly shorter than the other, she also had to order him a heel lift to make up the difference.[7]

Orthopedic Massage

Orthopedic massage is a relatively new branch of bodywork that attempts to firmly anchor massage therapy to the medical sciences. Historically, the treatment of soft-tissue (muscles, tendons, fibrous tissues, fat, blood vessels, nerves, and synovial tissues) injuries fell within the scope of a branch of medicine called orthopedics. Although most soft-tissue injuries are minor, prescription drugs or surgery are often the first protocol. Unfortunately, many of these conditions do not always respond well to either of these methods and since many people are wary of this type of intervention, they've had little option other than to simply wait until the pain resolved on its on.

Because of this there has been a growing gap between doing nothing and taking medication or getting surgery. However, in recent years, other professions have surfaced to meet the needs of this growing void. Among the most prevalent of these professions are chiropractic, physical therapy, and massage therapy. Lately, there has been a dramatic increase in the use of massage therapy to treat soft-tissue pain and injury. Whereas before it was viewed as being beneficial for general treatment, today massage therapy has evolved to a level where it has become an effective method of choice for treating numerous specific soft-tissue conditions.

An orthopedic massage therapist can be seen as an injury specialist in the field of massage and bodywork therapy. This modality is perhaps the most scientific in the somatic family and evidence of its exacting process can be seen in the four stages of an orthopedic treatment.

The four stages of an Orthopedic treatment

- Assessment
- Matching the treatment to the injury
- Treatment Adaptability
- Rehabilitation[8]

Assessment

Because of the highly specific nature of orthopedic work, it is imperative that the therapist determine the correct nature of a condition. The important process of assessment begins the moment patients and therapists meet. How patients walk, how they sit, how they hold their purse, how they breathe, or how they cross their legs can reveal a world of information about their condition. Dr. Travell always took notice of the patient's shape, size, gait (walking pattern), and posture and became so proficient at recognizing patterns that she could often diagnose problems in seconds.[9] There are several methods of evaluation that can be used to create an effective plan of treatment.

MUSCLE TESTING   By testing the strength of a muscle's contraction, the therapist can determine specific areas of dysfunction. For example, pain, stiffness, or loss of mobility of the arm or shoulder may warrant testing of the deltoid muscles. If you place your hand at the top of the arm where the arm meets the shoulder, you will be directly over the deltoids. First, patients are simply asked to raise their arm straight out to the side. Once their arm makes a right angle to the rest of their body, the deltoid is fully engaged. At this point the patient is asked to hold their arm there and resist while the therapist tries to push the arm down in the opposite direction. A healthy deltoid muscle will "lock" and will be able to provide a firm resistance. A muscle whose integrity has been compromised, however, will provide a resistance that is weak and feels mushy in comparison. It may "lock" momentarily before giving way or it may simply give immediately (Figure 7-4).

RANGE OF MOTION TESTING   Another method of isolating problem areas is by checking a joint's range of motion. For example, to test the range of motion of the neck, back, and upper shoulders, the patient can be asked to perform a "neck roll," a full circle with the head, beginning with the chin tucked to the chest and eyes looking down. From there he or she can roll the head around to the side, trying to get the ear as close to the shoulder as possible. The movement continues, circling around until the nose is pointing straight up to the

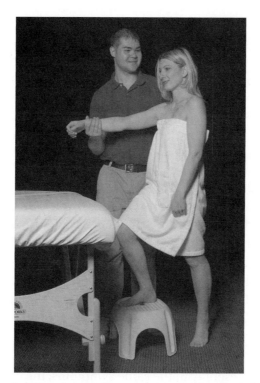

Figure 7-4 Prior to the treatment, muscles can be tested to check their degree of damage. This helps the therapist decide how to approach the treatment.

sky. The head is then allowed to circle to the left shoulder and then down to the nose, where the movement began. This simple test can reveal restrictions and imbalances in the patient's musculature while giving insight into what techniques may need to be used in the massage therapist's efforts to help release and relieve those painful restrictions. Similar tests can be conducted on the various articulations and joints of the body.

POSTURAL ANALYSIS   By examining a person's posture (postural analysis), a skilled therapist will be able to determine areas of muscular imbalances and dysfunctions. A hip that's higher on one side will often cause the body to compensate by lifting the opposite shoulder. This is because the body is constantly trying to right itself and sometimes the only way it can do that is by shifting another part of the body. A similar pattern of compensation can occur when the pelvis is rotated too far forward. This not only increases the arch in the lower back, but in the neck as well. This puts a tremendous strain on the entire back because these muscles have to constantly fight in order to keep the body upright. Some therapists may use a grid in order to more clearly observe the imbalances.

GAIT ANALYSIS   A skilled therapist will be able to determine imbalances and dysfunctions in a client's body by simply observing the way he or she moves (gait analysis). This method of testing provides a more complete picture of the body's "story" because it not only reveals patterns of strain, it also reveals how that strain affects the way the client uses his body. It can also reveal if a client is moving in a way that's actually causing injury. By correcting a patient's unhealthy patterns of movement, the therapist can provide much longer-term relief than just treating the muscles involved.

MATCHING TREATMENT TO INJURY   Since there is no single massage modality that will treat every pain or injury, the therapist must selectively decide which ones will be most beneficial, which ones will be ineffective, and which ones may actually be harmful. For example, deep friction across the muscles of the wrist in the case of carpal tunnel syndrome would aggravate the condition. The same stroke applied along the length of the muscle's fibers, however, would be beneficial. It is important that the massage therapist be highly aware of these fine details.

Treatment Adaptability

Even if two people present with the same symptoms, the causes of each condition may be very different. Because of this it is important that the therapist be flexible and not adhere strictly to any one style or principle. It is also important to get away from recipes or routines that can prevent the patient from receiving the individualized care and attention that they need. What works for one client may be ineffective for another so the therapist may have to experiment with a variety of approaches to find the one suitable for the specific case, provided that the practitioner has been well-trained in other methods and techniques.

Rehabilitation

One of the leading causes of failure to achieve positive results in treatment is caused by attempting to rush the repair of a soft-tissue injury. While most systems have a clear method of treating a condition, emphasis on the rehabilitation process is often lacking. After an injury, it is important that the damaged tissue has had time to repair before it is manipulated. Stretching an injured muscle too early can cause a lot of pain and may damage the area further. For example, in carpel tunnel syndrome, stretching the muscles of the wrist before the tissues have had a chance to normalize may turn out to be a very painful mistake because the stretch would actually pull on the very nerve that is being compressed by the surrounding tissue.

In addition to normalizing the damaged tissue, the orthopedic massage therapist will focus on other aspects of rehabilitation, including strengthening and conditioning. These stages are important for complete recovery because injuries often leave behind a wake of other dysfunctions. This stage of the treatment protocol helps the injured muscle become reintegrated into the body's natural mechanics.[10]

The Session

The session for a deep tissue, neuromuscular, or orthopedic massage can vary greatly, depending on the therapist and the setting. In a chiropractic office, the treatment may hone in on key areas and can be as short as 15 minutes. At a spa, healing arts center or clinic, the treatment may be an hour or longer and may include the whole body.

This kind of work is done in layers, slowly melting away the top protective layer so that the deeper issues can be addressed below. The initial warm-up phase will utilize the techniques of a Swedish massage to ready the body for deeper work. Once a contracted muscle is discovered, slow, compressive strokes can be applied along the length of the muscles. This stimulates nerve receptors to recalibrate the muscle's length, encouraging it to relax and elongate. If a trigger point is discovered within the muscle, direct pressure is applied to alleviate it. After the muscle has released, a slow, steady stretch is applied that stimulates other nerve receptors that help balance the muscle's tone. If the stretch is applied too quickly, a mechanism known as the stretch reflex will kick in to tighten the muscle to keep it from being damaged by overstretching. When pressure is applied slowly, however, the stretch reflex is bypassed and the muscle relaxes.

Because of the intense pressure that may be employed in any of these treatment modalities, some soreness may be felt a day or two following the treatment. Afterwards, however, the area should feel much better. After any type of massage, especially if deeper work has taken place, it is always advisable to drink lots of fluids to help wash away the toxins that were released during the session. In many cases, this type of massage has been proven to be more effective than physical therapy or painkillers.

It must also be remembered that although muscular conditions form in specific locations, the condition of one muscle is usually a reflection of the whole body. While stretching throughout the day is one of the most significant ways to keep muscular dysfunctions at bay, it is also vitally important to integrate a healthy program of diet, stretching, and exercise to keep the entire system strong and vibrant.

Benefits

- Restore function and mobility after injury or surgery
- Alleviate muscle tension
- Improve range of motion
- Alleviate postural distortions
- Enhance performance

Conditions Helped by Deep Tissue, Neuromuscular Therapy, and Orthopedic Massage

- Low-back pain
- Neck and shoulder pain
- Frozen shoulder
- Tennis elbow
- Whiplash
- TMJ disorder
- Carpal tunnel syndrome
- Headaches
- Scoliosis

Contraindications and Precautions

Under the following conditions, deep massage should not be administered:

- Severe trauma
- Fever
- Skin disorders
- Recent injury/surgery
- Severe hypertension
- Broken bones
- Hernias
- Severe bruises
- Burns
- Varicose veins

Training of a Practitioner

Training of a deep tissue practitioner can vary greatly. Practitioners may claim to be deep tissue therapists right out of school because they simply "work deeply," or after years of experience, continuing education, and specialized training where they've come to understand and incorporate the skills and principles of many other modalities. Because of the looseness with which this term is often used, neither would be wrong. However, when seeking a deep tissue practitioner it is advisable that the therapist has had a minimum of 500 hours of schooling behind them with preferably some specific training in the techniques of deep tissue work.

For neuromuscular therapy, many schools, have the training built right into their core curriculum, while other schools may offer it as continuing education courses and certification programs. The NMT (Neuromuscular Therapy) Center in Florida, for example, offers training and certification in various states across the United States. In addition to the basic training that a massage therapist receives in school, the NMT Center requires 80 additional hours of specialized study in their Neuromuscular Therapy Program. The material is separated into four sections: 1) Torso/Pelvis, 2) Cervical/Cranium, 3) Upper Extremity (the arms), and 4) Lower Extremities (the legs), and each section covers anatomy, physiology, common conditions, and treatment protocol. Examination for certification is only allowed after all sections have been completed. [11]

The **Orthopedic Massage Education and Research Institute (OMERI)** founded by Whitney Lowe, who is a forerunner in this field of study, offers a three-day training program for orthopedic massage. Their coursework is divided into three sections: 1) the pelvis, neck, and back; 2) the lower extremities; and 3) the upper extremities.[12] The Center for Pain Management offers three different levels of orthopedic study: an introduction to orthopedic massage, a 3-day workshop, and a 5-day intensive.[13] Both schools offer workshops in select cities across the States and offer students the opportunity for certification upon completion of their courses. These are just a few of the many options from which to choose when either looking for a pathway for learning somatic forms of massage therapy and bodywork or seeking qualified therapists in these specialty areas.

MYOFASCIAL RELEASE

The historic thread of **Myofascial Release** dates back to the late nineteenth century where it shares common roots with osteopathic medicine. There, through a common founder, Andrew Taylor Stills, the idea of myofascial work was born. But while Stills raised and developed osteopathic medicine into a full fledged system, his successors were the ones to bring Myofascial Release to maturity.

Similar to the way in which one lineage within the martial arts grew into different branches, there evolved two distinct styles of myofascial work—one hard, one soft. The hard, direct style was adopted by Rolf and her contemporaries in the 1950s and went on to become what is known as Structural Integration. This form of hands-on work is discussed fully in Chapter 8: Somato-Psychic. The soft style was nurtured by the German physiotherapist Elizabeth Dicke, who shaped and molded the young form into what she called **Bindegewebs Massage**. With only a subtle touch it offered powerful results. This work involves lightly "hooking" the skin with the fingers and dragging it to create a mild stretch on the underlying fascia. Later this also came to be known as connective tissue massage (Figure 7-5).

Many people later adopted these techniques into their own systems and helped to continue shaping the relatively young modality. One of these people who fed and nurtured the adolescent system was John F. Barnes, who went on to become a giant in the field of bodywork. Barnes, a physical therapist, developed his own style of Myofascial Release that married both the hard and soft branches into one system. His work was hugely successful, and *Massage Magazine* ended up naming him as one of this century's most influential professionals in the therapeutic world. Barnes's system has impacted the training of tens of thousands of massage and bodywork therapists through books, seminars, and

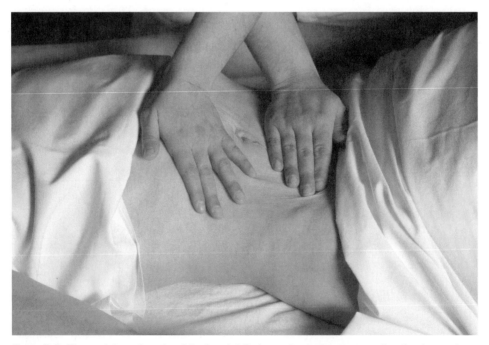

Figure 7-5 Therapist performing Myofascial Release technique on a client's stomach. Myofascial techniques stretch the tissue as opposed to pressing deeply.

workshops, and his influence has helped make Myofascial Release one of the most recognized forms of specialized massage modalities today.[14]

Theory and Principles

Despite the complexity of the human body, every structure is composed of only four types of tissues: muscle, nervous, epithelial, and connective. Out of these, **connective tissue** is the most abundant and is composed of three basic ingredients: 1) collagen, 2) elastin, and 3) ground substance. **Collagen** fibers are the longest molecules known and are stronger than steel.[15] They can hold 10,000 times their own weight and are responsible for the strength and resiliency of a tissue's structure. **Elastin** fibers are like long bands that allow the tissue to stretch and absorb shock. **Ground substance** is a clear, thick, fluid similar to raw egg whites. It surrounds every cell in the body and lubricates tissues, allowing them to slide over one another. These three substances combine in different quantities to form blood, bone, ligament, tendon, and fascia.

Fascia is a loosely woven fabric of collagen and elastin that forms into strong, translucent sheets. These sheets form networks throughout the entire body to limit, contain, and support our inner environment—essentially blending the entire organism into one unit. Its reach is so pervasive that it covers nearly every structure in the body. Every organ is held and protected by sheets of fascia. Every muscle and nerve is wrapped in fascia and bundled into larger groups by fascia. Fascia encases fat tissue and interweaves it through every muscle (Figure 7-6).

The fascia surrounding the muscle is also the same substance that transforms into tendons. It is a continuum in which fascia turns into tendon, tendon turns into bone, bone turns back into tendon, and tendon turns back into muscle's protective covering. In this way, they are all interconnected. From the top of head to the tip of the toe, fascia intertwines, penetrates, suspends, and connects nerves, arteries, veins, fats, muscles, and organs. Because of this it has been dubbed the "great organizer."[16]

One of the most interesting discoveries in Myofascial Release has been the discovery of the body as a tensegrity structure. The word *tensegrity* is derivative of the words *tensional integrity*. This type of structure maintains its shape by a balanced network of continuous tension. Arranged according to the idea of tensegrity, well known contemporary artist Kenneth Snelson's tensegrity sculptures are held up not by the metal rods but by the cables providing a constant stream of opposing yet balanced tension, a winning combination of push and pull.[17]

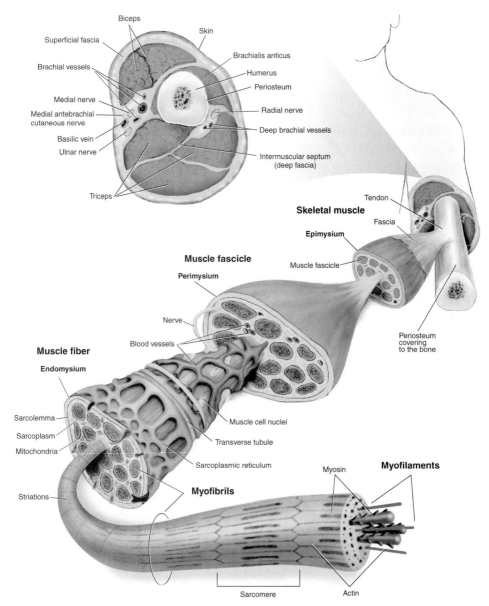

Figure 7-6 Planes of fascia for compartments—cross-section of the arm. This white, protective sheath wraps around every muscle, organ, and bone in the body.

In the human body, the fascia acts as cables providing the tension necessary to hold the entire structure together. In this type of structure, the position of each bone is determined by the length of the fascia that connects them together. By controlling the position of the bones, fascia determines our body's posture. As is the nature of a tensegrity structure, when one area is affected, the entire system becomes affected as well. This means, for example, that if there is a tightness or constriction in the lower back, it can easily lead to strain in the neck and shoulders.

As we age, become injured, and/or develop more and more scar tissue, collagen fibers grow closer and closer together and eventually stick to one another. This inhibits motion and distorts posture. Then, each time the muscle contracts it pulls and drags everything caught in its sticky web. It strains and stresses neighboring muscles and organs, wearing them out before their time. The science of Myofascial Release is designed to release these adhesions so that muscles and organs can function freely and naturally.

The Skin

The skin is our richest organ of sensation. In the fetus, the skin develops from the same tissue as the brain. As development unfolds, the skin moves to the outside, but it still maintains intimate contact with the brain via thousands of nerve innervations that relay information back and forth 24 hours a day, 7 days a week. It is also the organ that we live through more than any other because it is what gives us the ability to receive sensations from the outside world.

The skin forms around the body and provides protection for our muscles and organs. It is often thought of as separate from the body's underlying constituents, but it is more truthfully the outermost layer of the muscles, bones, and organs. Because of this connection, if the skin is affected, the underlying components will be as well and vice versa. Therefore, by freeing the skin of restrictions, underlying structures are released as well, including the superficial layer of the fascia.

Because the superficial fascia, just like the skin, is one continuous sheet of tissue, a restriction in one area will resonate throughout the entire organism. These restrictions often occur from injury, stress, or underlying muscular contractions. A pull of the skin even 1/8th of an inch can restrict motion considerably. Imagine how restricted the motion of your hand would feel if the skin over your wrist were held tight. Try this on yourself: Hold the skin down on the front of the wrist and try to bend the hand the other way. Immediately you can feel how tight the movement feels even though the underlying muscles are fine. Now imagine this type of restriction on the diaphragm, which only moves half an inch. Without this half an inch of free movement for even just a few minutes, your whole body would cease to function.

The Technique

Collagen fibers are designed to resist force and can withstand 2000 pounds per square inch of pressure. Because of this, quick or passing massage strokes only affect the most superficial layers and have no lasting effect. A common mistake that many massage therapists make is that they move much too quickly and don't give enough time for the fascia to release. A Swedish massage might affect the fascia, but most likely won't make any permanent changes in the fascia's condition. To make a real and lasting difference, a consistent pressure must be applied and held for *at least* 90 seconds. If this threshold is not met, the whole process will have to be started over. In general, it takes between 2 and 5 minutes of sustained pressure to really create lasting changes.

As resistant as fascia is, it takes surprisingly little pressure to initiate the movement. Just a few ounces are enough to ease the fibers apart. In fact, too much pressure may actually trigger a protective resistance mechanism from the body. This may be a difficult concept to grasp for therapists who are used to thinking that only deep, intense pressures can create change. Most massage therapy schools focus primarily on the body's musculature. While this approach and understanding is foundational and necessary, it must be understood that muscle is only one type of tissue in the body. And, like people, different types of tissues have different needs and personalities. Some must to be attended to very slowly and gently. Others can be engaged more readily or with greater intensity.

The Assessment

The condition of one's fascia can be measured with great accurateness both visually and manually. The visual method involves scanning the body's standing posture to determine which lines of fascia's pull have been compromised. These lines of pull have been well documented and are commonly referred to as myofascial meridians, or anatomy trains.

These lines, like tracks, encircle the body running up, down, left, right, over, and under—looping around and connecting the entire body into one unit. And it is these lines of pull that maintain the body as a tensegrity structure. An injury or restriction on one part of the line will often generate tension up and down the rest of that line that can be readily observed in the way a person stands or moves. A head that slumps forward indicates that the front line is pulling too much while the posterior line is being overextended. One shoulder that's higher than the other can indicate that either the line running down the side of the body is contracted or that the integrity of one of the diagonal lines running across the body has been jeopardized. Rebalancing these lines of pull can improve a number of issues, including dysfunctional walking patterns, rounded shoulders, other postural distortions, and even fallen arches.

Manual assessment of the fascia involves testing the elastic quality of the skin. The hand is placed gently on the body's surface and the skin is pushed up, down, left, and right to compare mobility in each direction. In healthy tissues, there will be movement in each direction with an end-feel that is springy. Exploration of fascia throughout the body will reveal that its thickness, mobility, and elasticity is different in different areas. The fascia of the wrist may feel tight compared to that of the forearm. The fascia of the stomach may feel tight compared to the lower back. The skin on the back may move more than an inch while the skin over the ankles may not move even half of that distance.

The Treatment

Each Myofascial Release treatment can vary greatly depending on a client's specific condition. Unlike Swedish massage in which a global approach to treating the body is employed, myofascial work is much more specific to the exact conditions and locations that are affecting the client. Because of this, the length of each session can range from 15 minutes to over an hour. It can incorporate the whole body, or just smaller, affected local areas or regions. Myofascial Release can be used as a stand-alone treatment or it can easily be integrated into other therapies, including chiropractic, physical therapy, occupational therapy, and other massage and bodywork therapy modalities. The treatment follows a back-and-forth protocol of evaluating, then treating, re-evaluating, then treating again. This process can be repeated as many times as necessary. Generally, it is recommended that the client receive a greater number of sessions, closer together in the beginning and taper off as the condition improves.

Depending upon the condition, different methods will need to be employed in the treatment. To free the superficial layer of fascia, there are several methods that can be utilized. **Skin-rolling** is often chosen as the initiating technique because of its versatility both as an assessment tool and as a method of treatment. This technique involves grasping just the skin, being careful not to pinch, and then rolling the flesh between the fingers and thumb. For example, when treating the back, skin-rolling can begin at the lower back, moving up between the shoulder blades, and even up the neck to the back of the head. When the therapist finds restrictions, it is important to move carefully since the areas can be quite tender and sensitive. With skin-rolling, the client may experience a burning or pinching sensation.

This technique will be easier to accomplish on some areas and harder on others. When the fascia is too tight and the skin is unable to be rolled, skin-rolling can be modified by taking the skin and just holding it, applying a mild pull. To intensify, a twisting motion can be supplied while maintaining the hold.

Often an intermediary maneuver following skin-rolling, **cross-handed stretches** can be applied to large or small areas and are useful for releasing fascia along specific lines of the body. With the forearms crossed and fingers pointing in opposite directions, contact is made with the full hands and pressure is applied with just enough downward force to maintain consistent contact without slipping. As fascia softens and fibers lengthen, **adhesions** release and patterns of strain in the body are freed. A sensitive therapist will be able to detect these shifts and follow the flow of unwinding to the next location.

Arm and leg pulls loosen restrictions at the deepest levels and will affect fascia anywhere along its line of pull. The leg pull is done with the client lying on the back and the therapist taking a snug hold of both ankles from underneath. A mild pull is introduced to one leg, then the other. The therapist goes back and forth, evaluating and gently testing each side. From this position, an expert therapist will be able to extend his or her sensitivity high up into the body to feel for restrictions at the ankles, knees, hips, and even up into the spine.

To release holdings at the ankle, a firm but gentle pull that affects just the ankle is applied. Here the therapist's mental state is very important. Their mind must be focused on releasing just the fascia around the ankle. If the therapist's mind wanders to the hips, their pull will reflect the thoughts of the mind. To release the knee, the same process is applied with just enough force to affect the knee and the mind solidly directed to the area being worked. To release the hips the pull is mildly strengthened and concentration now encapsulates the various structures of the hips. At the hips, different angles can be assumed to accommodate the variety of ways in which the legs can move. Each position must be held for the requisite 2 to 5 minutes before moving on to the next.

The arm pull is performed in similar fashion, with the therapist being careful not to exert too much pressure on the wrists. This pull, if done properly, can extend into the elbows, shoulders, neck, chest, and back. At certain angles, this pull can even extend into the hips. Note: This technique should not be done if the client has loose joint capsules or if the shoulder dislocates easily.

Treating Scars

Myofascial release is one of the best methods for working on scars whether they are from accident or surgery. It is important, however, that the scar is well healed or else there is risk of reopening the wound. For surgeries, the physician can determine the wait-time before treatment can begin. For injuries or accidents, the wait-time will vary, depending on the wound's depth and severity.

There's a lot more to scars than meets the eye, and what they look like on the surface is only half the story. The other half is what's going on below the surface. Scar formation is usually accompanied by adhesions (internal scar tissue) that fan out in all directions from the scar. When this happens, the area hardens and becomes constricted, blocking the flow of blood and nutrients while decreasing mobility. With myofascial work, these adhesions can be released and scar tissue can be mobilized, making them more pliable, yet at the same time stronger.

In treating the scar, the very same techniques can be used that were applied on the fascia. Skin rolling can be done up, down, left, right, and diagonally until all the restrictions are released. If the scar can't be rolled, it can be held and bent in each direction.

When scars are deeply indented, neither of these techniques may prove effective. In this case a cross-handed stretch can be applied directly on the scar. This can be done along the length of the scar or on either sides of the scar with the thumbs. Direct pressure into the scar can also be used to break up adhesions. While staying on one spot, the pressure can be focused in different directions according to need. This process can be repeated up and down the scar until all restrictions have been released.

It is important to note that these areas may be sensitive because of the amount of adhesions that often surround a scar. Because of this it is imperative that the therapist remember to keep in close communication with the client. The sensations associated with the releasing of adhesions can range from feeling just a mild stretch to feelings of burning and pain. The area may also flush with blood and turn red—usually a tell-tale sign that positive changes are occurring. Working on scar tissue is a step-by-step process and will take several sessions before the final results are achieved.

Conditions that can be benefited by Myofascial Release
- Chronic muscle pain and tension, including neck and back
- Recurring injuries
- Poor posture
- Jaw pain
- Scoliosis
- Scarring from surgery or injury
- Headaches
- Poor range of motion
- Fibromyalgia
- Carpal tunnel syndrome
- Frozen shoulder

- Plantar fasciitis
- Sports and other injuries
- Spasm/spasticity
- Neurological dysfunction
- Rehabilitation
- Head trauma

Contraindications and Precautions

- In cases of malignant cancers, acute rheumatoid arthritis and **aneurysms**, myofascial work should be avoided.
- Areas of bruising, opens wounds, and fractures should be avoided. Unaffected areas, however, can still be worked.
- Arm pulls should not be conducted if the patient has loose shoulder capsules or if his or her shoulder dislocates easily.
- Before working on scar tissue it is important that the area be well healed.

Training of a therapist

Myofascial Release has become such a popular modality that courses can readily be found in many of today's massage and bodywork therapy schools all over the country. These specialty courses are offered either as part of the school's larger certificate or licensure program in massage therapy or on a postgraduate level as separate individual workshops or certification seminars in the school's continuing education program. Certification training programs in Myofascial Release are also offered all over the country by independent practitioners and seminar companies specializing in this modality. These trainings are often open to those who already have a background in massage and bodywork therapy. Although training for Myofascial Release can be much more intensive, courses generally run about 20 hours over a few days. No separate licensing program for this discipline exists, but many schools will award a certification upon completion of their training. Unless specifically exempt from state law, those who practice Myofascial Release in states requiring a massage therapy license will need to have one in order to work legally.

SPORTS MASSAGE

Jack Meagher, the physical therapist who is most widely given credit for bringing **sports massage** to the United States, first became interested in the system while stationed as a soldier in France during WWII. There he received massages from a German POW in order to enhance his performance for camp football games. His experience was so positive that he later claimed that this type of bodywork could boost performance by an impressive 20 percent.[18] Although intrigued, it wasn't until much later that he decided to pursue the study seriously. Following the war he returned to pro baseball, but his career was abruptly interrupted by an old war injury. This set Meagher off in a new direction to heal his damaged body. For years he worked to develop the theory and practice of sports massage and eventually, with his own treatments, he was able to overcome his injury to such a degree that he returned to baseball semi-professionally [19] (Figure 7-7).

Although countries in Europe's Eastern Bloc had been utilizing sports massage for some time to improve athletic performance, it wasn't until the 1980's that the medical community in the United States began to appreciate the advantages that sports massage could offer. As more and more news of sports massage's effectiveness reached the athletic community, research studies were conducted to scientifically determine its value. In one such study, a group of professional cyclists was asked to pedal to the point of exhaustion then perform 50 leg extensions after a 10-minute break. During the break, half of the cyclists

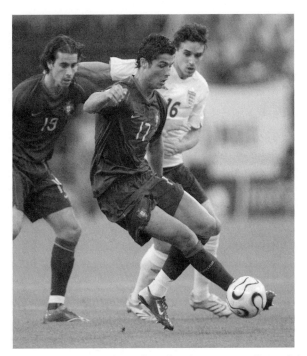

Figure 7-7 Professional sports team in action. Sports massage therapists are now an integral part of professional sports due to their assistance in alleviating the stress and strain on the body of major league athletes. *Image copyright 2009, Jonathan Larsen. Used under license from shutterstock.com.*

received sports massage while the other half merely rested. The results revealed that in only 10 minutes, the legs of the cyclists who had been massaged were 11 percent stronger than the ones who received just a short break. In the world of sports, where fractions of an inch or hundredths of a second determine who is first place 11 percent is an enormous edge.

Johnny Parker, strength and conditioning coach of the New York Giants from 1984 to 1992, heard of the recent developments in sports massage and decided to give his team a leading edge. His efforts gave his players a decisive advantage. The implementation of sports massage into his athletes' training regimen helped them to achieve and sustain peak performing levels over the course of the long, grueling season. The Giants were able to play harder, longer, and with fewer injuries. It improved their energy, boosted their drive, and sustained their ability to play again and again at full force. Being strong in their bodies gave the Giants the sense of confidence and spirit that the team needed to make it to the top, and during his tenure as the strength and conditioning coach, Parker helped take the Giants to the Superbowl three times. They won it twice in 1986 and in 1990. According to Parker, there is no doubt that sports massage gave his team a distinct advantage. Soon, other teams followed suit. At one point, the Chicago Bulls employed six different massage therapists—each with their own individual specialties that ranged from preventing injury to alleviating muscle fatigue and relieving muscle spasms.[20] Today, having qualified traveling sports massage therapists as part of the team is common practice.

Since its inception, sports massage has represented one of the fastest growing fields in massage therapy. In 1985, the American Massage Therapy Association (AMTA) formed the National Sports Massage Certification program, which led to the formation of the National Sports Massage Team (NSMT). Up until the late nineties, members of the AMTA's National Sports Massage Team offered their services to the some of the greatest athletes in the world at events like the Olympics, the Goodwill Games, and the Iron Man.[21] Since that time the AMTA has discontinued the NSMT, leaving it to their state chapters to coordinate sports massage teams, provide training and continuing education venues, and organize participation with sporting events in their respective areas of the country. Not all state chapters have sports massage teams. In addition to treating the professional athlete there is also a growing demand for the services of well-trained and versatile sports massage therapists in today's world as more and more people, particularly the Baby Boomers, live longer and more active lives, participate in all kinds of physical activities and sports, and recognize the need to maintain an active and healthy lifestyle.

Theory and Principles

The differentiating factor between sports massage and other modalities is its emphasis on preventing injury. Most of the other modalities come into play after something has gone wrong. In sports massage, however, one of the major goals is to see problems before they become issues—before the athlete ever feels pain and has to slow down. If an athlete feels pain, it can affect his performance and his entire life. The issue goes much deeper than just the body. Many athletes identify themselves with their sport and when the ability to use their body becomes impeded, a major part of their life can seem crippled. Ultimately, it can negatively affect a deeper sense of who they are.

But even without traumatic injuries such as the straining of muscles or the tearing of a ligament there are other issues that can drastically affect the way an athlete performs. The chronic stress of intense training can lead to a thickening and rigidifying of support tissues in the body. This eventually decreases range of motion and inhibits mobility. For athletes, full mobility is crucial to their game and its loss can kill their careers. As muscle fibers become more and more constricted, the circulation of blood becomes less and less efficient. As the muscle's supply of oxygen and nutrients dwindles, metabolic waste builds and stagnates. Muscles harden, movement slows, and the body becomes less responsive. Overall the athlete feels bulkier, less dynamic, and can even feel less alive.

Exercise and physical activity is good for the body, but it comes with a set of responsibilities. A certain level of maintenance and upkeep is required. As muscles pump to produce action, metabolic waste is formed. This waste, if left unresolved, will stagnate and decrease the work potential of the muscle. It slows down healing and blocks the flow of fresh nutrients from coming in and feeding the hungry muscles.

Sports massage helps to not only normalize these conditions, it also helps to prevent them from happening in the first place. According to John Jerome, the author of *Staying Supple*, "Athletes—the ones who last for very long anyway—eventually come to understand that the single physical asset most critical to continued and successful hard use of the human body isn't strength, speed or endurance, but suppleness."[22]

Also, while many athletes know that increased training leads to improved performance, they often neglect an important phase of their regimen—the recovery. This crucial aspect of effective training can hugely impact an athlete's success. In fact, the speed and quality of the recovery will directly impact the speed and quality of an athlete's development.

Three Categories of Sports Massage

Keeping the athlete in peak physical condition requires several different approaches, each depending upon the time and place. There are three basic categories into which sports massage can be divided. The most popularly known form falls in the category of event massage. As its name suggests, this is the type of massage administered to an athlete at the actual competition or performance. The next category is maintenance massage. These treatments are done in between events and can be a regular part of the athlete's training regimen. The goal here is to smooth out any bumps from the previous event and to get the body in shape for ones that are coming up. The last category is rehabilitation massage. This is for when an athlete becomes injured and is on the road to recovery. The aim here is to help an athlete get back on track as soon as possible.

EVENT MASSAGE   In an event massage, the specific goals for each session will depend upon the athlete, sport, or type of event because different sports engage and stress different groups of muscles. Knowing this will determine the focus of each session. For example, when treating a runner, the concentration is placed on the legs, hips, and lower back, but if it is a baseball pitcher that needs the work, his session will be more focused on the arms and shoulders.

Event massage can take place before, during, or after an event. If the session is done prior to a competition or performance, it is known as a pre-event massage. This treatment has an entirely different agenda than a massage that is given to an athlete after the event, known as a post-event massage (Figure 7-8).

Pre-Event Massage   The pre-event massage is a preparation for action. The goal here is to fire up the body and bring it to optimal performance levels by loading and energizing the muscles with oxygen and nutrients. It is also designed to ready the body to handle the rigors of an all-out performance. The pace is brisk and enlivening and involves the application of quick, pumping compressions, joint-loosening jostles, and stimulating percussive movements. While loosening and releasing joints and muscles, it is at the same time activating. As blood and fluids course through arteries and veins, a wake-up call is sounded to every cell in the body, making it more dynamic, more alive. This is akin to a robust pep-talk before the game.

Post-Event Massage   A full-out competition or performance can take a grueling toll on an athlete's body. The post-event massage is intended to bring the athlete's body back from a state of action and dynamics to one of rest and restoration. The most immediate concern that sports massage therapists must consider when athletes finish their performances or competitions is

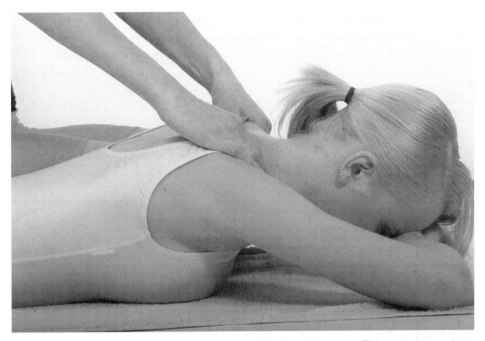

Figure 7-8 Sports massage at events is done with the clothes on. This can occur at a wide range of sporting events such as marathons, baseball games, bike-a-thons, or swim meets. *Image copyright 2009, Edw. Used under license from shutterstock.com.*

whether or nor they are even in a state to receive the treatment. If they display signs of severe strain, sprain, dehydration, hyperthermia, or hypothermia, immediate medical attention may be required. During this initial screening process other potential issues should be considered, such as blistering and stress fractures.

The therapist should also make sure that the athlete has had an adequate cool-down. This is an integral phase of an event because it prevents the pooling of blood in the extremities and ensures that blood takes its normal course of returning to the heart. It also helps to bring the heart rate back down to near resting levels. These are important functions for the body to undergo and an athlete should not be massaged before they've had a proper cool-down.

Once it has been established that it is safe to work on the athlete, the treatment can begin. Goals here include:

1. Relaxing any areas of tightness.
2. Reducing spasms, cramping, pain, and soreness.
3. Increasing circulation to flush out metabolic waste.
4. Facilitating faster recovery and return to training.

This session should be mild and soothing with a slow, rhythmic pace to bring the body back down to a normal, resting state where healing and repair can begin. Friction and other deep strokes must be avoided because the athlete's musculature may be too sensitive after an event. The muscles, after firing for so long and so hard, can feel raw and the last thing needed is intense pressure boring into swollen, overworked muscles. An improperly trained therapist who treats athletes as if they are just coming from a day at the office as opposed to a marathon can actually do harm by applying pressures that the body isn't ready to handle. This may result in damaging two things—the integrity of the tissue and the athlete's trust of the therapist.

It is important to note that a pre- or post-event massage does not replace the need for an adequate warm-up or cool-down. These are still necessary components of an athlete's regimen.

MAINTENANCE MASSAGE   The goal of maintenance massage is two-fold: 1) To take care of any issues caused by the last event and 2) to prepare for the next one. It is imperative that the therapist find out when the next event or training session is in order to determine the type of work that needs to be done, especially if deeper work is being considered. Within 24 hours of an event (before or after), deep work should be avoided.

There are four components of a maintenance massage session:

1. Intake
2. Assessment
3. Treatment
4. Follow up

REHABILITATION MASSAGE   This aspect of sports massage has to do with helping athletes get back in the game after being on the injured list. There are several mechanisms that get triggered in a rehabilitation massage that are conducive to a speedy recovery. These include the improved cleanup of metabolic waste (which can impair the healing process) and the more efficient delivery of vital nutrients and minerals. It should be noted that this aspect of sports massage closely resembles the work of orthopedic massage.

Goals of the rehabilitation massage include the following.

1. Increase Circulation: Increasing circulation means the increase of blood and fluids flowing through the body. As a result more nutrients are being fed to the damaged area and there is less buildup of toxic waste in the body to slow down the healing process.

2. Reduce Pain: The increase in circulation has an added benefit of decreasing tissue sensitivity that can be caused by the buildup of metabolic waste.

3. Increase Mobility: The body seals a wound by laying down layers of tissue that eventually form a scar. Since the body is trying to seal the wound as quickly as possible, the tissue is laid down in a haphazard formation, which can result in reduced movement and flexibility than the tissue had before. By working directly on the scar and aligning the scar tissue to flow with its surroundings, function and range of motion can be markedly improved.

4. Decrease Muscle Spasms: Injuries often give rise to a combination of overused muscles that become tight and contracted, along with weak, underdeveloped muscles that need to be strengthened and that can lead to muscle spasms. This can be a direct result of the injury, or it can be a secondary condition that arises from compensation. **Compensation** occurs when one side of the body becomes injured and the other side tries to do its work. For example, when a person breaks a leg, twists an ankle, or injures one side of the body the opposite side has to work much harder. As a result, a lot of strain, pain, and muscle spasms are often experienced.

Precautions   Because each category of sports massage is designed to fulfill a different phase of the athlete's needs, each type comes with its own specific checklist of precautions that must be attended to. This is one of the unique aspects of sports massage. For the pre-event session, the massage therapist must be careful not to do anything that might hamper the athlete's upcoming performance.

Deep Work   Deep specific work should not be done right before or after an event. Intensive work, while often necessary, sometimes requires a recovery period of its own during which the athlete may feel sore, weak, or ineffective for a day or so. Competing or performing while in this state can lead to pain and the inhibition of muscle reactivity, which can seriously throw off the athlete's timing. It can also have the psychologically dampening effect of bringing the athlete's attention to a trouble spot, which can cause anxiety before and during the performance. Competition is as much mental as it is physical and if the massage therapist is not careful, he or she can tamper with the finely calibrated balance of both elements.

Oil   Oil should generally not be used prior to an event unless it can be completely wiped off because it can interfere with the evaporation of sweat, stain uniforms, or cause athletic equipment to slide. In a post-event, maintenance, or rehabilitative treatment, oil can be used as needed.

Ice   The use of ice can cause muscles to stiffen and become unresponsive. It can also inhibit pain sensations, which can be dangerous to the athlete before an event. Pain is the body's indicator that something is wrong. When damage occurs to the body, the nervous system sends lightning-fast signals to the brain. These signals are interpreted as pain. The use of ice, however, can stun the nervous system and cause these signals to weaken and slow down. In fact, the athlete may not even feel the injury and continue behaving as if nothing happened. If an athlete continues in this fashion, the injury can get much worse. What may have started as something small and fairly treatable can become severe or even irreparable.

Talking/Distractions   Prior to an event, talking with the athlete should be kept to a minimum. Athletes tend to have very specific warm-up rituals and they need room to focus. Even talking about areas of tightness or bringing problem areas to their minds may throw them off their game.

Timing   It's important that the athlete not get too relaxed prior to an event. The pre-event treatment should be short (15–20 minutes) and upbeat. Any more risks overworking the athlete and actually depressing their performance.[23]

Intake

In order for the treatment to be as successful as possible, it is important that the therapist find out a few things before beginning. What is the reason for getting a massage? What are the specific and desired outcomes? Some clients will want to accomplish very specific goals. A dancer may feel restricted in a certain position or movement. A runner may have a specific pain in the hips that needs to be alleviated. Others may feel a general sense of tiredness or soreness. Also, questions about what the athletes are experiencing right then and there are important. Are they experiencing any stiffness or soreness? Are there any problems with injuries or limited range of motion?

Assessment

The next segment is the assessment. One way to start is to look at the athlete's standing posture. This can give a ton of information about how an athlete is using or misusing his or her body. Certain over- and underdevelopments can be picked up readily by the eyes of a well-trained practitioner. The sports massage therapist can also stretch, mobilize, or palpate the body in order to assess the athlete's muscle condition and range of motion.

Although these methods can establish a pretty clear picture of the athlete's story, the most comprehensive way to assess his or her condition is to watch him or her in action. By observing the way a runner runs, or the way a golfer swings, the therapist can get the most accurate assessment of the situation. It's the difference between watching an accident unfold as opposed to studying the pictures and tire marks afterwards. Being on location allows the therapist to suggest real-time changes that the athlete can translate into immediate corrections. This is exponentially better in terms of effectiveness and enhancing performance than just suggesting something back at the office, which can easily be forgotten or misinterpreted. Out in the field, therapists get to see how their athletes compensate, what happens when they get tired, what movements are causing them pain, and what can lead to trouble in the future.

Treatment

The treatment will vary dramatically depending upon the athlete, the sport, and specific concerns. The sports massage therapist must be aware of the finer distinctions of how different sports will affect the body in different ways. Concentrated training and repetitive motions of the same joints and muscles in one sport take a toll on specific areas of the body. Therefore, certain patterns of imbalance are common within that particular sport.

For example, running is a high-impact sport that affects different people in different ways. If there is an imbalance in the system, the lower back, the back of the legs, the calves, and the feet can take a tremendous pounding. It is important to check for spinal and pelvic misalignments as even a small imbalance can add up to major problems over the course of many miles.

In cycling, the entire weight of the athlete is supported by the bicycle, unlike in running or skiing. This predisposes a greater risk for muscle imbalances to develop, since the "stabilizer" muscles do not get a chance to develop like the others muscles do. Also, the athlete is postured with the torso bent over the handle bar while the neck is craning backwards to hold up the head. Here the back is completely unsupported by the lower body and is therefore constantly engaged. Tight-fitting cycling shoes also tend to be a problem as they cramp the feet, and the hands often become sore from both supporting the body and absorbing vibration from the road.[24]

Athletes of field sports like soccer, lacrosse, basketball, and tennis require similar bodywork as runners, but with some modifications. While running exerts a consistent linear effort, field sports requires bursts of top-end speed, rapid lateral movements, and radical changes in direction. This puts greater stress on the stabilizing muscles, hips, knees, and ankles. The hard pounding can also generate a great deal of tension in the feet.[25]

Follow Up

It is important for athletes to understand that it is nearly impossible to participate in sports and not be injured at some point. It is equally important for them to understand that there are many means and measures available to ensure that they get to enjoy their activity for as long and as fully as possible. This requires active participation in their own recovery process by following the recommendations laid out by their sports massage therapist. And by seeking regular, preventative treatment, they'll be able to reduce their chances for harm.

Keeping athletes at the top of their game or taking them to the next level may also necessitate changes in other factors, including their training, diet, and lifestyle. This may require the introduction of other professionals such as a coach, a nutritionist, and a counselor to help further guide them on their way.

Sports Massage Techniques

Like most of the modalities within this spectrum of bodywork, the techniques of sports massage are actually a composite of techniques derived from the classic Swedish system, Myofascial Release, neuromuscular therapy, and orthopedic massage.

The long, gliding strokes inherited from the Swedish system encourage circulation, and this in turn warms tissues to make them more soft and pliable. Techniques of Myofascial Release free fascial sheets from one another and improve the muscle's ability to glide. This is an important function in athletic endeavors because it increases the efficiency at which a muscle can contract while at the same time improving a muscle's range of motion. While Myofascial Release deals with the outer layer of a muscle, NMT deals with issues within the muscle itself. Neuromuscular therapy seeks to relieve congested areas within the muscle (commonly known as knots) that create pain, tension, weakness, and poor functioning. In addition, the strong medical roots and specific scientific logic of orthopedic massage therapy lend themselves well to this type of work—especially during the assessment and rehabilitation phases of treatment. The techniques of all of these modalities must be mastered to become a complete sports massage therapist.

While the effleurage of Swedish massage is the staple of many other systems, it is often not used in a pre-event session because of its tendency to promote relaxation. It can, however be liberally used in other sessions. Compressions are often an effective way to begin a sports massage session.

Performed lightly it can be an effective technique to evaluate the condition of the underlying musculature. With added pressure it can be used to warm the muscles up and loosen joints in a noninvasive way. In pre-event sessions the compressions are quick and lively. After an event, pressure can be deeper and more sustained to help the body wind down.

The circular, kneading movements of petrissage is an excellent tool for spreading muscle fibers and increasing circulation to specific areas without going too deep. With simple modifications, this stroke can easily be done over clothes. When friction is applied before or after an event, it must be light and nonspecific. Deeper work at this sensitive time may actually be damaging to the athlete's body and performance. During the maintenance or rehabilitation phases, however, deeper work may be applied and even necessary.

The slow, rocking movements of jostling, shaking, and rocking can help loosen joints and large groups of muscles, while a faster motion excites the nerves and awaken the body. Tapotement has a similar effect. If used for a short duration, this technique stimulates the nerves and brings the body to attention. A longer duration will have the opposite effect of sedation. In a pre-event session, this technique is kept brief. In addition to these techniques, any number of stretches and joint movements can be used that are designed to open and ready the body for action. These techniques, sometimes known as body mobilizations, can be used throughout all of the sessions.

Benefits

- Helps break through barriers by restoring fatigued, contracted muscles to their fullest potential.
- Improves circulation, muscle functioning, and recovery time
- Enhances mental clarity and alertness.
- Removes waste products that block nutrients and impede recovery, thus increasing the athlete's reservoir of energy.
- Restores the length and suppleness of muscles.
- Heals micro-tears in the muscles.
- Detects potential problems and irregularities long before they become conditions.
- Reduces the potential for injury by keeping muscles strong, supple, and flexible.

Training of a Practitioner

The quality and length of sports massage trainings can vary greatly all the way from a few hours of lessons taught as part of a massage therapy course to a 30- to 50-hour sports massage specialty training within a massage therapy program. Today some schools are even offering much longer sports massage specialty tracks as part of their full program. Sports massage trainings are also offered as separate weekend workshops and seminars, as well as more intensive and longer certification training programs for continuing education credit. Massage therapists can choose to practice a general type of sports massage or specialize in a specific sport. Some schools cater to this type of concentration and offer courses designed specifically to treat dancers, runners, cyclists, golfers, and so on. Since athletes specializing in different sports have such different needs when it comes to sport massage treatment, it is essential for practitioners of sports massage to be able to recognize these needs and be able to administer the appropriate techniques for the most effective treatment. Without this specialized training, massage therapists may do more harm to their athletes than good.

MANUAL LYMPHATIC DRAINAGE

When **manual lymphatic drainage** first appeared in Europe in the 1930s , it stirred quite a controversy in the medical community. At the time the lymph system was considered dangerous and was unexplored. It was largely an unexplained phenomenon, and massaging the **lymph nodes** was something that was absolutely not done for fear of spreading viruses or bacteria. At one point, children with swollen lymph nodes in the neck were considered diseased and were operated on right away to remove the offending tissues. The same general theory of the time led doctors to hastily remove spleens and appendixes without consideration of how their loss would negatively impact the rest of the body.[26]

The first steps toward deflating these myths came in 1932 when Dr. Emil Vodder and his wife Estrid (both massage therapists) were treating English patients who were visiting Cannes on the French Riviera. Due to Britain's notoriously damp climate, the majority of the vacationers were fighting off chronic colds and they all presented with swollen lymph nodes in the neck. Although it was considered taboo at the time to treat lymph nodes, even for physicians, Vodder was compelled by an intuition that kept egging him on. He stepped into what some would consider a forbidden zone in medicine at that time—to treat the lymph nodes—and to his happy surprise, the colds vanished.[27]

This was a groundbreaking discovery, and for the next three years, Dr. Vodder and his wife studied and discovered the mysteries of the **lymphatic system**. During this time the pair developed a method of treating the lymphatic system through a series of gentle massage techniques. This treatment came to be known as manual lymphatic drainage. In 1935, Dr. Vodder introduced their work to the public and exposed the true nature of this overlooked system along with their highly effective method of treatment.

The Vodder's work showed that the lymphatic system was responsible for a host of functions that are vital for the body's survival. The lymphatic system serves a huge role in the body's ability to fend off disease and illnesses. It also cleanses and purifies the body in a way that no other system can and it supports the healing process by carrying nutrients, vitamins, and hormones to areas in need. Some called it the "neglected child of medicine." Others claimed that it was our most important system. And still some others saw it as *the* source for good health. Parisian newspapers simply called it "revolutionary."[28] From this point on, Dr. Vodder and his wife spent the next 40 years reeducating the world.

Theory and Principles

The lymphatic system is a network of vessels that parallels the **circulatory system**'s network of arteries and veins and actually picks up where the arteries and veins leave off. The circulatory system is responsible for transporting blood all throughout the body. Essentially it is composed of two major elements—the heart that pumps the blood and the vessels that hold and transport blood. The vessels that take blood away from the heart to feed muscles and other tissues are the arteries. The vessels that return blood back to the heart are the veins. The arteries and veins can be considered the highways of the circulatory system. When blood reaches its intended destination, it exits the arteries through tiny capillaries that branch out from the arteries like the roots of a tree. The walls of the capillaries are so thin that fluid is able to pass right through them and into the surrounding area. Ninety to ninety-eight percent of this fluid is then reabsorbed by the capillaries and returned to the heart through the veins.[29]

The leftover fluids that the capillaries were not able to pick up must be handled by the lymphatic system which becomes automatically activated when pressure builds from its accumulation. When this fluid is taken into the lymphatic vessels, it is called **lymph**. Although this only accounts for 2 to 10 percent of the leftover fluids, this can have a major impact on the way the body functions and feels. Often what is left behind include proteins and other large debris that the capillaries simply can't handle. Due to the way proteins are constructed, they have a propensity to attract water. This means that if they are left behind for too long, they will attract so much water that the whole area swells, creating a condition called edema.

Edema

There are 3 stages of edema. The first stage is completely reversible, the skin is still soft to the touch, and there are no permanent changes caused by the fluid buildup. At this point, pressing into the flesh with the fingers yields only small dimples that fade away. In stage 2, the affected area begins to feel more like butter. The area becomes tougher because tissue is being laid down by the body in order to provide extra support for the excessive amounts of fluid in the area. Unfortunately, this is not a real solution to the problem. Pressing the fingers into the area now will leave behind small indentations that linger.

When the edema reaches stage 3, it is considered irreversible. More and more tissue has been laid down and too many structural changes have taken place. People at this stage of edema can show extreme physical changes. While the condition cannot be cured, it can however, be eased (Figure 7-9).

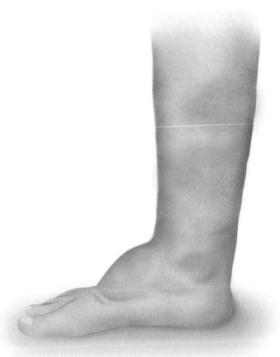

Figure 7-9 Edema can cause uncomfortable and painful swelling of the arms, fingers, legs, or other parts of the body. Lymphatic drainage helps the fluid filter back out of the affected areas to decrease the swelling.

Functions of the Lymphatic System

As the body's major defense mechanism, the lymphatic system is called upon any time the body is under attack. The lymphatic system is responsible for producing natural killer cells—powerful agents in the body's ongoing war on disease. These cells act exactly in the way that their name implies and have amoeba-like capabilities to squeeze through tiny slivers in capillary walls to intercept intruders. These cells are *the* major force for upholding the body's immunity. Basically, the more abundant they are, the stronger the immune system. Manual lymphatic drainage can boost the production of these guardian cells by as much as 30 percent.[30]

In addition the lymphatic system has an enormously important job of clearing toxic waste and debris that can disrupt every function in the body. Excess fluids contain the remnants of dead cells, waste, bacteria, and viruses. The lymph system acts as the pipelines of a sewer system to drain this mess away and the more that can be drained away, the cleaner the body becomes. But like all drains it can become clogged and, like any clog, it can damage the surrounding environment if left unmanaged. It can also become a breeding ground for germs and bacteria.

Anatomy of the Lymphatic Vessel

When lymph enters the lymphatic vessels, it is moved into a small chamber within the vessels called lymph angions. Angion literally means "heart" and was named so because it acts as a pump for circulating fluids much like the muscles of the heart. At either end of the angion is a valve that only allows lymph to move in one direction. The lymphatic vessels are made up of thousands of these tiny chambers and valves. Because of the one-way valve system preventing fluids from going the wrong way, there is no reason for worry over whether the fluids are being pushed in the wrong direction to make the swelling worse. However, nothing positive will result from it.

Each lymph angion is coated in a layer of smooth muscle that spirals around it. Stretch sensors are built into the angion walls and become activated as fluid pressures build. This triggers the muscles into a spiraling contraction that flushes the fluids into the next chamber. A vacuum is created in its wake and as lymph is pumped out from one end, more lymph is sucked in from the other. This push-pull dynamic creates a chain reaction that advances lymph all throughout the body in wavelike contractions.

Eventually all lymph reaches what is known as the terminus. This is the point where lymph pours back into the heart to rejoin the bloodstream. But before lymph is able to be readmitted into the circulatory system it must go through hundreds of relay stations along the way called **lymph nodes**.

There are 400 to 700 lymph nodes in the body and their size can range from the head of a pin to the size of an olive. One half of all the lymph nodes are located in the abdomen and there are a large number in the neck as well. The rest are scattered throughout the body, resting in naturally protected nooks and crannies like the armpits, the groin, the crease of the elbows, and the backs of the knees. The primary function of the lymph nodes is to filter and purify the fluid that flows through them. Lymph is a viscous liquid similar to egg white that normally moves very slowly. The process of purification that occurs by passing through the nodes actually thickens the fluid and slows it down even more. This is where manual lymphatic drainage comes in. With proper application of this massage modality, the lymph can be made to flow up to 20 times more efficiently.

When lymph nodes are backed up, however, they harden and become hindered in their duties. If these clogs occur in the head, neck, or face, it can result in nose and throat infections, migraines, oily skin, swelling, and acne. By clearing out the waste, lymphatic drainage flushes the sinuses, cleanses the pores, and detoxifies the skin, leaving behind a healthy, happy glow. Because of this ability to rejuvenate the skin, manual lymphatic drainage is valued by the beauty and spa industry. It is also highly valued for its ability to diminish cellulite deposits as well as prevent their further growth[31] (Figure 7-10).

The Technique

In order to treat the lymphatic system, it was necessary to develop new techniques to specifically target its unique properties. There are four factors that must be gauged in order to properly administer a manual lymphatic drainage treatment. These include

1. Pressure
2. Direction
3. Rhythm
4. Sequence

Pressure

Massage therapists who have not learned manual lymphatic drainage tend to assume that the motion and pressure of this technique is similar and will yield similar results to that of traditional effleurage (a gliding stroke used in Swedish

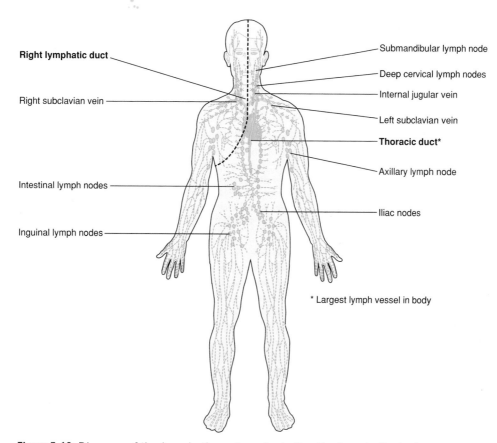

Right lymphatic duct

Right subclavian vein

Intestinal lymph nodes

Inguinal lymph nodes

Submandibular lymph node

Deep cervical lymph nodes

Internal jugular vein

Left subclavian vein

Thoracic duct*

Axillary lymph node

Iliac nodes

* Largest lymph vessel in body

Figure 7-10 Diagram of the lymphatic system, including the lymphatic ducts.

massage). Common sense seems to dictate that effleurage would be the most appropriate means of flushing fluids in the body. However, there are factors that make using effleurage for this specific purpose a much less effective approach.

Unlike blood vessels, lymphatic vessels reside very close to the surface of the body. The lymph system is designed so that it almost encases the entire body and removes excess fluids as they rise to the surface. Seventy percent of all lymph vessels are actually located in or just below the surface of the skin. Traditional massage techniques are aimed at reaching the muscles below the skin, so these strokes generally go beyond the lymphatic system. Effleurage may actually be too deep and the stroke performed as it normally would be for a Swedish massage can actually squash the lymphatic vessels. Pushing too hard can even break the filaments that hold the vessels in place. Luckily, these replace themselves within 24 hours. Pressure for lymphatic drainage should be calibrated to access just the right depth so the hands don't slide over the skin and yet it should remain light enough so that nothing below the skin can be felt (e.g., muscle, bone, etc.). This amounts to only 1 to 4 ounces of pressure.

Direction

Like highways and ocean currents, there are predictable routes that lymphatic vessels follow, and to effectively administer a manual lymphatic drainage treatment, a therapist must know how to navigate the lymphatic currents. This requires knowing the order in which the lymph system must be activated and the location of where each section of the vessels must be drained to. The contents of this journey have been studied and charted into maps and diagrams that reveal the location of the lymph nodes and the direction of proper lymphatic flow. If these routes are not followed, the treatment will be of little value. This is due in large part to the one-way valves running up and down the system's vessels.

Rhythm

The rhythm and pace of a manual lymphatic drainage treatment has been specifically calibrated to stimulate the lymphatic vessels in just the right way to open the gates and initiate the pumping chain-reaction. This is another factor that predisposes traditional strokes like effleurage to be ineffective for lymphatic drainage. In order for the angion "pumps" to be activated an initial pump must be supplied in order to "kick start" the whole process. The technique for stimulating the lymph system is akin to administering CPR to thousands of tiny little hearts. Each stroke lingers for just a second or two so that lymph can be sucked up into the vessels and when the pressure is released, the gate closes behind them. An effleurage on the other hand supplies only a smooth, continuous pressure that does little to initiate the chain reaction.

Sequence

The area nearest the node is always drained first and then the work continues further and further away from the node. As fluids move out, a vacuum is created in their wake that draws more fluids in. Only the proper sequencing will create this beneficial chain reaction throughout the body.[32]

The Treatment

The end of the lymphatic road is the beginning of the session. The terminus (the area that lymph dumps back into the bloodstream) is located high in the chest just underneath the collarbones. To start, the hands are placed gently above the collarbones where very light, semi-circle motions are applied. At this position, the stroke is repeated five times moving just the skin. Afterwards, the therapist repositions his or her hands a few inches higher on the neck and again the same five strokes are applied. The therapist continues in this fashion, working systematically up the neck applying the same crescent-shaped strokes at each interval.

At the top of the neck the hands climb sequentially up the underside of the jaws both stimulating nodes that are there and flushing the lymph down the chain to the neck and to the heart. The strokes continue from the base of the jawline and climb to the chin and mouth. Then, back by the ears, another procession of delicate, pumping strokes ascends to the nose and then another line starts, this time from the temples to the eyes. This progression continues until the entire head and face is cleared. The sensation of a manual lymphatic drainage session is much different than that of a regular massage. The pressure used is as gentle as what you might use to rock a sleeping baby, but because it engages the part of the nervous system that induces rest and relaxation, it can be a highly tranquil experience.

The next line of work begins at the cluster of nodes nestled protectively where the torso meets the arm. This area must first be cleared in order to make way for the rest of the appendage. The arm is placed over the head to access this delicate area and in the same, slow, monotone rhythm, the work progresses all the way down to the hands. Along the way the strokes alternate, with pressure being applied with the full hand, or just the fingers; with both hands, or just the thumbs. The session progresses to the chest and then moves to the abdomen with the same care and concern for delivering the fluids to their proper nodes. Here the lymphatic currents become more difficult to navigate as different areas of the chest and abdomen must be drained to different nodes. In order to drain the legs, the nodes tucked into the groin area must first be cleared before the thighs and then the calves can be drained.

Benefits

- Decreases edema
- Strengthens the body's immune functions
- Clears the sinuses
- Improves healing time
- Helps the body fight colds and 'flu
- Prevents the growth of cellulite and reduces its presence

- Improves oily skin, acne, scars, and other skin conditions
- Post-surgical care—especially when lymph nodes have been removed due to tumor or cancer

Contraindications

This is a very gentle system, so there is little to worry about as far as damaging delicate tissue or going too deep. However, there are times when spreading fluids throughout the body can be harmful or even fatal. Under the following conditions, manual lymphatic drainage should not be administered.

- Acute inflammation: This is often caused by bacteria, viruses, poisons, and allergens; therefore it would be unwise to send these contaminants coursing deeper into the body.
- Thrombosis and phlebitis: If these conditions are agitated it can lead to the formation of free-floating blood clots that can cause fatal damage.
- Malignant tumors: Lymphatic drainage for someone who has aggressive malignant tumors may spread the cancerous cells. On the other hand, receiving manual lymphatic drainage after a having been treated for the cancer with toxic allopathic methods such as chemotherapy would be beneficial.
- Major heart problems: In congestive heart failure, there is already too much stress on the heart. Since the lymph system dumps back into the heart, lymphatic drainage would put too great a strain on the already weakened organ.[33]

Precautions

It is highly recommended that clients afflicted with any of the conditions listed below first receive the approval of their primary health-care provider before receiving manual lymphatic drainage treatments. Although they are still eligible to receive manual lymphatic drainage, certain precautionary steps may be required before treatment can begin. Once the necessary safety measures are taken, manual lymphatic drainage may be administered to clients with the following conditions:

- Kidney problems
- Bronchial asthma
- Thyroid problems
- Medications/Chemotherapy
- First trimester of pregnancy
- Menstruation

Training of a Manual Lymphatic Drainage practitioner

Training to become a manual lymphatic drainage practitioner generally requires students to have completed a course of study at a massage therapy school for a minimum of 500 hours before they are admitted to a program. The program at the Dr. Vodder School of North America is 160 hours long and is administered in four sections: 1) Basic, 2) Therapy I, 3) Therapy II, and 4) Therapy III. Each section is five days long and exams in oral, written, and practical forms must be passed before students can continue to the next section. Classes are offered in select cities across the United States, and certification is provided upon completion.[34] Other schools such as the Academy of Lymphatic Studies and the Upledger Institute offer similar programs.

SUMMARY

This chapter introduces the somatic level of massage therapy and bodywork which includes modalities with the intent to affect changes mainly in the physical body. It provides an understanding of how the modalities of Swedish Massage, Neuromuscular Therapy, Trigger Point Therapy, Orthopedic Massage, Myofascial Release, Manual Lymphatic Drainage, and Sports Massage each fit into the somatic level of massage including how they differ, and how they are similar to each other. A basic overview of the history, the theory and principles, process of assessment, as well as a description of the techniques involved are presented for each of these modalities of the somatic level. This chapter also acquaints the reader with what the general experience of undergoing a treatment session is like and identifies who are the best candidates to seek this form of treatment and what conditions are most benefited. Also presented is a list for each of these modalities of their general benefits, contraindications, and/or precautions. A brief discussion about training, licensing, certifications, and requirements is also included.

CHAPTER REFERENCES

1. Grabowski, S. R., & Tortora, G. J. (2002). *Principles of anatomy and physiology*. New York: John Wiley & Sons.
2. Beck, M.F. (2006). *Theory and practice of therapeutic massage*. (4th ed.). Albany, New York: Thomson Delmar Learning
3. *Professional membership*. (2006). Retrieved October 13, 2006, from http://www .amtamassage.org/membership/profmship.html
4. *Professional membership*. (2006). Retrieved October 13, 2006, from http://www .amtamassage.org/membership/profmship.html
5. Finando, D., & Finando, S. (2005). *Trigger point therapy for myofascial pain*. Rochester, VT: Healing Arts Press.

6. Claire, T. (1995). *Body work: What kind of massage to get and how to make the most of it.* Laguna Beach, CA: Basic Health Publications, Inc.

7. Claire, T. (1995). *Body work: What kind of massage to get and how to make the most of it.* Laguna Beach, CA: Basic Health Publications, Inc.

8. Lowe, W. W. (2003). *Orthopedic massage: Theory & technique.* Edinburgh: Mosby.

9. Finando, D., & Finando, S. (2005). *Trigger point therapy for myofascial pain.* Rochester, VT: Healing Arts Press.

10. Lowe, W. (2003). *Orthopedic massage: Theory & technique.* Edinburgh: Mosby.

11. *Course descriptions.* (2006). Retrieved September 25, 2006, from http://www .nmtcenter.com/courses/

12. *Orthopedic massage certification program.* (2006). Retrieved September 25, 2006, from http://www.omeri.com/omcp.htm

13. *Course descriptions.* (2006). Retrieved September 25, 2006, from http://www .orthomassage.net/course_descriptions

14. *Myofascial release.* (2006). Retrieved July 23, 2006, from http://en.wikipedia.org/ wiki/Myofascial_Release

15. Riehl, S. (2001). *Beginning myofascial release.* [VHS]. Real Bodywork.

16. Riehl, S. (2001). *Beginning myofascial release.* [VHS]. Real Bodywork.

17. Kenneth, S. (2006). Retrieved July 23, 2006, from http://en.wikipedia.org/wiki/ Kenneth_Snelson

18. Levine, A., & Levine, V. (1999). *Bodywork and massage sourcebook.* Los Angeles: Lowell House.

19. Claire, T. (1995). *Body work: What kind of massage to get and how to make the most of it.* Laguna Beach, CA: Basic Health Publications, Inc.

20. Levine, A., & Levine, V. (1999). *Bodywork and massage sourcebook.* Los Angeles: Lowell House.

21. Claire, T. (1995). *Body work: What kind of massage to get and how to make the most of it.* Laguna Beach, CA: Basic Health Publications, Inc.

22. Johnson, J. (1995). *Healing art of sports massage.* Emmaus: Rodale Press Inc.

23. *Intro to sports massage* [Swedish Institute Handbook]. 2006.

24. Johnson, J. (1995). *Healing art of sports massage.* Emmaus: Rodale Press Inc.

25. Johnson, J. (1995). *Healing art of sports massage.* Emmaus: Rodale Press Inc.

26. Wittlinger, G., & Wittlinger, H. (2004). *Textbook of Dr. Vodder's manual lymph drainage* (Vol 1., 7th ed.). Stuttgart: Thieme.

27. Wittlinger, G., & Wittlinger, H. (2004). *Textbook of Dr. Vodder's manual lymph drainage* (Vol 1., 7th ed.). Stuttgart: Thieme.

28. Wittlinger, G., & Wittlinger, H. (2004). *Textbook of Dr. Vodder's manual lymph drainage* (Vol 1., 7th ed.). Stuttgart: Thieme.

29. Riehl, S. (2000). *Lymphatic drainage massage.* [VHS]. Real Bodywork.

30. Riehl, S. (2000). *Lymphatic drainage massage.* [VHS]. Real Bodywork.

31. Riehl, S. (2000). *Lymphatic drainage massage.* [VHS]. Real Bodywork.

32. Riehl, S. (2000). *Lymphatic drainage massage.* [VHS]. Real Bodywork.

33. Riehl, S. (2000). *Lymphatic drainage massage.* [VHS]. Real Bodywork.

34. *Therapists & Health care practitioners: Training.* (2006). Retrieved September 28, 2006, from http://www.vodderschool.com/therapists/training.cfm

Somato-Psychic Layer of the Massage Therapy and Bodywork Continuum

CHAPTER GOALS

1. Develop an understanding of how the modalities of Rolfing®, SOMA Neuromuscular Integration®, Hellerwork, the Alexander Technique, and the Feldenkrais Method® fit into the somato-psychic approach of massage.

2. Recognize the significance of these modalities, how they differ, and how they are similar to each other.

3. Develop a basic understanding of the theory and principles of the somato-psychic approach.

4. Develop a basic understanding of the process of assessment that the somato-psychic approach utilizes.

5. Develop a basic understanding of the techniques involved in the somato-psychic approach.

6. Become acquainted with the general experience of a session in the somato-psychic approach.

7. Identify who should seek this form of treatment and what conditions benefit most from the somato-psychic approach.

8. Become aware of contraindications and precautions of the somato-psychic modalities.

9. Become knowledgeable about the training, licensing, certifications, and requirements that the practitioner needs in order to practice this system.

INTRODUCTION TO THE SOMATO-PSYCHIC LAYER OF MASSAGE THERAPY AND BODYWORK

Modalities that focus their treatment on the **somato-psychic layer** blur the line between bodywork and psychotherapy. Here the mind and body are viewed as two parts of the same entity, two doors to the same building. The somato-psychic approach views the body as a reflection of the mind; therefore, dysfunctions of the physical form are evidence of disorder in the mind. We are a compilation of learned physical and emotional postures held in response to stress, and the body is the tell-tale diary that reveals how we've faced both the challenges and opportunities that we've been given in this life. The way that our bodies are either locked, contorted, and twisted, or open, free, and balanced is a reflection of the life that we've lived and the experiences that we've encountered.

Practitioners of the somato-psychic approach are the architects and engineers of bodywork. The creators of this system were visionaries—their aim wasn't only the better functioning of the human organism; rather it was the full actualization of the human potential. Their goal was to encompass the entire scope of human possibilities, and the physical body was seen as merely the gateway for change.

Although the founding member of each modality comprising the somato-psychic approach was infused with his or her own distinct passions, a common love of the ideal brought the founding members onto the same path. They looked beyond themselves and saw that the major obstacle for human beings in achieving their potential was their own selves. Like many others, they saw mechanical inefficiency and squandered potential, yet what makes them stand apart is that they went beyond the range of everyday optimism to create and implement real methods of change. In studying the human body they realized that it was capable of so much more grace and fluidity than most allow or would even acknowledge. They realized it would only require simple corrections in positioning and mechanics to unleash the storehouse of human potential, and they found that by improving the most exterior functioning of a person, that person's entire life could be transformed.

They saw the body as a metaphor and the mind as the body's blueprint. They realized the body could disclose our inner world and communicate the textures of our emotional life. They understood how the body could convey practical information about how we handle stress and aggravation and how it can reveal a much deeper reality like how much love and affection we received as children. They learned that the physical body is a mirror of the life that we live. Without knowing it, we expose everything and anyone trained to do so can "read" the story that our bodies readily tell.

Students of this approach study lines of tension, efficiency of motion, restrictions of movement, relationships to universal forces, and the dynamic interactions that allow for the unified functioning of the human machine.

The Modalities

The somato-psychic layer of touch covers two branches of bodywork commonly referred to as structural integration and functional integration. While structural integration seeks to alter the *form* of the physical body, **functional integration** seeks to create change in the *course* of the physical body. Although these two lines of thought were distinct schools in the past, an intermingling of functional and structural has produced offspring that express the best of both parents. Structural integration utilizes deep manipulation of the body to create more economical alignment. It first began through the study of the physical body as the primary motivator of change, but as the form evolved it began to include the greater nuances and textures that interplay in the experience of a human being. Explorations of the mind and its vast psychology revealed a greater richness of the self than had been previously acknowledged and penetrating new insights were made into the need for healing to take place on a number of levels.

Ida Rolf, the originator of structural integration, infused her work with internal analysis, but it wasn't until the next generation that direct change in the psychology was actively pursued. **SOMA Neuromuscular Integration** and **Hellerwork** are some of the bold, evolutionary advancements in somato-psychic work that have helped usher it in to the modern world by recognizing and attending to aspects of the self that were not appreciated or even acknowledged in previous generations. While still fully utilizing the genius of Rolf's traditional 10-step process, the pioneers of the somato-psychic approach embraced modern ideas of psychology and spirituality to achieve new territory for bodywork.

The functional integration component of this layer strives for the same goals and principles as structural integration, but this approach seeks physical and psychological advancement by correcting the body in motion. According to this system, many of the physical ailments that we suffer today are direct responses to our habitual misuse of the body, caused by our poorly developed range of movement options. By creating a new language for the body, functional integrators allow for a greater diversity of movement options, thereby providing greater freedom of choice.

This concept goes against the conventional ways of approaching an injury that are disempowering because people are taught to think in terms of what needs to be done to them rather than what they can do to help themselves. Provided with healthier alternatives, patients become empowered to make better and better decisions for themselves.

Allowing the body to move once again with its natural ease and grace heightens its sense of balance, calm, and wholeness. And by creating a stable and nourishing construct in which the mind and the emotions can reside, a new world of inner peace can be enjoyed. Outlook becomes more expansive. Perspective becomes more encompassing. Thoughts become crisper and sharper. Vision becomes brighter and more focused. Stress inevitably comes, but goes away much quicker. Once free from pain there is a greater sense of ability and with this comes a confidence of being able to achieve one's full potential. In short, it becomes a new body with a new life.

ROLFING®

Ida Rolf's life's work was to answer the question, "How do we reach or achieve our highest self? What conditions must be met? What's standing in our way?" An idealist to the core, she searched tirelessly for the answers and, as is common to all visionaries, she not only saw what was present, she also saw what was possible. What is even more significant, however, is that she understood how that possibility could be attained. Similar to how the sculptor Michelangelo could see the figure craving to be freed from its marble prison, Ida Rolf could see the perfection inherent in the human form. Her life's work was dedicated to liberating this potential.

History

Although Dr. Rolf could have made her mark anywhere, her own issues with spinal arthritis, as well as the ailments of her sons, drew her intellect toward researching the human body. She spent years exploring a variety of alternative therapies, including homeopathy, chiropractic, **osteopathy**, yoga, and the exciting work launched by one of her contemporaries, F. M. Alexander—the Alexander Technique. The common thread that tied together these varied approaches was their core premise that form and function share an intimate and interdependent relationship. It was this central idea that would go on to form the underlying structure of Ida Rolf's major work.

At first her work was only seen as an adjunct to chiropractic and osteopathy, but Rolf knew that her techniques could play a much more significant role in the healing and balancing of the human body. But even with a Ph.D. in biochemistry from the College of Physicians and Surgeons of Columbia University, as a woman in the male-dominated world of science she faced heavy resistance before she was taken seriously.[1]

It wasn't until the 1960s, when Fritz Perls, founder of Gestalt Therapy and the director of the Esalen Institute, gave her the opportunity that she needed to put her work on the map. By relieving his severe attacks of chest pain, Rolf was able to earn Perls's respect and, more importantly, his support. The Esalen Institute afforded Rolf the critical springboard to launch her work. After all the years that she dedicated to developing and perfecting her system, she had finally found the fertile ground to plant her seeds of knowledge. She taught every summer at Esalen until 1972, when she reestablished herself in Boulder, Colorado. There she founded the Rolf Institute, whose mission till this day is dedicated solely to the practice, teaching, and expansion of her life's work.

But even after all that she had fought for and after all that she had accomplished, when Rolf reached the age where one's mortality is an urgent and impending reality, she became fearful that she had not done enough and worried that her life's work would be lost. However, by the time of her passing in 1979 she had already trained over 200 Rolfers and personally integrated thousands of people, including Georgia O'Keefe, Cary Grant, and Greta Garbo.[2] Her work is still carried on by not only the Rolf Institute in Colorado but also at institutes located in Munich, Melbourne, and Sao Paulo. Today there are over 1350 Rolfers and Rolf Movement Practitioners worldwide, and Rolf's fingerprint can be found in the many types of bodywork involving deep tissue or fascial work.[3]

Theory and Principles

Fascia

Ida Rolf was an invigorating force in bodywork. She pioneered the idea that in order to create permanent change in the body, fascia, an interconnecting network of fibrous tissue that wraps and connects every organ and muscle in the body, must be directly addressed. Prior to her work, fascia was never rigorously studied or attended to. Mostly it was seen as an obnoxious matter that one had to get through in order to get to what was really important.[4] Muscle was already known as a dynamic agent that provided shape, form, and mobility and everyone knew that bone provided muscles with a solid foundation on which to work. But no one had ever really given fascia the credit it deserved until Rolf recognized it as a critical and widely overlooked component in determining the health and function of the body.

There are two layers of fascia. The superficial layer is located just under the surface of the skin and envelops the entire body to hold and contain its contents. This layer can easily be damaged by injuries, accidents, and surgery. The deep layer is denser and more resilient. When fascial health is high, muscles, organs, and tissues glide over one another like layers of silk, but after trauma, illness, or injury, the layers become sticky and adhere to one another. Instead of gliding smoothly past one another, internal structures pull and tug on each other causing tension, friction, and wear and tear. Over the years fascia becomes tight, distorted, and rigid. The network that once provided support and protection now confines and constricts. The fascia becomes part of the problem.

The function of fascia is to integrate all tissues yet keep them separate. Unlike muscle, which is highly active and mobile, fascia is more stable. Muscle is like the pulp of an orange. Fascia is like its translucent skin. It provides shape and support to the body. Because the fascial web extends and intertwines throughout the entire body, a distortion in one section will ripple through the rest of the system.

These distortions are what make up what Rolf called the **random body**. In this state there is no unifying principle allowing for cohesive functioning of the body. In one person the random body may play out with the head tilting to one side, the hips twisting, the back locking and the feet turning out. Each component is out of sync and every step is an expression of tension and inefficiency. Balance is precarious and energy is wasted. In another person the head juts forward, the shoulders hunch forward, and the feet are turned in as if the body was caving in on itself. Energy is constantly expended to keep from tumbling forward. The organization of the body is haphazard and chaotic, causing it to be unstable, unreliable, and uneconomical. Greater and greater amounts of energy are required for upkeep and maintenance.

In a random body muscles become deformed and their role becomes distorted. Muscles were meant to contract then relax, but the disorganized system creates a state of constant tension. The muscles begin to emulate bone not only in function, but in quality as well. Instead of being the soft, mobile, and dynamic mechanisms that they were meant to be, they become hard, contracted, and rigid. The enwrapping fascia shortens along with the muscle and it too becomes hard and rigid. Eventually it traps muscles into a contracted state. What had previously been an agent of support and protection has now become an imprisoning cage, straining the body and pulling it into awkward, degenerative postures.

But because the fascia is pliable it can be pushed and pulled into a better organization. Its jigsaw pieces can be ordered to form a unified whole that is coherent. The body can be revitalized and rejuvenated. A new relationship can be established. The body can learn to work with astonishing efficiency, but only when given the opportunity. This is the real work of **Rolfing**—allowing that opportunity to be expressed.

The Weight of Gravity

A simple reason accounts for the distortion seen in so much of the human population. Since the moment we are born until the moment of our passing, we are engaged in a lifelong struggle against the most powerful universal force acting on the planet—gravity. It is a force so all-pervading that we rarely even recognize its dominion over us. As a friend it can brace and reinforce. As an enemy it will tear down piece by piece. No matter how strong the body or how determined the mind, inevitably as the days, weeks, months, and years pass by, gravity's relentless persistence will dominate. No one can win against a force that never rests.

Defeat in the human body is reflected by shoulders that slump, spines that twist, or gaits that jilt. As the body assumes these postures of defeat again and again, the mind follows suit. It affects the way we think, the way we feel and the way we move. The body tires, the mind limps, and the emotions stagnate.

The evolution of the human biped was an act of war against gravity (Figure 8-1). Rolf saw herself as an agent of this evolutionary process that dared to challenge this potent force. However, Rolf didn't envision victory in this war. That would have been silly and futile. She saw instead a way that this force could be harnessed. She saw how this power could pass harmlessly through the human body simply by embracing and aligning itself to the universe's own laws of mechanics.

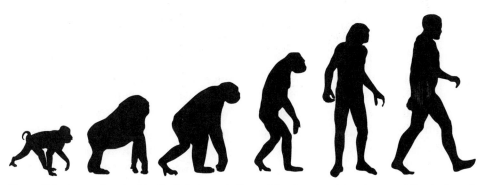

Figure 8-1 According to Ida Rolf, the evolution of the human biped was an "act of war" against gravity. *Image copyright 2009, ImageZebra. Used under license from shutterstock.com.*

In studying the universe she found that a patterned order was required for survival. Rolfing satisfies the need for this order by drawing together the units of the body into a balanced composition. When people bring themselves into order, they revitalize themselves. They waste less energy. This is law. The greater the order, the greater the energy.[5]

"We seek to create a whole that is greater than the sum of its parts."

—Ida Rolf

Emotions Embodied

Science clearly indicates that to every emotional state there is a unique combination of measurable physiological factors within the body. As the waves of emotions change from minute to minute, day to day, week to week, the chemical composition of the body alters along with them. As momentum builds and the emotional chemicals amass, more and more of the body literally becomes that emotion.

A child who grows up angry grows into a body that embodies anger. His chin juts out, his head sits forward, and his shoulders draw up in a chronic interplay of defensiveness and aggressiveness. A hand pressed to his shoulders reveals a rock-hard mound of unyielding tension. His personality is just as unyielding and equally as rigid. Emotionally, he is as tense as his body and unable to cope or adapt. The people around him worry. As he gets older his doctor worries about heart attacks, high blood pressure, and ulcers. His life is an exemplification of anger. It is no longer his life. His life belongs to anger.

Anger translates to tension in the body. When the body tenses, muscles contract. When the muscles contract for extended periods, they permanently shorten. As the body becomes tight, rigid and entangled, the person's emotional range grows small and limited. The mind becomes as restrictive and stubborn as the body.

According to Rolf, the physical personality is no different than that of the psychological personality. The physical is merely the material expression of the psychological just as the words on this page are the material expression of an idea. Because the two are intimately related and inseparable, change in the physical body will cause change in the psychological body. This physical restructuring translates into the mental and emotional realm. Just as cleaning off a messy desk can clarify one's intents and purposes, reorganizing one's physical body will lessen clutter and confusion in the psychological body as well.

Differentiation and Integration

Differentiation is one of the primary goals of Rolfing and leads to integration. It is the functional separation of layers of muscle and tissue enabling them to "unglue" from each other so that they can work independently and are then free to integrate. When muscles are differentiated, each part of the body is allowed to realize its full potential. Each muscle achieves greater definition and its relationship to the rest of the body is clarified. As a result, muscles are properly integrated and their work becomes simpler, easier, and more focused. The body wastes less energy and there is less chance of injury by doing something it wasn't designed to do.

Assessment

To the trained eye, clues to the underlying patterns of the body can be deciphered by examining its contours just as an expert seaman can read the currents of the ocean by observing its surface patterns. The Rolfer's job is to redirect the wayward currents into a more focused stream. They look beyond the surface to see the body as a mass of potential waiting to be actualized.

An initial appraisal is conducted to evaluate the body—its curves, its imbalances, and its structural asymmetries. If a house was tilted on one side, a builder wouldn't just jack up the one side. That would only provide artificial relief. Instead he would repair the foundation and make the necessary adjustments so the house can stand firmly on its own. Just so, a Rolfer's job is to look at the whole picture and correct the underlying imbalances (Figure 8-2).

In order to obtain the most accurate assessment of their posture, clients are asked to disrobe to either their underwear or bathing suits. From there, a photograph is taken in order to capture the evidence of their misalignment so that they can compare and see how much progress they have made when they reach the end of the sessions. It also serves as a visual guide that the therapist can study, as well as use to show the clients where rebalancing and realignment is to take place. Similar photos are taken after each session to track the progression of the body's transformation.

Through these visual logs, remarkable changes in the person's physique can be observed. The superiority of a structurally integrated form is immediately and intuitively recognized. Instantaneously the body gives off the distinct sense of grace, power, and poise. Symmetry cannot only be seen—it can be felt. Without even knowing why or ever having studied the human form, the inherent sense of rightness carried by a body in perfect alignment is distinct (Figure 8-3).

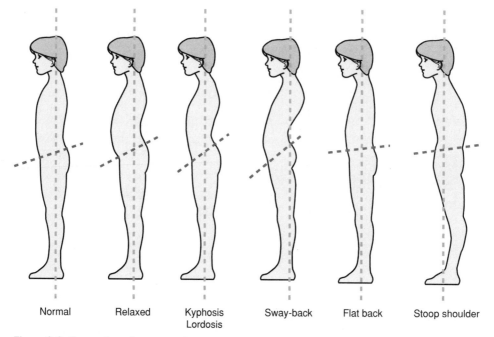

| Normal | Relaxed | Kyphosis Lordosis | Sway-back | Flat back | Stoop shoulder |

Figure 8-2 Examples of poor postures.

Technique

With fingers, elbows, fists, and forearms, intelligent pressure and friction are applied to shift the body's underlying structural features into a more stable state. Fascia, like wax, becomes soft and pliable when warmed by movement. Layers are slowly peeled off and pieced back together. The body is melted, molded, recast and integrated. It is shaped, sculpted, and given new form. Lines, angles, and definition are carved into blocks of muscle and bone. The fascia is stretched to create new boundaries that distinguish rather than separate.

The sensation of Rolfing is unique because its focus is on the tissue surrounding the muscle rather than the muscle itself. No oil is used to allow for the maximum amount of grip and friction and it feels more like being stretched like taffy as opposed to being kneaded like dough. The pace is much less rhythmic or undulating than other forms. Because Rolfing works deep into the body, people automatically assume that the work is painful, but Rolf herself worked on 4-month-old infants and on 90-year-old grandmothers. Any resistance to change, however, can be uncomfortable.

Taken piece by piece, the techniques closely mirror those of Myofascial Release. Much of their tools and actions are identical; however, their aims are completely different. Although both systems seek to release fascial

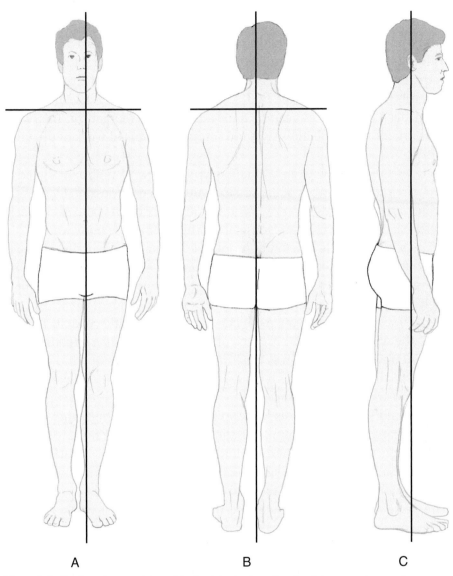

A   B   C

Figure 8-3 Posture is considered to be ideal when the body's mass is evenly distributed around the central axis that passes through the body's center of gravity.

holdings, the work of Rolf and her heirs is infused with streams of spirituality, philosophy, and psychology. Whereas myofascial work can affect a person at levels beyond the physical, that is not its strength nor is it its intention. Primarily myofascial treatment seeks to relieve pain and improve range of motion.

The Session

The transformational process that takes a random body and forges it into a unified whole has been formatted into a progression of 10 sessions. Each session builds upon the previous one and is synchronized to the natural unfolding of the body. The early sessions focus on releasing the superficial layer of fascia that encases the entire body, the body's "stocking." As the superficial fascia is stretched, deeper structures become freed and begin to reorganize. This is the groundwork for the more intensive and internally focused work of the later sessions.[6]

Each session begins with an evaluation, and homework may be assigned at the end to reinforce the work of the session. Although each session focuses on a specific part of the body, every session usually incorporates the neck, back, and pelvis so that clients enjoy a sense of having their whole body worked on. Pauses may interlace the session in order to evaluate the occurring changes and so that the therapist can check with clients to see how they're feeling. While every session has a specifically predetermined focus, each treatment is uniquely modified to accommodate the needs of the individual client.[7]

The first session works to open the chest to allow a greater capacity for respiration. The ribs, often adhered to each other and surrounding structures, are freed so they can open. This gives the lungs space to stretch out and expand. The increased capacity for breath results in greater oxygenation, which fuels the body and boosts its functioning.

The second session involves work on the aspect of the body that has the closest relationship to the ground—the feet and ankles. The feet are considered diplomats of the body sent to negotiate the terrain below. Processing of these areas establishes a greater sense of steadiness and support. They become like anchors attaching each step firmly to the ground.

The third session integrates and reinforces the earlier work. In addition, the shoulders, ribs, and pelvis are aligned. At the end of this session, the structure is decompressed and greater breath capacity is achieved. This is a critical juncture of the work and the patient is given the option to wait for a longer period before proceeding to the next phase, which involves integrating the core. Some practitioners have referred to this as the point of no return. Because of the sensitive nature of the emotions that are associated with this level of the body, work must progress proficiently towards resolution. Stopping in the midst of this next portion can leave issues exposed and unresolved.

The next four sessions focus on the deep fascial layers and the tissues close to the spine. Establishing a balanced pelvis is central to the work and is considered the keystone to the whole architectural framework. A distortion here can instigate complications throughout the whole system. If the objective of Rolfing were boiled down to a single motivation, it would be to align the pelvis horizontally while sitting the last lumbar vertebrae properly on the sacrum.[8]

By the seventh session, breathing has improved because the fascia around the neck, face, and skull that can constrict airflow through the nasal passages has been released. Following the end of the core-body session, many patients report the easing of emotional distress. While the work of the first seven sessions concentrates on the individual compartments of the body, the aim of the last three sessions is to integrate the entire body into a fluid whole.[9]

Throughout the process, clients are taught new ways of relating to their surroundings. Sessions may involve guided visualizations to help release particular areas of holding. They are taught new ways to look at their movement in relation to gravity and are given exercises that reinforce the work of each session. This educational process helps to maintain their newly aligned structure. After completion of the tenth session, additional, regularly scheduled maintenance sessions are recommended for a period of 6 to 12 months to help assure the positive changes and benefits gained become permanent.

Benefits

As with all modalities of the somato-psychic layer, benefits are achieved at both physical and psychological levels.

PHYSICAL BENEFITS

The following are some of the major physical benefits Rolfing clients may experience:

- Muscles, returning to their originally intended form and function, become strong, supple, and more capable.
- The body moves with greater ease and efficiency as fascial restrictions are eliminated.
- The internal organs are decompressed and as a result all of the body's functions (digestion, respirations, circulation, etc.) become improved.
- The body becomes longer, taller, and more defined and radiates a more youthful appearance.

PSYCHOLOGICAL BENEFITS

The following are some of the major psychological benefits Rolfing clients may experience

- an increased understanding of who they are and what their relationship to the world around them is meant to be.
- a greater feeling of ease derived from the neutralization of the tension created by constantly struggling against the force of gravity.
- a feeling of being more grounded, stable, and substantial.
- a greater feeling of trust, freedom, support, and openness.

To many, this process is life changing. For the first time they actually feel and understand what it means to be grounded, and this triggers a sense of wholeness and vitality. At the same time, clients may enjoy a freedom of expression that they've never experienced before. The transformation of some bodies may be visible throughout the process, but other bodies that are not ready may change little upon completion of the series. Years may pass before the body accepts the changes and realizes the new possibilities. Much of this depends upon the state of the client. While Rolfing can bring them to the verge of change, it is up to them to take the last step.

Who will benefit most from this type of therapy?

PERSONS WITH POSTURAL DEVIATIONS   Although almost anyone can benefit from Rolfing, those that have obvious postural deviations will show the most improvements. Whether the head is jutted forward, the back is hunched, the hips are twisted, or the feet are flat, dramatic changes are not uncommon—even if clients have been experiencing their problem for all or most of their lives.

Some postural deviations can be caused by damaged, shortened, or genetically deformed bones. Although these cannot be corrected with Rolfing, their negative effects can be vastly reduced. The body was meant to be a symmetrical unit, therefore when a deviation exists the body must compensate by creating unnatural patterns of strain and holding. Throughout the 10-session series, these negative patterns will be released and the client will be taught new ways of using their body that reduces pain, stress, and tension and allows greater mobility.

DANCERS   Because of the scrupulous focus on alignment, many dancers often look to Rolfing as the ultimate form of bodywork. And since their livelihood depends upon being open and moving freely, Rolfing is well suited to their needs.

Contraindications and Precautions

- Anyone with acute pains, illness or those with heavy addictions should defer Rolfing due to the intensive nature of the work.
- Persons with heart disease, cancer, closed-head injuries, or post-surgical conditions should seek a physician's permission before beginning any type of deep manipulation.
- The same contraindications as for Swedish massage should be observed.

Training of the Practitioner

Education

Schooling involves 650 hours of training, half of which is spent in lectures and the other half split between observations and practical hands-on work. Since this form of bodywork requires understanding of both the body and the mind, students must undergo a rigorous program of study that includes anatomy, physiology, kinesiology, and psychology. To become a Rolfing Movement Integrator, students must undergo an additional year of training.[10]

Licensing and Certification

To be called a Rolfer, practitioners must be trained and certified by one of the Rolf Institutes located in Boulder, Colorado; Melbourne, Australia; Sao Paolo, Brazil; and Munich, Germany. Licensing in massage therapy is a state-by-state issue and Rolfers must also hold a current license in massage therapy to legally practice in most states where the right to touch another person is generically outlined and mandated through state legislation. However most Rolfers do not consider Rolfing to be a form of massage therapy.

Other Requirements

Due to the intensive nature of the work, practitioners themselves must be in good health, possess physical **stamina**, and be fully committed to Rolfing.

SOMA NEUROMUSCULAR INTEGRATION

While one look at **SOMA Neuromuscular Integration's** family tree will provide a brief overview of the basic outline of this somato-psychic modality, to truly understand this form one must study its distinct nature. In some ways the distinguishing characteristics can be seen as a refinement of its parent model, Rolfing. However, its path seems to have moved it into a more scientific and intellectually based study than its sibling, Hellerwork. Whereas Hellerwork shines in the depth and complexity of its treatment sessions, Soma is brilliant in its approach to assessment and became one of the first systems of touch therapy to focus on a body-mind approach integrating specific soft tissue manipulation with psychological principles.

History

Bill Williams, Ph.D., and his wife, Ellen Gregory Williams, Ph.D., both trained in psychology, founded Soma in 1978. Together they created new ways of seeing and assessing the body and encouraged a more thorough exploration of the client's psychological realms. They viewed the body as a hologram, an exact three dimensional physical expression of a human's inner world including the thoughts, emotions, intuitions, spirit and whatever else makes a human being distinctly human. This allows a practitioner to read and come to know the whole human being though the body. In addition, viewing the body as a hologram provides greater access to more of the dimensions of a human at once then when dealing with only one or some of the parts. They also introduced a more flexible model of treatment that catered to greater personalization and individuality. They also developed new ways of affecting change and techniques for those changes to be more permanently embraced. Because of the greater emphasis placed on the importance of understanding and attending to the mental and emotional aspects of a person, this modality can be considered a deeper exploration of the somato-psychic layer of touch.

As a dedicated student and fellow researcher of Ida Rolf, Bill Williams realized that Structural Integration was so new and had such a dense body of knowledge that it could be developed in a new direction that Rolf herself had not explored. Due to his background of psychology and energy, he was compelled to delve more deeply into the internal world than Rolf, a biochemist, had desired. So Williams, with Rolf's blessing, created a sister system that has qualities distinctly its own.

Theory and Principles

Soma is an ancient Greek word that refers to the integration of body, mind, and spirit.[11] Its goal is to create structural and emotional changes by rebalancing and integrating the body's neuromyofascial system.[12] Although based on the same 10-session series as Rolfing, Soma's unique qualities readily distinguish it from its predecessor. In Soma, the process doesn't end with structural change. In fact, transformation of the body is merely the framework and sets the stage for the real journey to take place. It's not just about changing the body. It's about changing the body to transform the emotions. The real goal here is self-discovery.

Personalization

In the original Structural Integration, differentiation and integration of the client was of primal importance. In Soma, differentiation of the therapist is just as imperative. Soma acknowledges and appreciates the unique strengths of an individual and embraces each therapist's growth and development. If the therapist has a background in movement, exercise, or counseling, that becomes a principal element of the practitioner's approach. The therapists aren't simply taught to integrate others. They are also taught to integrate themselves. This fosters a community of sharing where practitioners can refer freely back and forth between each other.

Notebook

Generally speaking, the more people become engaged in an activity, the more they feel attached to it. In order to establish greater ownership of the changes that take place during treatment, clients are encouraged to participate as much possible. The first step for clients to become actively involved in their own transformation is simply becoming more aware of not only the treatment but also of their physical and psychological reactions to the treatment. In order to foster greater levels of self-awareness, clients are presented with a notebook in which they can journal their progress. This way they become part of the journey every step of the way.

The notebook also serves another vital function—to promote greater communication with their therapist, an important element when traversing potentially rough terrain. In addition, the notebook also contains useful techniques for self-relaxation and movement explorations.

The Three Brain Model

The process of differentiation is a process of optimization. When a function is required of a muscle in an undifferentiated body, it is unable to extend or contract to its fullest ability because it is stuck to other muscles and tissue in the surrounding area. It is only when the muscle is separated and given independence from the others that it is allowed to function at full force. Williams saw what a dramatic difference differentiation made on the physical body and he wondered what would happen if the same process was applied to the mind. He then developed the Three Brain Model.

Williams distinguished that there was not just one "brain" but three, each with different functions, capacities, and purposes (Figure 8-4). The left brain is the brain of logic. It is the brain of language, spatial details, and linear thinking. It is responsible for creating plans, policies, maps, and action-item lists.

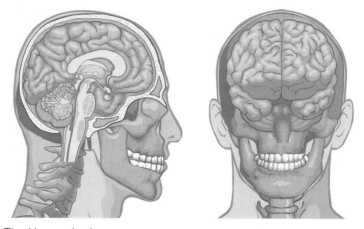

Figure 8-4 The Human brain. *Image copyright 2009, Oguz Aral. Used under license from shutterstock.com.*

In short, it is the brain of modern-day progress. This is the slowest of the three brains and is only capable of processing 16 bits of information per second. Because of its strict limits, this component always operates in a lag. This means that whenever we are in this mode we never really capture the absolute present. And since we are only taking in such a small part of an event, we never really enjoy the full experience.

Although left-brain logic is highly prized in today's culture, it wasn't originally intended to be engaged all the time like it is today. Its main function is to weigh, judge, and measure, and it was meant to be activated only when these actions were necessary. The only way that this brain can actually perceive is by comparison. It wasn't programmed to feel a sense of satisfaction or even to seek happiness. The only fulfillment it knows how to seek is to have more than something or someone else. Because of this it can never be satisfied. A person dominant in this hemisphere may always chase the picture of accomplishment without ever really attaining it. And because it can handle so little information, it quickly burns out, leading to nervous tension, anxiety, and feeling rushed, as if we never have enough time.

A vastly more powerful brain is the right brain. This is the brain of driving force. It gives energy to ideas and gives them wings to fly. This is the brain of daydream, reverie, and intuition. This is where we go to rest. Whereas the left brain looks to sort, define, weigh, and measure, the right brain reaches out to encompass, understand, integrate, and appreciate. Its capacities are limitless. This brain has the power to perceive beyond ordinary logic because it works in nonlinear ways. It reaches into the space of genius and is the brain that is responsible for flashes of inspiration and moments of brilliance that seem to come from nowhere. Because of this, the right brain is the favored realm of artists and thinkers. Compared to the left brain, the view from here is like seeing from another planet. Deepak Chopra eloquently describes this state as the "quiet moment between the thought."

The core, or the third brain, is also known as the central nervous system (CNS). This aspect is responsible for regulating all life functions such as digestion, respiration, blood circulation, and so on, as well as motor skills like riding a bike, playing tennis, and driving. It is also responsible for our lightning-quick reflexes. It has millions of responsibilities each day, which means that the amount of information that this brain can handle is astronomical compared to the left brain. Whereas the left brain can only handle 16 bits of information per second, the core is a monster that can engulf four volumes the size of War and Peace in the same span of time.[13]

While each brain has a time and place where it is most useful, we often become stuck in just one perspective and we end up approaching everything from that same mindset regardless of the situation. This is as ineffective as using one tool to do every job— like using a toothbrush to clean your teeth, wash the dishes, and scrub the floor. When we lose our ability to shift freely from one mode to another, we lose our freedom—we lose our ability to make a choice. But, according to Karen Bolesky of the Soma Institute, "When we choose how we respond and from which brain, we begin to experience life with greater energy and vision."

Assessment

In order to effect change at deeper levels, Williams realized that more facets of the human being had to be explored. He realized that it wasn't enough to look at just the physical structure to understand the true nature of the form. For lasting changes, Williams conjectured, he had to go inside that structure to allow its inner workings to be exposed.

Holographic Body Reading

Holographic Body Reading, an invention unique to Soma, is one of the new ways of "seeing" that was developed by Williams. It interprets the body as a hologram by viewing it as an exact physical expression of a human's inner world. This makes it easier to grasp how strain in one area will create a complex network of imbalance throughout the rest of the mind/body system. By providing a clearer and more thorough visual blueprint of the body's interrelating components, a more accurate and individualized roadmap to healing was conceived. This method of observation has been a valuable tool in quickly facilitating the ability of novice students to assess clients accurately.[14]

Drawing Interpretation

In addition to the photographs taken at each session to mark progress, clients are asked to engage in creating spontaneous drawings of how they feel before and after the 11 sessions. Although the physical landscape revealed in a photograph can be difficult to detect to the lay person, the subjective drawings created by clients provide an immediate and visceral representation of their internal world that can be more easily understood. These drawing interpretations, at times more telling than the photographs, provide a glimpse of the client's emotional world that often doesn't get to be expressed.

Somagraphy

It has long been understood by certain groups in the medical world that specific parts of the body pertain to specific emotions. Somagraphy is a tool used for identifying these somato-emotional regions in order to better comprehend the full spectrum of what the patient is experiencing. Often, methods like this can communicate vital information that even patients themselves may be unaware of.

The Sessions

The sessions are oriented in a similar fashion to that of Rolfing; however, each session is infused with the unique personally and psychologically engaging qualities of Soma. Each session is highly personalized according to what the client needs that day.

People seek Soma because they want to experience a shift in their lives, but like all transitions, the process can be uncomfortable, alarming even—especially when the deepest aspects of the body are being unlocked. Core work essentially shifts a person's entire foundation, thus the client is required to take on new meanings and come to terms with a new identity. These core sessions must be progressed through quickly because of the disorienting amount of emotion(s) that can be released. Before or after these core sessions, the amount of time lapsed in between treatments is relatively unimportant. Clients can choose to wait a week, a month, or even a year before their next session in the series. The beauty of this process is that the body remembers what it has learned. Even long after the sessions are complete, the body continues to assimilate the new knowledge. The body, remembering the lessons learned, applies them to the world again and again.[15]

The 11th Session

Based on the principles of SOMA Neuromuscular Integration, Somassage can either be the eleventh session of a Soma series or it can be a stand-alone treatment for those who are seeking just a singular or introductory treatment.

As the eleventh session, its role is to further the process of integration and to remind the body of all the changes that have taken place in order to reinforce the new principles of balance, alignment, and mechanics. It is like any change at the core level, it takes time to adapt to the new protocol. Somassage is used as a maintenance treatment and does not seek to facilitate any new structural changes. For this reason it is recommended that a full year is allowed for the SOMA series treatments to set in before any further structural work is pursued.[16]

As a regular stand-alone treatment for those who have not been through the SOMA series, **Somassage** is an energizing, full-body session designed to introduce elements of better alignment. It lengthens the body while working to integrate its connective tissue and increase global awareness of the body's connectedness.[17] Any changes, however, will be temporary since the foundational construct to retain those changes obtained through the SOMA series have not been established.

Benefits

The physical benefits may mirror those derived from Rolfing; however, because Soma also directly addresses a client's mental and emotional components, the benefits in these areas may be greater and more exact. Post-SOMA series bodies are more fluid, relaxed and energetic. They function with greater efficiency, rebound faster from injury and illness and are better able to generate and access their inherent power. Post-Soma series minds experience greater clarity and self-consciousness and tend to be more creative.

Contraindications & Precautions

One caveat that Soma practitioners will offer to their clients is that first and foremost the client must desire change, because this process will create it. If the client is not ready, he or she could feel violated. Otherwise the same contraindications and precautions for Rolfing should be observed.

Training of a Practitioner
Education & Certification

The SOMA Institute is located in Buckley, Washington. Courses during training include standards like anatomy and physiology, as well as more specialized education on social and psychological integration and neurofascial anatomy. Additional training can be attained in the Soma Advanced Bodywork Intensive.

Completion of its 656-hour training course is required to receive certification for SOMA Neuromuscular Integration and for Somassage. Although no separate license is required to practice SOMA Neuromuscular Integration, practitioners must abide by the particular laws of their state regarding touch which usually means they must fulfill their states' requirements for a license in massage therapy.[18]

HELLERWORK

Hellerwork is one of the new breeds of somato-psychic bodywork and incorporates the structural theories of Rolfing with the functional principles of movement therapy. At the same time, modern psychology is applied to achieve greater understanding of the body-mind construct and to attain deeper, more encompassing levels of healing. A trademark of this approach is its highly developed sessions that involve a multilevel method of peeling away the physical and underlying psychological components of an issue. Like the rest of the members of this tightly knit somato-psychic family, in this modality the mind-body is viewed as such a densely interwoven concept that either of these aspects can be used as the doorway for change to enter. However, to elicit the greatest response, Hellerwork holds open both doors at the same time.

History

Hellerwork is the life's work of Joseph Heller, a Polish immigrant who developed a detailed understanding and appreciation for the effects that stress had on structure as he was working as an aerospace engineer in a jet propulsion laboratory. His focus transitioned from machines made of metal, oil, and plastic to bodies made of flesh, blood, and bones in the mid-1900s when he was swept into the currents of the humanistic psychology movement. In these new waters he became involved with cutting-edge thinkers and pioneers of a new formula for the workings of the human being. A new passion evolved in him—one that involved the human body and its mysterious mind.

   Heller's unique practice of bodywork was crafted under the tutelage of some of the foremost healers of his time. Under Ida Rolf he developed a solid foundation of her 10-session transformative series and went on to become the first president of the Rolf Institute in 1976. With Judith Aston, pioneer in the field of human movement, and founder and developer of Aston Patterning®, he learned to propel the perfectly aligned structure into the most efficient lines of force and the most effective patterns of movement. And, in his studies with Brugh Joy, a progressive medical doctor, he was opened to the understanding of the powerful role that energy could play in healing.

Through the interplay of these various approaches, Heller's work fused into his own unique model while still maintaining and expressing the core principles of his previous teachings. In his studies with practitioners of various approaches, he realized that in order to create long-term change, it wasn't enough to deal with just the physical component of a dysfunction if there were underlying emotional adhesions that weren't being addressed. Also, it would do no good to fix something if the patient was continuously subscribing to habitual, pain-inducing patterns of movement. Therefore, it became imperative that work on restructuring the body was accompanied by both a reeducation of movement and a releasing of psychological tensions.

Theory & Principles

While structural integration states that the body speaks volumes, Heller went a step further to listen more intently to what the body was saying. In conventional communication, the body's experience must be translated into a verbal expression of that experience. In Hellerwork, practitioners train not only to listen to the body's raw, uncensored voice but also to "speak" to the body in a language it can immediately understand.

Dual Responsibility

One of the most profound aspects of this approach is the concept of dual responsibility. This is a team approach to healing that involves the client just as much as it involves the therapist. For the most profound changes to occur, clients' desire for change must match the therapist's desire to help them. Specifically for this reason, clients are asked to examine their own internal world so that they can take an active role in their own healing. Since obtaining an accurate picture of one's internal landscape depends much on the client's willingness to be open and forthright, a safe bubble of trust and honesty must be developed between client and therapist.

During this process it is important that the therapist never lose sight of how much courage it takes for their clients to delve into themselves and explore some of their fundamental issues. The therapist is essentially asking the client to excavate buried issues and this often requires them to face aspects of their lives that are uncomfortable, frightening, or even painful. Not everyone is willing to look at themselves in such an honest light. In a world where so many people look to others for change, it takes a certain strength, maturity, and determination to take a path that puts responsibility on one's own shoulders.

Although this can be seen as a more difficult path, it does come with rewards that match the efforts invested. With greater participation comes greater ownership. Not only do clients develop a deeper understanding of their bodies and emotions, they also end up having a stronger appreciation for the process. And since they were an active force in creating those changes, they end up feeling a much higher degree of responsibility for sustaining their new form. It is empowering in the same sense that teaching someone to fish is an infinitely greater act than just giving them something to eat.

Psychological Adhesions

In this layer of the massage and bodywork continuum, realigning the postures and patterns of the psychological body is just as important as creating changes in the physical body. While other somato-psychic forms of bodywork seek to create changes in the psychology by directly working on the physical, Hellerwork directly engages the psychological body to create change. This multilayered approach to the human being is the magic of Hellerwork. In this modality it is believed that only such an approach can create enduring changes, so restoring just one component without working on the others is seen as incomplete.

While adhesions in the physical body are unraveled with the hands, knuckles, and elbows, adhesions in the mental body are eased apart with carefully projected queries and commentaries. Even if the client is unable to provide an answer then and there, a seed has been planted that can blossom later. These "seed" questions burrow into the client's psychological body and, as they sprout, they beg the client to examine fundamental ideas of not only who they are but also, more importantly, who they can be. This process kneads away psychoemotional tension, and the very act of answering the questions often produces a relief that can only come from knowing where one stands on key issues.

The Session

Each session in this system revolves around a specific theme and the succession of themes is based on the timeline of our lives. The first three sessions explore the issues of our infancy; the following sessions delve into the subject of our adolescent years; and the final sessions explore the issues we must face in our adult life.

The theme of the first session is "inspiration." Since this is the first act that we perform when we are born into this world it makes sense that the work starts here. Air is a connective medium between us and our environment. This session explores how the client draws in the world around them, both literally and figuratively. Is breathing comfortable or does the client struggle? Is it open and even or constricted and choppy? Not only will this session explore the physical act of drawing air into the body, it will also explore sources of psychological, emotional, and spiritual inspiration with questions like, "What inspires you?" "How important is inspiration in your life?" And "When was the last time you felt inspired?"

The dialogue compels clients to step out of the monotonous stream of everyday thought to really examine what's going on in their lives. This process of reflection, even if only entertained for a moment, is a process of expansion. As the mind softens to examine the contents of the moment, the body responds by letting go. To examine oneself requires releasing one's wall of tension and temporarily abandoning one's self-imposed psychological borders in order to mingle freely with the world. It allows for the exploration of one's life and the context in which it is taking place. It is a moment of freedom from the confines of our own minds. Although the immediate outcome of this process may only produce a small change, even the slightest shift may be just the nudge clients need for positive changes to snowball into a landscape-shifting avalanche.

The next session, "Standing on Your Own Two Feet," deals not only with the obvious physical component of the legs and feet but also with the psychological topic of self-sufficiency. Work in this session is geared for greater "understanding" of our connection to our foundation. It's about our relationship to the ground below us that provides the support we need to either stand tall or propel us forward. Here we learn that to be self-sufficient and to "stand up" for ourselves, we need a firm foundation.

The third session, "Reaching Out," deals with the arms and the sides of the body. In this session the themes of giving, receiving, asserting ourselves, making contact and asking for what we need are explored. The sides support the arms but they are also an expression of how we stand by others in our relationships. When we are connected to our sides, the arms have a solid foundation on which to reach out to either give or receive support.

The core sessions strike upon primal concerns, and here the work begins to reflect topics of our adolescent years. In session four, "Control and Surrender," work is done to develop a greater sense of security about the surrounding environment and the people around you. It's about not being uptight while still "keeping it together." The idea is to develop a sense of a controlled surrender.

"The Guts" contain some of our deepest emotions and this is the subject of session five. This is the birthplace of convictions and intuition and this session is about becoming more aware of our "gut feelings." This is also the place where we receive and process both physical and emotional nourishment. For example, how our bodies handle food often parallels how we handle love in our lives.

"Holding Back," the theme of session six, is not only about the back of our body, but also about all the things that stifle us, limit our self-expression, and curb our creativity. This is where we bear our psychological burdens. All the emotions that became internalized—anger, sadness, worry, and so on, even excess joy,—become lodged in the muscles and tissues of our backs until they are released.

Session seven, "Losing Your Head," is about aligning the head properly over the shoulders while exploring ways to get out of our racing minds so that we can connect with the rest of our body. It's about restoring full range of motion to the muscles of our face that often grow so tense that we become restricted from the full freedom of expression we were meant to have.

Until now the work has been compartmental, but the goal here is to put it all together. The concluding sessions work to facilitate balance, alignment, and uniformity. Each structure is brought into proper relationship with the others and the system is integrated into a cohesive whole. Having faced issues of the developmental years, it is now time to define issues of maturity and adulthood.

Session eight is about balancing the lower half of the body—the pelvis that houses the womb and the legs that reach down to connect with mother earth. Here we are dealing with the feminine principle in everyone, both male and female. The feminine energy radiates and draws in rather than directing and seeking. It is about developing our receptive nature, learning to trust our intuitions, and becoming more understanding of processes.

The ninth session explores the theme of masculine power. The physical component is the upper body, mainly the chest and arms. These are the components of doing. They are our real and metaphoric tools of activity, insight, direction, and penetration. Although some things in our lives need to be attacked head on, this session teaches that we don't have to do it with stress and strain. Our culture, however, seems to believe otherwise, reflected in popular phrases such as "no pain, no gain." Here more powerful ways are explored of utilizing the masculine energy—ways that can only be achieved through ease, continuity, and grace. The lesson here is relaxed productivity.

The tenth session is about "Integration." As the name implies, this isn't about adding anything new; rather, it's about properly utilizing what already exists. Physically, the points of integration in the body are the joints. Freely moving, healthy joints parallel the definition of maturity. In children the joints are unstable and in the elderly the joints are rigid and stiff, but in the mature adult they are strong and stable yet free and open. This session looks at the entire body and work is done to allow each part to move freely so that it can operate as a cohesive whole.

The eleventh and final session is called "Coming Out." This session is a sort of debriefing before the client steps back out into the world. Generally, it is an interactive communication session with no bodywork. Together client and therapist review the process and address any issues that may still be lingering. This session is about looking back to move forward. This is a transitional point where the torch of responsibility is being handed down from therapist to client, but along with the burden of responsibility come the fires of empowerment. The integration that occurs here goes beyond the limits of the client's own personal body. The final lesson is about integration with the world.

Although completion is an emphasis here, it is really just a beginning. And like any journey, the participants have expanded their perspectives, forged new bonds, and developed a greater understanding of themselves and the world around them. This final session is about sustaining these bonds long after the journey is over.[19]

Afterwards, most people experience a fairly strong shift in their physical and emotional postures and patterns. Not only do they look more "together," they feel lighter and more energetic. They may also experience a sensation of being unburdened or unchained. The beauty of overcoming barriers, especially deeply ingrained ones, is that the self learns from these experiences and utilizes that knowledge again and again to catalyze change elsewhere. It sparks an empowering attitude that cascades through the rest of their lives.

Movement Education

Part of the 60 to 90 minute session is dedicated to a reeducation of movement, with the client standing, sitting, or walking. Coaching new patterns of movement is done through easy to remember but effective suggestions and visualizations that help clients rebalance their movement for optimal alignment and fluidity. Depending upon the practitioner, a variety of other methods can be utilized, for example video feedback, in order to enhance the process.[20]

Benefits

Both the physical and emotional/psychological benefits of Hellerwork mirror those derived from Rolfing and SOMA Neuromuscular Integration.

Contraindications

The same precautions as for Rolfing and SOMA should be observed.

Practitioner Training

To explore others, one must first explore oneself, and to develop as a therapist, one must first develop as a person. Because of this perspective of Hellerwork, students must first undergo the 11-session series before they can begin their training. They must study their own patterns and come to greater understanding of their own manifestations in order to work with people at deeper levels. And because a certain level of emotional maturity is required with this work, students must be 21 years of age or older before beginning their schooling.[21]

Education & Certification

Completion of a 1250-hour training program is necessary to become a certified Hellerwork practitioner. Training sessions are available in a variety of structures and are offered internationally. They can be in the form of intensive residential programs, weekend sessions, at-home mentorships, independent studies, or a combination of all of the above.[22] To maintain a practicing level, 36 hours of continuing education are necessary every 2 years. Practitioners can also take advantage of additional trainings offered by the association throughout the year.[23]

THE ALEXANDER TECHNIQUE

"For 100 years the Alexander Technique has been the performer's 'secret weapon' to breathe better, move and even bow better."[24]

The Alexander Technique is a branch of the somato-psychic layer of bodywork that seeks to achieve more intelligent and economical use of the self by directing the body in more effective patterns of movement. F.M. Alexander discovered that when simple reconfiguring was applied to the body's machinations, the body held itself in such a manner that many of the physical and emotional ailments disappeared. Along with the Feldenkrais Method, the Alexander Technique represents the functional integration portion of this layer. While the goal of optimizing the use of self is similar to that of structural integration, in this realm the dynamic principle of function is more important than the static element of form. Through what he termed "Better Use of the Body," Alexander created a system that strives to allow the body to be utilized to its fullest potential.

History

In the midst of his career as a Shakespearean actor, Frederick Mathias Alexander (1869–1955), founder and developer of the Alexander Technique, became plagued by loss of voice and slumps in energy that occurred in the middle of his performances. Inhibited by an ailment that doctors couldn't find rhyme or reason for, Alexander's career and livelihood were jeopardized, so he scoured the world of conventional medicine, but found nothing that could resolve his issues.

Guided by an intuition that told him his posture was the key, he took matters into his own hands. He toiled for ten years meticulously studying the correlation between form and function. By observing himself in a three-part mirror, he discovered that his loss of voice and drops in energy were directly related to specific postures and misalignments. Again and again as he intentionally placed his body in familiar postures, he witnessed himself experiencing the very same conditions that he experienced on stage. As his neck tightened and his head shifted back, his chest billowed out, and his throat became compressed. He lost energy quickly and his voice ran hoarse and dry. Then, to his amazement, he discovered that a series of simple adjustments in his posture allowed him to move with a new reservoir of energy while giving him command of a steady and projective voice.[25]

Although Alexander developed this technique to improve the quality and duration of his own acting career, he realized many others suffered ailments caused by the exact same problem—misuse of their body resulting in poor posture. With the remarkable efficacy of his work, he quickly gained an admirable following. Among those that subscribed to his method were George Bernard Shaw, John Dewey, William Temple, and the Archbishop of Canterbury. He is even credited with liberating the creative capacities of Aldous Huxley. With such esteemed members of the world society lavishing his method with gracious tribute, the Alexander Technique became fashionable and spread quickly throughout the world.

As successful as Alexander was, his work was almost lost due to the heavy casualties suffered in the Second World War. Among the deceased were many of Alexander's students. But in the 1970s, the pulse of the Alexander Technique quickened again and became revived with Nikolaus Tinbergen praising the technique during his acceptance of the Nobel Prize.[26] Today, the Alexander Technique is one of the oldest methods of bodywork still practiced in the western world.

Theory & Principles

The Whole Person

Alexander found that each step, each breath, each movement, was not just the segregated act of one limb or one component, rather it was the engagement of the entire being at every level. It involved muscles, nerves, thoughts, and emotions. For a person to do one thing, every part of that person had to be involved. In this light, the idea of creating change becomes an intimidating undertaking, but Alexander discovered the central control mechanism that could reign over the entire animal. Via the proper calibration of the head, neck, and torso he found that he could lead the entire body. He called the management of these body components primary control. Rather than being a rigid and static position, primary control is a dynamic relationship that is in constant fluctuation. It is the mastery of this core component that is the foundation of Alexander's work.[27]

When this technique properly exercised the head floats up gracefully, perching forward at the top of the spine as the neck releases. The spine and torso should be long, floating up and away from the legs. The pelvis also floats up with the rest of the torso and the head to lift and lengthen away from the legs, which are reaching down to connect solidly with the ground. The chest and back should be expansive, filling out to the sides, and the ribs just hang comfortably upon the structure. (Figure 8-5)

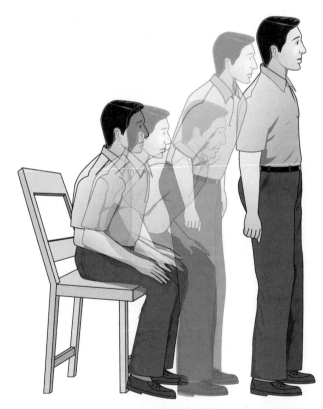

Figure 8-5 An Alexander Technique demonstrating the stages of getting up from a chair properly.

In this position, air flows the most freely from lung to throat to outer world and back again. With full oxygenation, blood enjoys a richness of energy and the body is given new vitality. Nerve impulses and commands pass without interference through the spinal canal and into the organs allowing full composition of power to reach each muscle fiber, cell, and tissue. Organs are no longer compressed and are given the freedom to function fully, becoming more efficient producers of energy and cleansers of waste. Brain functioning, including the accuracy of memory and the speed of thought processes, become heightened. In short, the whole body-mind becomes more alive.

Inhibition and Direction

Alexander's initial experiments in activating what he called "proper use" was met with the almost overwhelming strength of his own habits. He found that he could accomplish nothing through sheer force. He realized that he could no longer trust his perception of what was natural and right for his own body. Instead he had to go against his mechanical unfolding and direct the body by projecting a somato-psychic command. Stopping himself just as his body was about to reenact a habitual pattern, he would say to himself, "Allow the neck to be free to allow the head to go forward and up so that the back may lengthen and widen." This process of restraining the old pattern came to be called "inhibition."[28] Only after inhibition can the process of reconstruction begin.

Following inhibition, a new directive is given to the body to coordinate better use of the self. These directives are based on Alexander's Four Principle Commands:

1. Think longer
2. Think wider
3. Let the back open
4. Let the legs separate from the torso

These directives are to be accomplished all at once and one after another. While thinking longer one should think wider and at the same time the back should be allowed to open while the legs are allowed to separate from the torso. This way each direction builds upon one another rather than replacing the one before, so that all are accomplished simultaneously.

The Mind and Body

Like everyone else, Alexander was bred to believe that the mind and body are separate entities; however, during the course of his research and experimentation he came to the all-important revelation that the distinction existed only in theory. Although at first the suggestion of allowing the head to float forward and up was just a thought—nebulous and without form—with each successive practice the previously distinct ideas of thinking and doing became fused until thinking became indistinguishable from doing. Again and again the experiential evidence was clear— physical form was merely the solidification of thought. To give an understanding of this principle, Michael Gelb, author of *Body Learning,* provides a simple exercise:

"Direct your attention to your right hand without moving it at all in space. Focus on the index finger of the right hand as if you were intending to point the finger still further in the direction in which it is already pointing, but remember not to move it at all. Look at whatever your finger is pointing towards and sharpen the thought of your finger pointing towards it. This act of attention alone may have produced a change in the muscle tone of the finger . . . you will probably notice that the same subtle yet heightened degree of muscle tone can be maintained. When your attention is drawn away from your finger, the heightened tone decreases, although it is possible to bring it back at will . . ."[29]

The Teacher

Since this is a system of education, the relationship between the client and practitioner is that of student and teacher. Teachers should be the embodiments of the rules and principles of the technique. Their bodies should be long, graceful, and free flowing, moving with liquid precision as one unit. Each movement is the logical expression of the movement before it. They must not only be armed with theoretical knowledge, but with experiential knowledge as well. They must be able to feel where their students are locked or tight as if it was their own body. They must know how to communicate with not only the body but also the mind of the muscles as well. They must learn to develop fluency in the language of the body that can only be learned by experiencing the transformation themselves. Only then will they be able to effectively bring another human being to the state which they themselves have worked to achieve.

The Session

Although this is a gentle process, because of the focus and mentation required for the transformation it is both a physically and psychologically challenging quest that requires the proper calibration of opposing forces to achieve the ideal balance. This calls for a steady reservoir of time and patience.

The first step towards achieving the ideal is to become more aware of the body in space. These days we are so disconnected from our bodies that for many, developing the kinesthetic awareness to a degree high enough to accurately recognize the true positioning of their body is a leap in consciousness. Attaining a realistic recognition of one's positioning is critical to the process because to go anywhere, one must first know where one is. Only then can the real possibilities of change be explored. Here, students come to realize that not only are they performing suboptimally but, more importantly, that they can do better. They come to a point of empowerment—a point where they have a choice to either slide back into the old, harmful patterns of misuse or to choose a healthier, more effective path.

Each session typically lasts 30 to 60 minutes, with the student wearing loose, comfortable clothing, and takes place both on and off the massage table depending upon the training of the practitioner and the needs of the student. The length of the process is different for each individual. Some bodies progress quickly and efficiently while others take time to unwind. A series of about 30 sessions spaced 1 to 2 weeks apart is recommended, followed by a break to allow the work to take root and solidify. Afterwards, periodic refresher courses help crystallize the changes. While group sessions are offered, the lessons are more commonly one-on-one. The session can then be tailored to the individual's needs and the exercises will reflect activities related to his or her daily life.

A large part of the session is just feeling the body in space—becoming more aware of where we are and what we are capable of. Our long spines can stretch and lengthen to give us a posture that is erect and attentive, yet relaxed and responsive. We can feel our legs as extensions of the trunk, reaching all the way down to the ground beneath us. We can feel our chests become open and expansive as our shoulders relax and fall down to create a look and feel of grace, and calm readiness. We can feel our backs lengthen and loosen—supporting the body, but not straining.

Pain in the body is not always addressed directly. Since pain is seen as the result of inefficient and disconnected patterns of movement, the student is taught new patterns of movement that are efficient, connected, and pain free. To achieve this, the teacher utilizes a combination of active and passive mobilizations. Since the Alexander Technique is about learning to acquire better use of the body, most of the work is done during movement, including sitting, standing, and walking.

Throughout the session, the teacher guides the body with his or her hands into proper positioning while offering reinforcement through verbal coaching, such as, "Neck long, chest wide." Students may also be asked to think about their head as a balloon filled with helium or to visualize their back smiling.[30] When the positive pattern is appropriately performed, the small victory is celebrated with supportive praise such as, "That's it! "Nice and long!" "Good job!" Eventually the mixture of verbal and tactile messages become ingrained into the mind and the muscles while the healthy patterns of movement are methodically adopted into the student's daily life. Slowly but surely, the undesired patterns are displaced and fade away.

Benefits

Almost everyone exposed to the Technique inevitably feels taller, lighter, and more poised. Once the proper structural alignment is achieved, the body functions with marked improvement across all levels. Organs, now uncompressed, begin to function robustly. The lungs open to achieve higher levels of respiration, blood circulates with greater force and vitality, and the mind works with greater focus and intent. Less energy is siphoned off by sloppy, disjointed movements as more efficient use of the body is achieved. Motion becomes graceful and elegant as the body enjoys the freedom allowed by the adherence to an integrative principle.

Unity is achieved and from that unity extends power, grace, and presence.

Who the Alexander Technique will benefit

- The elderly, especially if they have trouble with everyday movements like getting out of bed, bending down, sitting, or standing up. The Alexander Technique can restore coordination and vitality.
- Performers whose bodies are their livelihoods (actors, dancers, musicians, etc.). This system can help them gain fuller use of their bodies (Figure 8-6).
- Those with physically demanding jobs requiring lifting, moving, and bending. Workplace-related injuries are often caused by poor mechanics.
- Persons with poor posture.
- Those wishing to sustain changes from other forms of bodywork.
- For those who want to take their inner lives to the next level, the Technique has been revered for unlocking the creative capacities of the likes of Aldous Huxley.

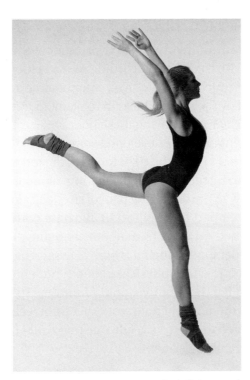

Figure 8-6 Performers who use their body to make their livings gain great benefits from Alexander Technique. *Image copyright 2009, AYAKOVLEVdotCOM. Used under license from shutterstock.com.*

Contraindications

Because of the gentle nature of this system, there are no contraindications. The teacher will work around whatever issue the student may be facing.

The Training of a Practitioner

It is only after long training as a student that practitioners can become teachers themselves. 1600 training hours must be completed over the course of at least three years. The minimum number of teachers is one for every five students. The American Center for the Alexander Technique (ACAT), which has trained almost half of all the teachers in the United States, limits their enrollment to only 12 new students per year.

The world of the Alexander Technique is regulated by several bodies of professional organizations. These include the North American Society of Teachers of the Alexander Technique (NASTAT), the Society of Teachers of the Alexander Technique (STAT) in London, England, and the ACAT in New York City. Standards are strict across the board and quality of training is a primary focus.[31]

THE FELDENKRAIS METHOD®

The **Feldenkrais Method** involves discovering new ways of making better and better choices with the body. According to Dr. Feldenkrais, this is hugely important because so much of the physical, emotional, and mental stress that we experience is caused by the poor choices in movement that we make on a daily basis. A determining factor in making these poor choices is the relatively small repertoire of movements we have developed compared to what is required of us. In other words, we aren't using the right tools for the job and therefore we end up compromising our integrity through a lifetime of incorrect use of the body, which leads inevitably to the damaging pain of stress, strain, and degeneration.

Feldenkrais developed his method to alleviate conditions arising from such stress, but his method wasn't just about changing the body. It was about changing the entire person through the body. He saw the body as a vehicle to reach not only greater levels of physical freedom but emotional and intellectual liberty as well. Like the other visionary founders in the somato-psychic layer of the massage therapy and bodywork spectrum, Feldenkrais was an idealist, and he considered the body as a gift, one that could be utilized to achieve his highest aim—self-empowerment.

History

Moshe Feldenkrais, a Russian-born Israeli, enjoyed an array of careers as an electrical engineer, nuclear scientist, and physicist, from which he amassed a formidable knowledge of universal laws and principles. He combined this experience with the practical knowledge of the human body earned from his extensive training in the martial arts, and this fashioned a deep and profound understanding of the human potential.

Although he came from a rich intellectual background, he was well grounded in his physical body. He was an avid sportsman and is credited with bringing judo to the western world.[32] It was this love of sport that actually led him to his defining moment. When suddenly crippled by a knee injury so debilitating that doctors weren't sure if he would walk again, an important and curious realization occurred that caused him to believe that this was something he himself could correct. At first, the injury got worse and this caused him to wonder if it was the way in which he reacted towards it that made it degenerate. He began to think that if the way in which he acted towards the injury could make it worse, then perhaps the opposite action could make it better.[33]

He began exploring with this line of thought and submerged himself deeper into human anatomy, physiology, and neurophysiology. He infused this newfound knowledge with his already extensive understanding of physics, engineering, body mechanics, and martial ,arts, and eventually was able to reeducate his body and regain full functioning of his knee. But even though he met with such extreme success, he wasn't fully sure how it happened, so he set out to understand the mysterious mechanisms of his healing. Although he had made a complete recovery, it wasn't until 40 years later that he was able to achieve the precise balance of knowledge and understanding to perfect his method.[34]

His work garnered momentum and inspiration from other influential bodyworkers of his time, and his theories are reminiscent of his contemporaries. He was a close personal friend of Ida Rolf, with whom he shared a common fascination for the science of form and function. And as an admirer of Alexander's work, he often recommended Alexander's book *The Use of Self* to his students. Once his system had sufficiently matured, Feldenkrais catalyzed the spread of his knowledge by utilizing the already established Esalen Institute of California as a launch pad for his work. He began a series of trainings in the United States starting in 1972, continuing until his death in 1984.[35] In his time he trained hundreds of teachers to carry on his life's work, and through his efforts the Feldenkrais Guild was formed that today not only trains new practitioners but maintains standards of practice as well.[36]

Theory and Principles

The great desire of Moshe Feldenkrais was to help people live life to their fullest potential by teaching them the art of learning. This is a different process of education than the verbal or mental learning that occurs in school, which he saw as incomplete and out of touch with the physical component of the human organism. True learning involved the use of not only the mind, but the entire body as well. This method of "body learning" is called **somatic education**.[37]

Change must begin by breaking down the ordinary everyday movements that one does a million times a day. That which is basic and taken for granted must be questioned. For instance, what happens when you go from seated to standing? Most people overexert themselves using more force than necessary, needlessly tensing and contracting the back of their necks in anticipation of the movement and then pushing down into the floor with their feet before the rest of the body is ready to follow. One action doesn't flow into the next and a disconnected, staccato progression unfolds.

By producing an expanded and refined repertoire of movement, a more unified functioning of the self is achieved. Muscles work with greater ease and relaxation. Sensations become pleasant. Feelings become light. Thoughts become more composed. The world is approached with more love and greater understanding. In short, we become better human beings.

The exploration of new physical paths triggers the exploration of parallel paths in the students' lives. Pain in the body is often dealt with indirectly since it is viewed as merely a sign that something is wrong as opposed to being the problem itself. A new thought process develops to look beyond the most superficial aspects of an issue. New awareness is brought to students' limitations and with this awareness comes the understanding that these limitations can be stretched to new forms and greater dimensions. Perception opens to encompass new possibilities and among these possibilities are choices that allow more freedom and greater mobility in not only one's physical body, but throughout one's entire life.

> "What I'm after isn't flexible bodies, but flexible brains. What I'm after is to restore each person to their human dignity."
>
> —Moshe Feldenkrais

Childhood Roots

Feldenkrais believed that nearly our entire repertoire of movement was learned during the first few years of our lives. Our methods of responding to stress become habitually developed and then quickly become concretized. We confine ourselves to just a few basic patterns and rarely deviate from those originals. Over and over again we program ourselves to respond in the same way even if the nature of the stress is different. This breakthrough insight came from a crucial opportunity afforded him by his wife, a pediatrician.

By observing children growing up he witnessed their natural, buoyant movements become sabotaged as they grew older. Our earliest postures, he found, are supplied to us from parents or other role models, and he realized that the physical pain and mental stress that we experience as adults are rooted in childhood development. Children naturally imitate adults that they admire and just as when they try on daddy's hat and tie or mommy's make-up, children try on their postures. (Figure 8-7) Feldenkrais saw how we disfigure our movements and allow poorly fitting postures to weigh rigidly onto our frames. Even if the postures didn't suit them or were uncomfortable, he noted they would still latch onto them and make them their own. We become used to these poor patterns of movement and we identify ourselves with and by them. This brought him to wonder—if we accept pain as a part of our daily lives and tell ourselves it's ok to suffer, what else might we tell ourselves? Feldenkrais

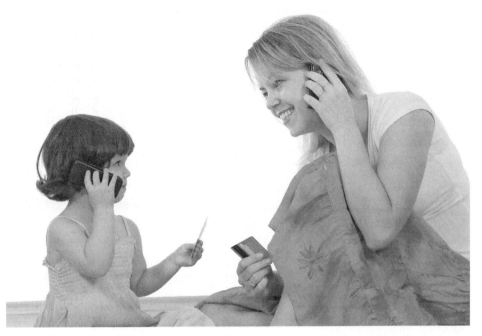

Figure 8-7 Our earliest postures are supplied to us from parents or other role models. *Image copyright 2009, Szocs Jozsef. Used under license from shutterstock.com.*

theorized that we became so limited in our range of movement that out of all the motions that our bodies are capable of producing we end up utilizing only 5 percent of our total potential.[38]

These habits of movement that we develop as children impact the way we approach our entire lives. The habitual postures affect not only physical health, but intellectual and emotional performance as well. Even though dysfunctional postures can lead to health problems, physical injury, and poor self-esteem, they have been so ingrained into our lives that we are no longer even aware of them.

Although we have formed a life-long relationship with these patterns, the nervous and muscular systems are so adaptable that they can unlock and even reverse long-established patterns. When the body is introduced to a superior form of movement, it is immediately recognized, and as the body and brain achieve greater levels of communication, new neural pathways develop. A burst of growth occurs as the brain recognizes a new ease and efficiency with which the body is moving. A greater cohesion is achieved between commander and soldier, alleviating a certain stress and tension that always accompanies vague and undefined relationships.

The Human Quartet

Feldenkrais saw the human being as a composition of four ingredients:

1. Movement
2. Sensation
3. Feeling
4. Thought

In every moment, he theorized, all four components are present and are actively intermingling. Because each unit is hardwired into the others, change created in one will ripple through the other three. For example, the feeling of anger will cause tension in the face and jaw, while creating terse and choppy movements. At the same time, the senses will be enlivened and thoughts will become focused and piercing. Or, if one is contemplating the negative aspects of life, the body will produce a posture that matches the depressing pictures in one's head. Sensations will be dull, the body will appear limp and ragged, and movements will be slow and laborious.

The Neural Connection

Although this process of change can begin anywhere, Feldenkrais came to believe that the moving component contained the richest potential for change. Early in his research, Feldenkrais intuitively came to believe that the power of the nervous system must be tapped in order to make real and lasting changes. The nervous system is what allows the brain to communicate with the rest of the body (Figure 8-8). When we are first born, the neural connections are so weak that we can't even lift our heads, much less speak or walk. These neural connections literally have to be built and developed through repetition. As we grow older, the neural connections grow stronger and so does our ability to perform normal functions like walking, talking, riding a bike, or driving a car. Unfortunately, as these normal functions become reinforced and ingrained into our systems, so do our negative tendencies.

During his own healing process, Feldenkrais worked heavily with the nervous system, and he came to the discovery that the nervous system was more occupied with movement than any of the other three components. He concluded that in order for the deepest possible levels of change to take place, the nervous system must be intimately involved.[39]

Another key factor for targeting movement was that it lends itself as the most accessible. Thoughts, feelings, and sensations are much harder to observe than movement, and many people don't even realize their emotional

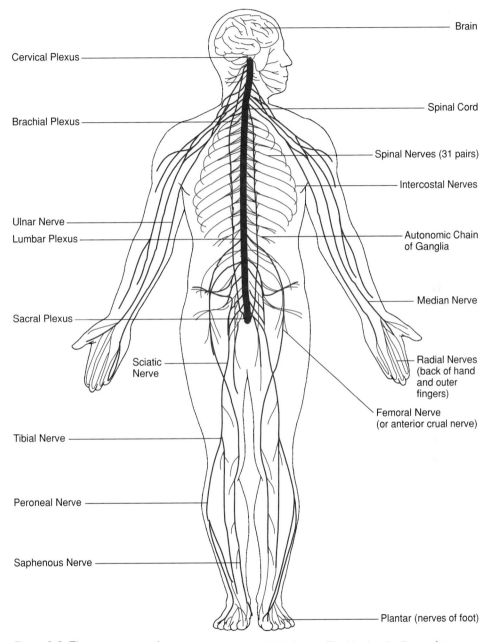

Brain

Cervical Plexus

Spinal Cord

Brachial Plexus

Spinal Nerves (31 pairs)

Intercostal Nerves

Ulnar Nerve

Lumbar Plexus

Autonomic Chain
of Ganglia

Median Nerve

Sacral Plexus

Sciatic
Nerve

Radial Nerves
(back of hand
and outer
fingers)

Femoral Nerve
(or anterior crual nerve)

Tibial Nerve

Peroneal Nerve

Saphenous Nerve

Plantar (nerves of foot)

Figure 8-8 The nervous system.   *Image copyright 2009, Patrizia Tilly. Used under license from shutterstock.com.*

or mental strain until they feel it physically. In order for people to engage confidently in a process of change, they need evidence that is concrete and recognizable.

> "So smart is the brain when we permit it that even after doing something a million times the wrong way, doing it right even one time feels so good that the brain-body system recognizes it immediately as right."
>
> —Moshe Feldenkrais, *The Humanist*

The Lessons

The Feldenkrais Method is not something that is done to you, rather it is something that is experienced. Unlike medical doctors, Feldenkrais practitioners are not authority figures. They don't tell you how to do things "right." They assist students in finding the unconscious blockages that blind their organic sense of what is right for their own individual bodies. As students get out of their own way, they are allowed to be the person they've always wanted to be.[40]

As with the Alexander Technique, the therapist is called a teacher, and like any good teacher their job is to provide a nourishing environment where boundaries can be stretched and redefined. They address disorganizations of the body and it is their job to tell the client what's working, what needs to be improved, and what needs to be dispensed with. They study the client's strengths and weaknesses, formulate a plan, and offer recommendations on how the plan can be implemented—but ultimately the work is up to the client.

Clients, considered students, are shown a new range of choices and are given options where no options existed to them before. With these newfound possibilities, it is their job to make the right decisions. Students learn to inhibit certain habitual neuromuscular activities while choosing more appropriate ones. So effective is somatic education that moving correctly just one time can permanently alter the body's programming. Each lesson learned is carried beyond the boundaries of the session and seeps into the minutes, hours, and days of the student's life. It is an organic process that gradually builds a momentum of healthy patterns while little by little weeding out patterns that are ineffective and detrimental.

2 Formats

Feldenkrais lessons are available in two formats, individual or group sessions. Both are done wearing loose, comfortable clothing. The one-on-one sessions came to be known as Functional Integration sessions while group classes are called Awareness Through Movement, or ATM.

THE FUNCTIONAL INTEGRATION SESSION   The individual session, Functional Integration, affords the student the full attention of the teacher; therefore, greater change at a more rapid pace can be expected. These sessions are tailored exactly to the individual's needs and the pace and content of each session will reflect his or her specific conditions.

The session begins with the student lying down on a low padded table. The first aspect of the session is to become aware of the body—its heaviness, its shape, its form, its positions, and its contours. Since it is only by recognizing the depths of how one moves that can produce real change, great emphasis is placed on becoming more aware of the minute details of one's unconscious movements. According to Feldenkrais, awareness equals control. Since you can't control something you are not aware of, the lesson begins here.[41]

Range of motion, flexibility, and areas of constriction are assessed and together the student and teacher analyze and discuss in detail the results of the student's movements. Inefficient patterns are brought to the student's awareness and, through gentle touch, new movements are suggested—never forced. The teacher guides the student's body through an arrangement of movements and weaves a new language to allow the body to express itself more fully. Throughout each movement, the attention is brought back again and again to the body. Gradually, a more dynamic range of possibilities is created, giving the client a more appropriate arsenal of choices to replace their old and ineffective patterns.

How long a client works with a practitioner depends upon the aim of the client. If the client is seeking relief from a specific issue, he or she may discontinue sessions as soon as the issue is resolved. Those who come to explore deeper levels of themselves may stay longer or take lessons on more a consistent basis. For those that are looking to enhance performance, reach the next level, or stay at the top of their game, the Method may be a regular component of their training.

AWARENESS THROUGH MOVEMENT CLASSES   Awareness Through Movement (ATM) classes last 30 to 60 minutes and are done in groups. Students are led through gentle movements that involve thinking, sensing, and imagining. These movements are often based on practical activities like reaching, lying, sitting, and looking behind, and they gradually develop from the simple and basic to the more complex and sophisticated.[42]

The full spectrum of exercises composed by Feldenkrais number over a thousand, but only a few hundred have been translated into English. Out of these, one exercise becomes the focus for the entire class.[43] The exercises are not exercises in their usual sense. The movements are small, tiny even. Each movement should be as easy as possible with as little effort as possible. Everything is slow, gentle, and infused with awareness. Although the movements are enjoyable and articulated with frequent breaks, the amount of concentration required can be fatiguing.

The teacher provides verbal guidance through a structured sequence of movements designed to explore the broad range of movement choices that a student has available. Often, visualizations are used to accompany the physical movements. No one is pushed beyond their level of ability, but they are encouraged to meet it. Working with one's own body and finding its own path through the movements is emphasized, and attention is constantly refocused to develop greater self-awareness.

Beginners start by lying on the floor in order to reduce the amount of interference from muscular tension that arises when sitting or standing. This allows them to be relaxed and more sensitive to subtle shifts of tensions within the body. First, the awareness is brought to the body. Here, with just a moment of sincere attention, areas of tightness and imbalance can be discovered.

Movements begin small and precise so that a simple turn of the head or raising of the arm absorbs the entire attention. The tiny movements bring small details of one's own body alive and one can feel the finer and subtler experiences of the body—the heaviness of a limb, the stiffness of a joint, or the effort of a muscle to produce even these miniscule movements. As the session develops, one begins to realize the dynamic relationship of one part of the body to another. A movement of the hips may cause muscles around the shoulders to tighten. A lifting of the head may be felt in the lower legs. Little by little the class progresses, weaving together broken strands of movement until the entire body works as a united whole.

The inherent but often forgotten relationship between students and their bodies can be revealed just after one session, but learning to master that relationship can take a lifetime. The process requires time, patience, and dedication. Because of this, lessons are often offered in a series of four to six sessions that meet once a week. Once the exercises are mastered, the students can practice them at home, but serious or chronic cases may take longer. Often a teacher will organize a series of classes to address a specific condition such as TMJ, low-back pain, or stress.

The Method is a gentle form of bodywork and pain or strain is not a requisite for improvement. If the student feels pain, he or she should bring this to the attention of the teacher. If a movement is strenuous or uncomfortable, the student needs to do less or take a break. Many people have come to equate force with effectiveness, but in this system it's not about strengthening, it's about integrating. It's about creating a seamless whole. Often students express surprise at how something so gentle can create such dramatic changes.

It's also not about doing it right or wrong. It's about exploring one's own, individual possibilities. This is how the greatest benefit will be achieved— when there is no worrying about "getting it." Last but not least, the lessons should be fun. It is in this open, dynamic, and evolving state that the ultimate goal of Feldenkrais can be realized.

Benefits

Integration carries with it a feeling of lightness and relaxed clarity and the benefits resonate throughout all the systems of the body. When the body works in concert, movements come with greater ease and efficiency. What may have been restricted and painful before now becomes free, fluid, and dynamic. When muscles fire properly and work in unison, their strength and ability multiplies. As the body learns to work together, discordant tensions become dissolved. The chest and diaphragm relax, which then allows the lungs to stretch and expand to full capacity. The whole body becomes enlivened and one's sense of vitality becomes heightened.

Overall daily tasks become much easier because less energy is siphoned off via muscle strain and tension. As alignment improves, much of the body's issues work themselves out. Relief is found from neck, back, shoulder pains, headaches, jaw pain, joint pain, TMJ, carpal tunnel syndrome, and so on.

Among those that have benefited from the Feldenkrais Method are Margaret Mead, the famous anthropologist, Julius Erving, the basketball star, Yo Yo Ma, the cellist, Peter Brook, the director, Yehudi Menuhin, the concert violinist, Whoopi Goldberg, the actress, and the first prime minister of Israel, David Ben-Gurion, who dubbed Feldenkrais a "national treasure."[44]

Who will benefit most from this modality?

- The elderly—especially if they have trouble with everyday movements like getting out of bed, bending down, sitting, standing up, and so on.
- Anyone who has difficulty moving on a day-to-day basis due to pain, weakness, imbalance, or decreased/limited range of motion.
- Those suffering from neurological disorders caused by stroke, cerebral palsy, and multiple sclerosis.
- People who have physically demanding jobs or jobs that require repetitive lifting, moving, bending, standing, cutting, and so on. Workplace-related injuries are often caused by poor mechanics.

- People with poor posture.
- Those wishing to sustain changes from other forms of bodywork.
- People looking to improve the way they look and feel.

Contraindications/Precautions

No contraindications. The Feldenkrais Method is a gentle, noninvasive form of therapy that will not interrupt or interfere with any other treatments, conditions, or medications. However, in the case of an acute or traumatic condition, it may be necessary for the client to work with another form of therapy prior to working with a Feldenkrais practitioner.

The Training of a Feldenkrais Practitioner

The Feldenkrais Guild of North America, established in 1977 by Moshe Feldenkrais, is the official organization of Feldenkrais practitioners and offers training based upon his teachings. Only those that have been personally trained by Dr. Feldenkrais or that have graduated from a Guild Accredited training program can use the following service-marked terms:

- Awareness Through Movement®
- Functional Integration®
- Feldenkrais®
- Feldenkrais Method®
- Guild Certified Feldenkrais Practitioner[cm]
- Guild Certified Feldenkrais Teacher®[45]

Although practitioners can be found internationally, schooling is only available in 11 states in this country. Training involves 800 to 1000 hours over a 3- to 4-year process. Students learn through lessons, lectures, discussions, and videos of Dr. Feldenkrais in which he discusses Newtonian mechanics, physics, neurophysiology, and movement development. Trainees must first acquire a deep understanding of their own movement in order to effectively transmit the knowledge to others. Eventually, trainees teach ATM and Functional Integration lessons under the professional supervision of a teacher-practitioner.[46]

CRANIOSACRAL THERAPY

Craniosacral therapy is a subtle form of bodywork that uses light touch and holding to affect the systems that are at the very core of the human body—the brain, spinal cord and the entire fascial system that surrounds and emanates from them. Because the technique is to tap into the craniosacral rhythm (CSR), caused by the movement of the cerebral spinal fluid that runs through the fascia, only small amounts of pressure are needed to create waves of change. Through this work, practitioners of craniosacral therapy are able to improve a wide array of conditions, including migraines, autism, nervous system disorders, learning disabilities, chronic fatigue, and more.[47] In addition, craniosacral therapy is also very useful in relieving the physical pain and emotional discomfort that has arisen from old traumas.

History

The roots of craniosacral therapy can be found embedded in the grounds of a branch of medical science called **osteopathy**. This form of medicine began in the nineteenth century with Dr. Andrew Still, a civil war surgeon who became disillusioned with conventional medicine when his three children died during an epidemic of meningitis.[48] Eschewing the unsanitary surgical conditions and crude pharmaceuticals of his time, Dr. Still developed an approach to health and healing that relied primarily on exercise, body manipulations, and lifestyle changes. At first, Dr. Still's work was received coldly by the medical profession and was dismissed as mere quackery, but eventually it came to be an accepted form of medical practice that still abounds today. The term *osteopathy* is really a misnomer because it literally means "bone disease." In reality, osteopathy benefits the whole of the body—not just the bones.

The next leap in the evolution of cranial-based therapy came with the work of Dr. William Garner Sutherland in the 1900s. At the American School of Osteopathy (now known as the Kirksville College of Osteopathic Medicine) there was a display case containing a skull that had been laid out into its separate fragments. Young Sutherland had passed by this display many times, but one day something about the separated pieces of bone caught his mind with a compelling thought. As a student of osteopathy he had always been taught that the structure of something was determined by the function it was created for. So what did it mean, then, that the bones of the skull appeared to be made to move? This observation conflicted with the accepted scientific knowledge that the entire skull was a fixed and immobile unit except for the obvious exception of the jaws. At the time, William Sutherland wasn't sure what he saw, but he knew he saw something significant. The full force of his discovery wasn't realized until years later when he took it upon himself to quietly study the phenomenon that had rooted in his mind.

In a quest for his own answers, Dr. Sutherland, a graduate by this time, devised a special helmet that exerted a controlled pressure on the various bones of the skull and wore this helmet while recording its effects. His wife, too, helped record her husband's behavior, moods, and bodily functions during the experiment and developed her observations into a book of her own. Based on the data he and his wife collected, Dr. Sutherland developed a sophisticated system of therapy, complete with its own methods of diagnosis and treatment. His studies had found it to be quite effective, yet he knew the skepticism with which his colleagues might view his work. Because of this, Dr. Sutherland published his findings under the pseudonym "Blunt Bone Bill."[49]

He also called his work **cranial osteopathy**—packaging it so that it would be viewed as an extension of osteopathy. Still, his work received a mountain of criticism, and it wasn't until almost half a century later that his theories on cranial bone mobility were given much credence and finally accepted as medical fact.[50]

Sixteen years after the death of Dr. Sutherland, another osteopath emerged that would take up the mantle of cranial-based therapy. In 1970, Dr. John E. Upledger had an opportunity to assist in a spinal cord operation being performed by a colleague. Upledger's job was to hold the spinal cord still while the neurosurgeon performed the operation. To both his surprise and embarrassment, Dr. Upledger found this seemingly small task to be quite impossible. The annoyance of the surgeon was obvious at Upledger's inability to perform what should have been a simple feat, but there was nothing Upledger could do.

The spinal cord, pulsing at a different rate from that of the heart and breath of the patient, slid beneath his hands as if alive. Until now, all of medical science stated that he shouldn't be feeling what he was feeling. There wasn't supposed to be a pulse in the spinal cord. But the facts were glaring and he realized that the medical texts were wrong—or at least incomplete. The spinal cord had a rhythm all its own. As far as doctors knew at the time, no other such "rhythm" existed. Dr. Upledger had stumbled across the unknown. As he witnessed the spinal cord pulsing beneath his hands, a quiet voice within him said that he had just experienced something vastly important. Later he came to believe that what he had come in contact with that day was nothing less than the very core of the human being—the point at which humanity's physical and spiritual components came together.[51]

Five years later, Upledger became a biomechanics professor at Michigan State University's College of Osteopathy. As part of a multidisciplinary team, he conducted studies on what came to be called the "craniosacral system." This team was able to scientifically conclude that the bones of the skull did indeed flex and shift with the tidal pressures of the cranial wave and they found that the spinal cord really did have a pulse of its own. They called this pulse the craniosacral rhythm (CSR) and found that not only could they evaluate a person's condition by listening to this rhythm, they could also treat a variety of conditions by making minute adjustments to the pulse. This work came to be called craniosacral therapy (CST).

As the years went on, the scope of illnesses that could be treated through craniosacral therapy became broader. With the success of his approach, Upledger sought to share his work with others. He began teaching nurses, physical therapists, and parents of brain-dysfunctional children, but ran up against the orthodox medical establishment, who branded him as a heretic for teaching nonphysicians. Eventually, in 1985, Dr. Upledger established his own school, the Upledger Institute, in Palm Beach Gardens, Florida, where his work continues to grow to this day.[52]

Theory and Principles

To understand craniosacral therapy, it is first important to understand how the craniosacral system operates. The outermost layer of the spinal cord forms a watertight sack that is embedded firmly in the inner lining of the skull. Contained within this sack is a clear, colorless liquid called cerebrospinal fluid, or CSF, that pulses back and forth from the brain to the tailbone. This rhythmic tide creates an expansion and contraction that forms the pulse of the craniosacral system and it is this rhythm that a therapist will use to both evaluate and treat.

This pulsation of fluid also creates a correlating expansion and contraction of the bones that form the skull. Although these bones appear to be rigidly locked together, Dr. Upledger's work at Michigan State University concluded that these bones actually have a small degree of movement. The key lies in the sutures of the skull that interlock to create a zipper-like fastening from one portion to another (Figure 8-9). As newborn infants, it is very obvious by the soft areas in the head that the skull has not yet fully formed. This malleability is necessary in order for of the head to pass through the birth canal without injury. Eventually, the skull hardens into what appears to be one solid piece. However, the connective medium gluing the bones together is composed of a pliant, cartilage-like substance that gives the joints a small range of motion.

These cranial sutures act like expansion joints found in roads, buildings, and bridges that allow for changes caused by variations in weather. This capacity for expansion and contraction allows the skull to absorb the increase in pressure by expanding when the level of cerebrospinal fluid rises and contracting as the fluids are reabsorbed. However, injuries, accidents, and illnesses can cause the bones of the skull to lose mobility and become locked into place. When this happens, the skull is unable to absorb the pressure of the expanding fluids and the pressure is then exerted on the brain. The brain is the major organ of

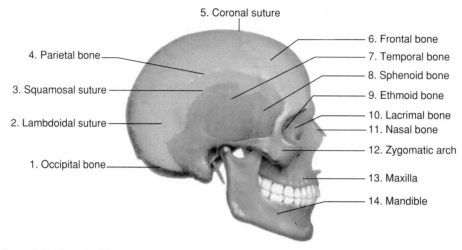

5. Coronal suture

6. Frontal bone
7. Temporal bone
8. Sphenoid bone
9. Ethmoid bone

4. Parietal bone
3. Squamosal suture
2. Lambdoidal suture

10. Lacrimal bone
11. Nasal bone
12. Zygomatic arch

1. Occipital bone

13. Maxilla
14. Mandible

Figure 8-9 The skull bones and sutures.

the central nervous system and is the control center for the entire body. The brain itself is actually so fragile that were it not protectively immersed in fluid, it would likely collapse.[53] Due to this high level of delicacy, even small changes in the brain's environment can cause major disruptions in its operations and, because it is such a central component for all of human functioning, even small disruptions here can have major reverberations throughout the whole body.

Controversy of Cranial Bone Mobility

In some countries, Upledger's theories on the movement of cranial bones are quite controversial. In the United States for example, craniosacral's theories have been considered impossible by the orthodox medical community because they believe that the bones of the skull are fixed and immobile. In other parts of the world, however, such as Italy and Israel, the general consensus acknowledges that the cranial bones do indeed have mobility. The key to alleviating this discrepancy lies in the condition of the skull examined. In the United States, anatomical studies have been traditionally conducted on dead specimens. In these examples, the connective tissue that stitch together the pieces of the skull had calcified and hardened, making it appear as if the skull was completely locked together. The studies of Upledger and company, however, were conducted on living, breathing, human beings where the tissues connecting the bones of the skull were still alive and pliant.[54]

Craniosacral Therapy's Wide Scope of Practice

In addition to being able to treat common ailments like neck and back pain, craniosacral therapy is also able to treat some unique conditions that are normally very difficult to positively affect through other forms of bodywork. Upledger's first work with severe headaches occurred when a World War II veteran who served in the United States Navy came for treatment. The sound of canon-fire blasting in his ears had left him with unrelenting headaches and ringing in the ears for 25 years. Upon examination, Dr. Upledger found that the bones on the left side of the skull were jammed inward. When this was released, the left side of the head actually expanded out and the veteran became exuberant. The veteran had suffered from these splitting headaches for a quarter of a century. After treatment they disappeared completely and never returned. Dr. Upledger repeated this experience again and again, reaching a success rate of 80 to 85 percent.[55]

With hyperactive and dyslexic children, Upledger's group observed that about half of the hyperactive children had signs of trauma during birth. During delivery, the baby's head is often pried backwards to hasten the birthing process, a maneuver that can damage a child's neck. When this type of birthing trauma was found and corrected, success rates were nearly 100 percent.[56] Later research led craniosacral therapy into the field of post-traumatic stress disorders, which included victims of rape, attempted murder, satanic cult abuses, beatings, and so on.[57] Today, this modality continues to grow and develop in its scope and practice, particularly by helping to bring to the surface and resolve the psychological memories and emotional aspects of post-traumatic stress disorders and other physiological conditions.

Assessment

The key to assessment in this modality is the ability to feel the craniosacral rhythm. This is accomplished by quieting one's internal noise and placing oneself in a receptive frame of mind. This allows the rhythm of the craniosacral pulse to fill one's awareness so that the nuances of the fluid's fluctuations can be more easily perceived. With the right kind of listening the therapist can hear distinct happenings all along the craniosacral system and even all over the body. The sensitivities of a craniosacral therapist are said to become so honed that they can actually detect traces of previous bodywork that the client may have received. These markings are known as signatures and are akin to an individual's fingerprints. It is said that each practitioner leaves his or her signature whenever they perform bodywork.[58]

Assessment of the craniosacral rhythm can be conducted at many locations. There are "listening stations" all over the body, but the pulse can be most strongly felt at the back of the neck and tailbone. Upledger's sensitivities had grown to the point where he could actually feel the pulse anywhere on the body. Advanced practitioners are able to do the same.

When assessing the craniosacral pulse, the therapist considers its speed, strength, symmetry, and elasticity. The average cycle of the craniosacral pulse is 6 to 12 "beats" per minute. Rhythms that are faster or slower than this can point to a potential imbalance in the system. For example, the rhythm of an individual suffering from brain damage may be slower while the rhythm of a hyperactive child may be much quicker.[59]

While listening, it is also important to keep in mind that the craniosacral pulse, like the breath and heartbeat, will vary from person to person. What's important here is that the distance, rhythm, and intensity of the pulse is balanced for *that* individual.

Techniques

To affect the craniosacral system, the weight of a nickel is all the pressure needed.[60] Admittedly, the amount of movement created with such little force will be quite tiny, but just as a slight shift in the plate tectonics at the core of the earth can induce massive tidal waves hundreds of miles from point zero, any shift in the sensitive structures of the craniosacral system can have far reaching effects.

Unlike many modalities where one technique can be applied to many different areas of the body, many of craniosacral's techniques are only applicable to one specific site. For example, using the earlobes to decompress the temples can only be done at that location. Also, unlocking the forehead requires a completely different approach than unlocking the base of the skull, which in turn is a completely different technique than releasing the sacrum. Sometimes bones deep inside the skull need to be accessed, and in these cases, the therapist actually has to go inside the person's mouth to create the necessary influence for change.[61]

One of the most important areas in this whole system is the base of the skull. This area connects deeply to the heart of the craniosacral system and can strongly influence the entire body. Here the therapist can perform a technique known as a release. With both hands gently cradling the client's head, the therapist's fingertips sink softly into the space where the back of the skull meets the back of the neck. While doing so, the therapist visualizes the bones at the back of the neck "unlocking" and stretching softly away from the head. In this system, such mental focus and intent is an absolutely necessary force. In fact, it appears that this directing of one's attention and intention may be *even more important* than the physical movement itself.

When a release has been successful, there are several signs that may appear. The area being worked can lengthen, become warm, and may improve in mobility. The whole body may visibly relax and breathing may be accompanied by a yawn or a sigh of relief. Also, releases don't just have to be physical. They can be emotional as well. Craniosacral therapy unlocks tensions that have sometimes been deeply held for a long time. When these tensions are released, they can also unleash emotions that have been trapped alongside it. Whenever a release occurs, the therapist allows the process to achieve full completion before moving on.[62]

The sacrum is another area that contains a great deal of importance in this system. Here the therapist arranges the hands into a "T" position underneath the client's body with one hand gently cupping the sacrum and the other softly bracing the lower back. Although this position appears invasive, clients will feel that the therapist's hands are more on the back of the body than anywhere that is sensitive.

Once locked in to the body's rhythm, the therapist may choose to simply follow along. This is called tracking. Often it will feel as if the body wants to go in a certain direction. When this happens, the therapist can choose to simply support the body's wish to move in a certain way or to perform a release here by simply holding the top hand steady and applying the slightest of pressure downward. Again, it is important to visualize the work. One's attention should be absorbed in the thought of the sacrum releasing from the bottom of the spine.

Sometimes the therapist will utilize techniques to achieve what are known as still points. Still points are when the craniosacral pulse is brought to a standstill. This stasis triggers a relaxation response of the nervous system and allows the craniosacral rhythm an opportunity to reestablish and correct itself. During a still point, a patient will often experience a strong pulsation known as a therapeutic pulse. The emergence of the therapeutic pulse is said to indicate the activation of a powerful healing mechanism within the body. While the therapeutic pulse is activated, the therapist should become still in order to allow the body's natural healing process to occur. [63]

Often the work of balancing the craniosacral system will also require work on areas outside of it. This is because many issues of the craniosacral system actually stem from somewhere else in the body like the hips, shoulders, arms, or legs. When work is done on these "outer" areas, the techniques are similar to that of Myofascial Release. Some may actually appear identical, yet the intent is different behind each system. In Myofascial Release, the intent is to balance the system of fascia that wraps, protects, and connects everything inside the body. In craniosacral work the intent is to balance and normalize the rhythm of the craniosacral pulse. However, in the process of doing craniosacral work, energy blockages and fascial restrictions are also released.

The Session

A craniosacral session is performed on a padded table with the client wearing loose, comfortable clothing. The first few moments of contact are made purely with the purpose of listening. Not only is the rhythm of the craniosacral pulse observed, the patient's breath, heartbeat, and overall condition are also evaluated so that the craniosacral rhythm can be assessed within the context of who this person is. This is important to remember because not only will rhythms fluctuate from person to person, the degree to which the cranial bones actually move will be different as well.

It is important that before beginning a craniosacral treatment the therapist be in a calm, focused state of mind. The therapist should tune in to the patient and silently ask the patient's inner physician to be the guide in the session. It cannot be stressed enough that the inner wisdom of the patient should dictate what the patient needs, not the will of the therapist. A release cannot be forced and it may not be in the patient's best interest to release something he or she is not ready to release. The therapist's intent should be for the highest good of the patient.

Throughout the treatment, the therapist will come back again and again to the rhythm of the craniosacral pulse. It will act as a lifeline to the inner workings of the patient's body. Through careful listening, the therapist can tap into this "lifeline" to find out where things are going wrong. There are many areas of the body where this rhythm can be "heard." One of the first places often explored is the sacrum. This point of access is not only the epicenter of many dysfunctions, it is also an important listening station where the pulse can be felt quite strongly.

The sacrum is the southern-most structure of the craniosacral system and has a symbiotic relationship with the neck. The spinal cord, which travels all the way from the head down to the pelvis, is protectively encased within the bones of the spinal column. The spine (commonly known as the backbone) is actually a composed of 24 separate bones. Together they form a flexible tunnel that can bend and twist while keeping its contents safe and protected. Throughout the length of this tunnel, the spinal cord floats freely except at two points —the top of the neck and near the top of the sacrum (tailbone). Because of this unique relationship, any disturbance of the sacrum will be automatically reflected in the neck. This means that issues like migraines, back pain, sinus problems, or even TMJ can actually be coming from down in the pelvis.[64]

The sacrum must be carefully and patiently observed to determine if it is operating properly. If it is tilted, rotated, or in some way uneven, there can be pain and dysfunction throughout the entire craniosacral system. Many times, these issues result from injuries sustained long ago. It may have been a childhood fall that can't even be remembered or a car accident that has been decades past. Overtime these injuries can create painful disturbances in the body.

To access the sacrum, the client is first asked to lift the hips slightly off the table so the therapist can slide the hands underneath. One hand braces the lower back while the other hand supports the sacrum. The therapist can use this position to "listen" to areas higher up in the craniosacral system . Quite often, the therapist will find that the sacrum's ability to move has been re-stricted. To decompress this area, the therapist can apply a gentle pull with the lower hand while the hand above it remains stationary, easing the tailbone away from the lower back. Although this is described as a pull, it is very subtle and comes more from intent than physical force.

Next the therapist moves to focus on the back of the head and neck. Working on this area is the reciprocal movement to the release of its counterpart, the tail-bone, and the work of performing a sacral release is not complete until this area is released as well. Here the therapist cradles the head in the palms of the hands while the fingers hook gently underneath the cranium just at the point where muscle meets bone. This technique decompresses the occiput from the spine. It is a highly important area because it connects deeply to structures at the heart of the craniosacral system.

Because all of the body's systems are connected together in vast webs of tissue and energy, restrictions and dysfunctions can stem from just about any-where in the body. A problem with the bones on the side of the skull may be caused by a dysfunction of the neck that may be coming from a restriction in the organs, which in turn may be caused by an injury in the hips. During treat-ment, the hands sometimes seem to have a mind of their own, floating back and forth over the client's body picking up hints and clues about the person's underlying condition. These clues must be followed like an invisible string to the source of the ailment.

Often, when the hands come to rest, the area may become warm and a slowly developing pulsation may occur. This is the therapeutic pulse at work. It is a somewhat mysterious phenomenon that achieves its name because it indicates that something positive is occurring in the patient. As the heat rises, so does the amplitude of the pulse. Like a well-orchestrated conductor and symphony, the two elements rise and fall together, climbing to a peak and then drifting back down until the heat cools and the pulse fades away. In the wake of the therapeutic pulse, when the release is complete, the tissue becomes no-ticeably softer to the therapist while the patient experiences a diminishment of pain. Curiously, the patient may even feel anger or fear, accompanied by a vivid memory of the past incident that caused the pain in the first place. This flashback, however, doesn't always come at the time of treatment. It may occur later that day or even in the days following the treatment.[65]

This phenomenon of recalling past pain and injury has come to be called tissue memory. Whereas the brain is normally considered the storehouse for memories, the flashback that occurs here indicates that the body's tissues themselves can retain memories separate from the brain.[66]

At the end of the session, the therapist nearly always applies a still point. This brings the whole body into a deep relaxation and smoothes out the work conducted. Then, just as gently as the session began, the treatment deftly ends. With such gentleness it is at first difficult to imagine the great magnitude of change that can be achieved with this system. However, it must be remembered that craniosacral work accesses systems of the body that are at the core of the human being and because of this, small modifications can have a huge impact everywhere else.

Benefits

- Migraine headaches
- Motor-coordination impairments
- **Colic**
- Autism
- Central nervous system disorders
- Orthopedic problems
- Traumatic brain and spinal cord Injuries
- Infantile disorders
- Learning disabilities
- Chronic fatigue
- Emotional difficulties
- Fibromyalgia and other connective tissue disorders
- Neurovascular or immune disorders
- Post-traumatic stress disorder
- Post-surgical dysfunction[67]
- Musculoskeletal problems

Contraindications

- Recent or acute strokes
- Cerebral aneurysm
- Brain stem tumor
- Acute head injury
- Internal bleeding of the head

Precautions

- Those on medications should consult a doctor first due to the changes in blood pressure that may arise.

- Working with infants should only be done by an experienced practitioner who is specifically trained in craniosacral work for infants, due to a baby's delicate system

Training of a Therapist

At the Upledger Institute initial level craniosacral training is a 4-day course that details and analyzes the anatomy and physiology of the craniosacral system. This level of training is geared towards understanding, feeling, and balancing the craniosacral system. Trainees are taught a 10-step protocol to locate and release major restrictions in the craniosacral system. Craniosacral 2 is another 4-day program available to those who have completed level one training. This course of study delves deeper into some of the more subtle and complex techniques and theories of craniosacral therapy. Here, the original work of Dr. Sutherland's cranial osteopathy is explored as well as well general protocols for treating infants and children.[68]

For advanced practitioners that have completed training in both these courses there are two levels of certification that they can receive. Level one certification requires basic knowledge of anatomy and physiology (from an accredited school or university), clinical experience of 75 craniosacral treatment protocols, and the successful completion of oral, written, and practical examinations. Level two certification can be applied for by those who have received the first level certification training. They must have at least 20 hours of study in one of the other courses offered by the Upledger Institute and must also complete case history write-ups along with 6 hours of presentation to an organized group. Maintaining these certifications require that the therapist complete twenty-four hours of continuing education courses approved by the Upledger Institute.

While initial craniosacral training can be found nationally and abroad, advanced certification can only be obtained at the Upledger Institute. Beginning the process of craniosacral training requires only that the applicant be at least 18 years of age. However, because craniosacral therapy training is not a licensing program, the therapist may be required to have additional training that allows them to practice bodywork in their state.[69]

SUMMARY

This chapter introduces the somato-psychic level of massage therapy and bodywork which includes modalities with the intent to affect changes in the physical body and at the same time deal with related issues of psychology. It provides an understanding of how the modalities of Rolfing, Soma

Neuromuscular Integration, Hellerwork, The Alexander Technique, and The Feldenkrais Method each fit into the somato-psychic approach of massage including how they differ, and how they are similar to each other. A basic overview of the history, the theory and principles, process of assessment, as well as a description of the techniques involved, are presented for each of these modalities of the somato-psychic approach. This chapter also acquaints the reader with what the general experience of undergoing a treatment session is like and identifies who are the best candidates to seek this form of treatment and what conditions are most benefited. Also presented is a list for each of these modalities of their general benefits, contraindications, and/or precautions. A brief discussion about training, licensing, certifications, and requirements is also included.

CHAPTER REFERENCES

1. Claire, T. (1995). *Body work: What kind of massage to get and how to make the most of it.* Laguna Beach, CA: Basic Health Publications, Inc.
2. Claire, T. (1995). *Body work: What kind of massage to get and how to make the most of it.* Laguna Beach, CA: Basic Health Publications, Inc.
3. Myers, T. Heirs of Ida Rolf. *Massage & Bodywork.* Jun/Jul 2004;19:18–19.
4. Myers, T. Heirs of Ida Rolf. *Massage & Bodywork.* Jun/Jul 2004;19:18–19.
5. Myers, T. Heirs of Ida Rolf. *Massage & Bodywork.* Jun/Jul 2004;19:18–19.
6. Claire, T. (1995). *Body work: What kind of massage to get and how to make the most of it.* Laguna Beach, CA: Basic Health Publications, Inc.
7. Levine, A, Levine, V. *Bodywork and Massage Sourcebook.* Los Angeles. Lowell House; 1999.
8. Claire, T. (1995). *Body work: What kind of massage to get and how to make the most of it.* Laguna Beach, CA: Basic Health Publications, Inc.
9. Levine, A, Levine V. *Bodywork and Massage Sourcebook.* Los Angeles. Lowell House; 1999.
10. Claire, T. (1995). *Body work: What kind of massage to get and how to make the most of it.* Laguna Beach, CA: Basic Health Publications, Inc.
11. *Soma Neuromuscular Institute Catalog.* Buckley, WA; 2008.
12. Bolesky, KL, Johnson SW, Grammarian JW, Nolte MW. Soma Neuromuscular Integration: how we define ourselves. [Soma Institute website] Available at: http://www.soma-institute.org/articles/Soma_Series_Compare_Article.pdf. Accessed March 3, 2008.
13. Bolesky, K. Three Brain Model Theory. [Soma Institute website] Available at: http://www.soma-institute.org/3brain.html. Accessed February 17, 2008.
14. Nolte, M. *Soma Institute*; 2008.
15. Osborn, K. Soma: from Ida Rolf's legacy to a new paradigm for Structural Integration. *Massage & Bodywork.* 2004, Jun/Jul;**19**: 20–28.
16. Osborn, K. Soma: from Ida Rolf's legacy to a new paradigm for Structural Integration. *Massage & Bodywork.* 2004, Jun/Jul;**19**: 20–28.

17. *Somassage*. Available at: http://www.soma-institute.org/somassage.html. Accessed February 17, 2008.
18. *Soma Neuromuscular Institute Catalog*. Buckley, WA; 2008.
19. *Hellerwork Client Handbook*. [Hellerwork Structural Integration website]. Available at: http://www.hellerwork.com/images/heller.handbook.pdf. Accessed February 22, 2008.
20. Hunton, J. Best kept secret in bodywork. [Hellerwork Structural Integration website]. Available at: http://hellerwork.com/archives/000925.html. Accessed February 22, 2008.
21. Become a professional Hellerwork practitioner. [Hellerwork Structural Integration website]. Available at: http://hellerwork.com/training.html. February 22, 2008.
22. Become a professional Hellerwork practitioner. [Hellerwork Structural Integration website]. Available at: http://hellerwork.com/training.html. February 22, 2008.
23. Vanderbilt S. Hellerwork: Structural Integration for mind, body, and spirit. *Massage & Bodywork*. Jun/Jul 2004;**19:** 20–28.
24. Kosminsky J, Caplan D. *Alexander Technique*. [video] Wellspring Media1998.
25. Kosminsky J, Caplan D. *Alexander Technique*. [video] Wellspring Media1998.
26. Claire, T. (1995). *Body work: What kind of massage to get and how to make the most of it*. Laguna Beach, CA: Basic Health Publications, Inc.
27. Gelb, MJ. *Body Learning*. New York: Henry Holt and Co; 1994.
28. Claire, T. (1995). *Body work: What kind of massage to get and how to make the most of it*. Laguna Beach, CA: Basic Health Publications, Inc.
29. Gelb, MJ. *Body Learning*. New York: Henry Holt and Co; 1994.
30. Gelb, MJ. *Body Learning*. New York: Henry Holt and Co; 1994.
31. Claire, T. (1995). *Body work: What kind of massage to get and how to make the most of it*. Laguna Beach, CA: Basic Health Publications, Inc.
32. Claire, T. (1995). *Body work: What kind of massage to get and how to make the most of it*. Laguna Beach, CA: Basic Health Publications, Inc.
33. Levine, A, Levine V. *Bodywork and Massage Sourcebook*. Los Angeles. Lowell House; 1999.
34. Claire, T. (1995). *Body work: What kind of massage to get and how to make the most of it*. Laguna Beach, CA: Basic Health Publications, Inc.
35. Claire, T. (1995). *Body work: What kind of massage to get and how to make the most of it*. Laguna Beach, CA: Basic Health Publications, Inc.
36. Strauch, R. An overview of the Feldenkrais Method. Available at: http://www.somatic.com/articles/feldenkrais_overview.pdf. Accessed October 16, 2008.
37. Strauch, R. An overview of the Feldenkrais Method. Available at: http://www.somatic.com/articles/feldenkrais_overview.pdf. Accessed October 16, 2008.
38. Strauch, R. An overview of the Feldenkrais Method. Available at: http://www.somatic.com/articles/feldenkrais_overview.pdf. Accessed October 16, 2008.
39. Levine, A, Levine V. *Bodywork and Massage Sourcebook*. Los Angeles. Lowell House; 1999.
40. Strauch, R. An overview of the Feldenkrais Method. Available at: http://www.somatic.com/articles/feldenkrais_overview.pdf. Accessed October 16, 2008.
41. Claire, T. (1995). *Body work: What kind of massage to get and how to make the most of it*. Laguna Beach, CA: Basic Health Publications, Inc.

42. Ehrman, R. Frequently Asked Questions. [Feldenkrais Educational Foundation of North America website]. Available at: http://www.feldenkrais.com/method/faq .html. Accessed October 6, 2008.

43. Levine, A, Levine V. *Bodywork and Massage Sourcebook.* Los Angeles. Lowell House; 1999.

44. Claire, T. (1995). *Body work: What kind of massage to get and how to make the most of it.* Laguna Beach, CA: Basic Health Publications, Inc.

45. About FGNA. Available at: http://www.feldenkrais.com/guild/about/aboutfgna .html. Accessed October 16, 2008.

46. Ehrman, R. Frequently Asked Questions. [Feldenkrais Educational Foundation of North America website]. Available at: http://www.feldenkrais.com/method/faq .html. Accessed October 6, 2008.

47. *craniosacral therapy/Somato Emotional Release* (2008) Retrieved from the Web Oct 23, 2007. http://www.iahe.com/html/therapies/cst.jsp

48. Claire, T. (1995). *Body work: What kind of massage to get and how to make the most of it.* Laguna Beach, CA: Basic Health Publications, Inc.

49. Claire, T. (1995). *Body work: What kind of massage to get and how to make the most of it.* Laguna Beach, CA: Basic Health Publications, Inc.

50. Sutherland, WG. *Father of Osteopathy In The Cranial Field* http://www.osteohome .com/SubPages/wgs.html Feb 25, 2008.

51. Upledger. *Your Inner Physician & You.* Berkley, California: North Atlantic Books; 1997.

52. Claire, T. (1995). *Body work: What kind of massage to get and how to make the most of it.* Laguna Beach, CA: Basic Health Publications, Inc.

53. Claire, T. (1995). *Body work: What kind of massage to get and how to make the most of it.* Laguna Beach, CA: Basic Health Publications, Inc.

54. Claire, T. (1995). *Body work: What kind of massage to get and how to make the most of it.* Laguna Beach, CA: Basic Health Publications, Inc.

55. Upledger. *Your Inner Physician & You.* Berkley, California: North Atlantic Books; 1997.

56. Upledger. *Your Inner Physician & You.* Berkley, California: North Atlantic Books; 1997.

57. Upledger. *Your Inner Physician & You.* Berkley, California: North Atlantic Books; 1997.

58. Claire, T. (1995). *Body work: What kind of massage to get and how to make the most of it.* Laguna Beach, CA: Basic Health Publications, Inc.

59. Claire, T. (1995). *Body work: What kind of massage to get and how to make the most of it.* Laguna Beach, CA: Basic Health Publications, Inc.

60. Upledger. *Your Inner Physician & You.* Berkley, California: North Atlantic Books; 1997.

61. Sullivan, M. *Cranio-Sacral Thearpy.* [DVD] (2004) Real Bodywork.

62. Sullivan, M. *Cranio-Sacral Thearpy.* [DVD] (2004) Real Bodywork.

63. Claire, T. (1995). *Body work: What kind of massage to get and how to make the most of it.* Laguna Beach, CA: Basic Health Publications, Inc.

64. Sullivan, M. *Cranio-Sacral Thearpy.* [DVD] (2004) Real Bodywork.

65. Upledger. *Your Inner Physician & You.* Berkley, California: North Atlantic Books; 1997.

66. Upledger. *Your Inner Physician & You.* Berkley, California: North Atlantic Books; 1997.

67. *Craniosacral therapy/Somato Emotional Release* (2008) Retrieved from the Web Oct 23, 2007. http://www.iahe.com/html/therapies/cst.jsp

68. *Your Source For Complementary Care Education* [Catalog] Upledger Institute; 2002.

69. *Craniosacral therapy Certification Program* [Pamphlet] Upledger Institute; 2008.

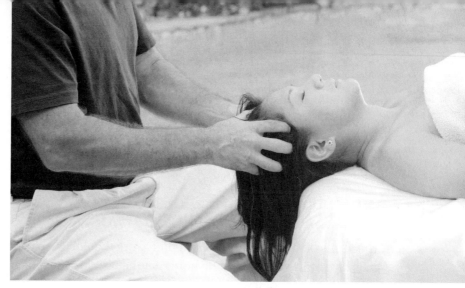

9
CHAPTER

The Bioenergetic Layer of the Massage Therapy and Bodywork Continuum

CHAPTER GOALS

1. Develop an understanding of how the modalities of tuina, amma therapeutic massage, acupressure, Zen shiatsu, Namikoshi shiatsu, Five Element shiatsu, macrobiotic shiatsu, Jin Shin Do® Bodymind Acupressure® and Thai massage fit into the bioenergetic approach of massage.

2. Recognize the significance of these modalities, how they differ, and how they are similar to each other.

3. Develop a basic understanding of the theory and principles of each of the modalities.

4. Develop a basic understanding of the process of assessment used in each of the modalities.

5. Develop a basic understanding of the techniques involved in each of the modalities.

6. Become acquainted with the general experience of a session in each of the modalities.

7. Identify who should seek this form of treatment and what conditions are most benefited by each of the modalities.

8. Become aware of contraindications and precautions related to each of the modalities.

9. Become knowledgeable about the training, licensing, certifications, and requirements that one needs in order to practice within each of the modalities.

INTRODUCTION TO THE BIOENERGETIC LAYER OF MASSAGE THERAPY AND BODYWORK

The forms of massage therapy and bodywork that focus on treating the bioenergetic layer of the human being hold that the visible aspect of any organism tells only a small part of the whole story, and therefore to truly understand the human entity one must learn how to look beyond the three-dimensional material structure of the physical body and include the energetic. When this perspective is taken, the foundational concepts of health and disease change and expand drastically. This expansion brings into awareness all existing levels of the total human entity and facilitates a new and deeper understanding of how to treat the "body."

Within the continuum of the Four Massage Therapy and Bodywork Levels, the **bioenergetic level** is the first to consider as part of its perspective the theory, assessment, and treatment of the qi or energy system as its primary focus of intention.

ENERGY AS A TREATABLE DIMENSION OF THE HUMAN BEING

The idea of treating the body, mind, and emotions through the use of touch is now fairly well accepted, but the idea of energy as a treatable dimension of the human being is one much less known and often misunderstood in the West. The bioenergetic branch of bodywork, which mostly encompasses various forms of Asian bodywork therapy, developed in an entirely different direction to the more familiar somatic and somato-psychic forms of therapy and requires a whole new language to describe and understand its workings. But even within the confines of this level of bodywork, there are ideas and vocabulary unique to each of the modalities in this category. However, regardless of the language used to describe it, by recognizing, understanding, manipulating, and balancing the energetic layer (energy system) of a human being, a broader and often deeper variety of conditions can be understood and treated. When the universe, including all aspects of human beings, is understood in terms of energy, even something as impalpable as thoughts and emotions are seen as having their role in unbalancing the energy system and thus contributing to disease.

The major force shaping the bioenergetic layer of bodywork is a system of healing that has been evolving for over 5000 years called traditional Chinese medicine (TCM). Whereas "humans" in the West are often seen as separate from nature, TCM views "humans" as an indistinguishable component of the world. To get a glimpse of just how deeply the Asian healing arts are rooted in the idea that "humans" are inseparable from nature, one only has to look at their medical vocabulary. Treatable conditions are described as "cold," "hot," "damp," or "dry." "Fire" is said to rise when someone experiences anger. A person who catches a cold is said to have been "invaded by wind," another of the six pernicious influences or energies that refer to the six climatic conditions of TCM. These include Wind, Cold, Fire, Dampness, Dryness, and Summer-Heat, and invasion by any of these six energies can work their way into the bioenergetic system and cause an energy imbalance that left untreated can lead to a serious condition. Because of this multileveled bioenergetic approach to understanding and treating the human being, most practitioners of these therapies must first study the philosophy and principles of traditional Chinese medicine.

The breadth of human history that TCM covers is quite long, and during that time various bioenergetic modalities have evolved that are grounded in this medicine—some that have stayed rigorously true to the original formula and can be seen to be closely related and others that developed their own unique theories and practices and are more like distant cousins.

TRADITIONAL CHINESE MEDICINE

Although TCM has been practiced for thousands of years, it is only in the last 20 to 30 years that it has been gaining popularity outside the borders of Asia. One of the major factors stunting its growth has been the language barrier. However, as cultural relations have developed, more and more of this knowledge has been translated, making its way into the rest of the world.

The integration of TCM into the field of **complementary and alternative medicine (CAM)** has been a rather slow process, in spite of the fact that most people who have encountered it usually recognize its tremendous worth—even if they don't understand it. One of the major factors behind the strength of the recent growth of this minimally invasive form of medicine is its effectiveness in treating a broad range of conditions. This coupled with its lack of side effects produce a win-win situation that many people recognize immediately.

Theory and Principles

TCM is a complex subject and requires a serious commitment to its study and practice, especially if one aims to use it as the basis of assessment and treatment for one of the many forms of Asian bodywork therapy, acupuncture, and/or Chinese herbal medicine. What follows here is just a brief taste to give the reader an idea of the subject and by no means is it meant to represent the true breadth, depth, and profundity of this great philosophy and field. (For those readers whose interests are piqued and would like to gain deeper insight into TCM, please refer to the bibliography at the end of this book.)

At the heart of TCM is the perspective that everything in the world is a form of energy. Dense matter like rock, wood, muscle, and bone form one end of the energetic spectrum while finer substances like air, gas, and even thoughts and emotions are found at the opposite. From this perspective, the only difference between a cloud, a desk, a thought, or an electric current is their density.[1] There is no real separation between tree and bird, water and earth, or man and universe. Even the space between two people is filled with a fine "mist" of energy. Everything is composed of one fundamental substance, whether it be a blade of grass, an airplane, or the cells of our skin. This fundamental substance is known as qi (pronounced "chee") and also known as ki in Japanese (pronounced "key"). Qi is both the fundamental unit of life and also the energy that motivates life. It is qi that makes up the body and it is qi that enlivens it. Qi is the air that we breathe and the food that we eat. It is the sky above and the ground below. The whole world is comprised of gradients of qi.[2]

The following describes in brief some of the most fundamental principles that are relevant and used in the practice of the various bioenergetic forms of Asian bodywork, especially those most closely related to TCM massage.

Yin and Yang

The traditional Chinese medical system is based upon the primary concept of **yin and yang**. This is the notion that a polarity of forces exists, actively changing throughout the day, season, and lifetime, but which overall maintains a necessary balance. If the world were a canvas, that canvas would be composed of qi. On this canvas, the background would be painted with the principles of yin and yang. Yin and Yang represent opposing, yet complementary forces that interact to give definition to the world. Yin is dark, still, and heavy. Yang is bright, dynamic and light. Yin is cold and contracting. Yang is warm and expanding. Yin is the grounding and nurturing energies of the earth. Yang is the blessing and the uplifting energies of the heavens. Yin is the encompassing and embracing aspects of woman. Yang is the conquering and penetrating energies of man.

Literally translated, yin refers to the shady side of a hill and yang refers to the sunny side.[3]

The concept of yin and yang isn't applied to permanently define and restrict something as either yin or yang, rather it is relative and utilized to understand the relationship between two parts of anything. Because of this, what was yin in one relationship can become yang in another and vice versa. For example the density of water is yin when compared to the fineness and freedom of mist, which is yang. Yet when water is compared to ice, the flowing, active, always-in-motion substance of water becomes yang relative to the density and fixed nature of ice, which is yin. Yin and yang are inherent in everything, therefore any yin or yang aspect or object can also be divided further into yin and yang. For instance, the temperature can be divided into degrees of hot and cold. Then cold, which is considered the yin of this pair, can be further divided into ice cold and cold, and so on; ice cold is yin and cold is yang. Ultimately, the real value of this principle in the practice of Asian bodywork lies in using it as a major diagnostic tool in helping to determine the energetic patterns of imbalance of patients (Figure 9-1).

The Five Elements

Whereas the theory of yin and yang reveals broad strokes, finer details can be determined by applying the principle of the Five Elements. Five Element Theory breaks everything down into five fundamental energies, substances, and qualities that comprise our existence—wood, fire, earth, metal, and water. Each element is host to a myriad of qualities and correspondences ranging from physical organs to emotional states to the seasons of the year. For example, a person can be said to be a wood or water type depending on his or her physical and psychological characteristics. Each type has its own advantages and disadvantages and each type is prone to certain diseases and ailments. With this approach, even something as nebulous as one's personality can be explained, understood, and treated by applying it to the Five Elements. As a result, the principle of the Five Elements can be used as another essential diagnostic tool for the bioenergetic bodywork practitioner. There are very specific correspondences to each of the elements that are

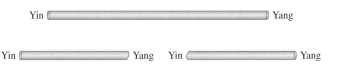

Figure 9-1 The principle of yin and yang is an important diagnostic tool in helping to determine patients' energetic patterns of imbalance.

clearly stated in the TCM literature, and these correspondences are the foundation of assessment using this profound TCM principle.

In addition, there are two special ways the Five Elements are ordered that have great diagnostic importance to the practitioners of Asian bodywork. The Five Elements together demonstrate the idea of a balanced tension (Figure 9-2). This is known as the Cycle of Creation and the Cycle of Control. Whenever this balance is disturbed it is reflected into the energy system and then manifests in the body as a pathological condition. The practitioner must look to these cycles to understand which related elements, organs, and channels, are out of balance. Once this is understood, the practitioner can take the necessary

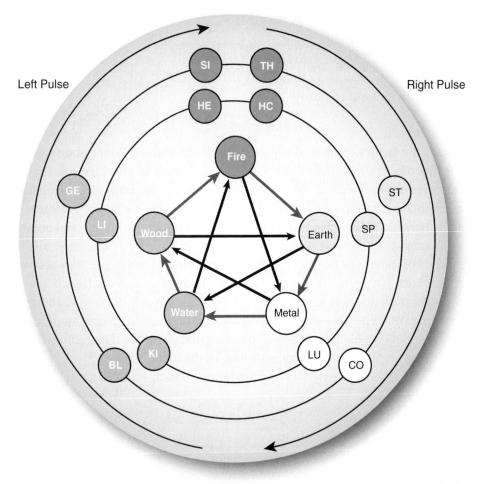

Figure 9-2 This diagram of the Five Elements is a graphic representation of the Cycle of Creation and the Cycle of Destruction.

steps by using one of the forms of bioenergetic treatment to bring the system back into its healthy, normal state of being.

The Organs

Further details of the body are expressed through the idea of the organs. Each organ has a sphere of influence that includes a very specific set of energetic, physiological, and emotional functions. Emotions, too, are considered a form of energy that can play an integral role in either the health or illness of an organ and therefore an individual. While emotions are often considered a secondary aspect of disease in western medicine, they are considered a primary factor in TCM where specific emotions are understood to affect the body and mind in very specific ways.

TCM describes the existence of 12 organs, which are divided into 6 yin and yang pairs. They also have an associated set of bodily tissues, sense organs, and energy channels. The six yin organs include: the Lung, Spleen, Heart, Kidney, Pericardium, and Liver while the Colon, Stomach, Small Intestine, Bladder, Triple Warmer, and Gall Bladder comprise the six organs that are considered yang. The yin organs are constantly operating and their main functions, from a TCM point of view, are to manufacture and store vital substances like qi, blood, and body fluid. The yang bowels operate intermittently and their main functions are to receive and digest food, absorb the nutrient substances, and excrete waste. Each organ pair is associated with one of the Five Elements, except for fire, which is associated with an additional pair.

When understood in the context of TCM, the influences, complexities, functions and correspondences of all the organs and channels serve as a foundation for better understanding the bioenergetic complex of the human being and assessing the patterns of imbalance that Asian bodywork therapists primarily focus on while treating (Figure 9-3).

Channels

Although the organs themselves are confined to a fixed location within the body, their sphere of influence permeates the entire body through the network of channels also known as the meridians. Channels are the pathways of qi and are actively engaged in transporting energy and nutrients, warding off disease, healing injuries, and naturally balancing disturbances in the body's equilibrium. The 12 primary channels are also known as the organ channels because of each channel's association with an organ. Although in textbook pictures and on classroom charts the channels appear to be discrete, inanimate lines skimming the surface of the skin, they are actually a living network of vessels and

Table of The Five Elements' Correspondences

Elements	Fire	Earth	Metal	Water	Wood
Climate	Heat	Damp	Dry	Cold	Wind
Seasons	Summer	Late Summer	Autumn	Winter	Spring
Yin or Zang Organs	Heart	Spleen	Lung	Kidney	Liver
Yang or Fu Bowels	Small Intestine	Stomach	Large Intestine	Bladder	Gallbladder
Tastes	Bitter	Sweet	Pungent	Salty	Sour
Sense Organs	Tongue	Mouth	Nose	Ear	Eye
Tissues	Vessel	Muscle	Skin & Hair	Bone	Tendons/ Sinews
Emotions	Joy	Worry	Grief	Fear	Anger

Figure 9-3 This table shows several of the most important and useful correspondences of the Five Elements of traditional Chinese medicine (TCM). Five Element Theory breaks everything down into five fundamental energies, substances, and qualities that comprise our existence and that are frequently used in TCM diagnosis and treatment.

branches webbing deep throughout the entire body, not unlike the arteries, veins, and capillaries (Figure 9-4).[4]

Through these channels, the influence of the organs reach out to every part of the body to protect and nourish it. However, if these pathways become damaged or blocked, the channels are no longer able to provide these essential functions. When this happens, the channels will often exhibit a palpable difference and may for example feel weak, empty, and lacking or may feel full, tight, and hot. (Hence the importance for bioenergetic therapists to develop really keen sensitivity and palpation skills.) The major role of bioenergetic bodywork practitioners is to restore the balance and harmony to the energy system and as a result resolve their patients' health complaints. Then their role is to help their patients maintain an overall improved state of health.

Points

When TCM was first developing, it was observed again and again that certain locations along the channels could be manipulated to influence the body. *The Yellow Emperor's Classic of Internal Medicine,* written almost 5000 years

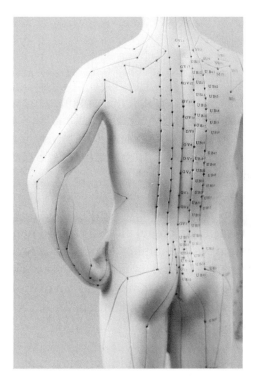

Figure 9-4 The acupuncture channels and points along the posterior parts of the body shown on an acupuncture model used for reference. *Image copyright 2009, Orrza. Used under license from shutterstock.com.*

ago, established the functions of 365 of these locations, which are considered the classical points of acupuncture.

Points are like the gateways into the energy channels. Because each point has a wide range of functions and capabilities, the same points can often be indicated to treat seemingly unrelated ailments. Points that ease pain in the back can be used to improve digestion. Points used to treat asthma can be used to boost the immune system. Points can provide pain relief directly in or around the area being pressed or they can have effects all the way at the opposite end of the body. Points pressed on the ankles and toes can help clear headaches and shoulder pain. Points on the hands and forearms can calm the heart and nourish the colon.

Correctly utilizing these points can have a powerful effect on the bioenergetic system, and the Asian bodywork therapist must have a firm grasp of their usage. Equally important, however, is knowing when not to use them. While certain points will have a calming, grounding effect on someone who is suffering from stress, the same points can induce premature labor in a patient who is pregnant. An unaware therapist can end up doing more harm than good if his or her training or knowledge has not been sufficiently developed.

Assessment

The way Chinese medical theory developed differs richly from the evolution of western science. Western medicine delved deeply into the body through dissection and microexamination of the human form. Asian spiritual perspectives held that the body was a sacred vessel that contained the soul; therefore, to cut it open was seen as an unthinkable act. So instead, they developed intricate ways of understanding the condition of the energy system and the body that required careful listening to the subtle textures in the heartbeat, the face, the tongue, and the abdomen.

Although there are many ways of assessing a patient's condition, two of the most powerful and most used ways are considered to be pulse and tongue diagnosis. Different areas of the tongue pertain to the different organs and their associated functions and areas of influence, including the channels (Figure 9-5). Markings in that organ's area of the tongue reflect the condition of that specific organ and energy complex. For instance, if the tip of the tongue is red, it can mean that there is a dysfunction or imbalance in the heart energy.

The shape of the tongue reveals different things as well. A swollen tongue points to blockages in the body that are causing things to back up and swell, often in the digestive system. If the coating on the tongue is thick and white, it can mean that the person is fighting off an infection.

The other widely used form of diagnosis in Chinese medicine is pulse diagnosis (Figure 9-6). There are three main pulse positions on each wrist and each

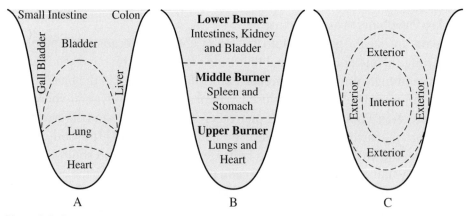

Figure 9-5 Practitioners of Asian (bioenergetic) bodywork, acupuncture, and Chinese herbal medicine learn to overlay and then view the surface features of the tongue with three different maps: 1) charting the internal organs, 2) dividing the body into three parts—upper burner, middle burner, and lower burner, and 3) viewing the body as interior and exterior, reflecting the movement of the disease.

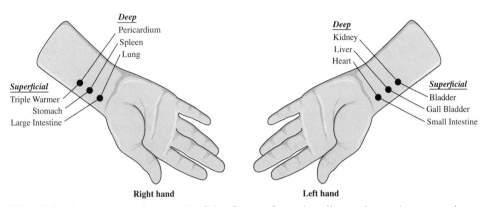

Figure 9-6 The modern placement of the fingers for pulse diagnosis most commonly taught today.

position has both a superficial (yang) and deep (yin) location, accounting for all 12 organs. At each position, the therapist gauges the pressure, speed, stability, and depth of each pulse to determine that organ's condition. For example, a strong, wiry pulse on the Liver position that feels like a guitar string points to overactive Liver energy, which can indicate stress, frustration, anger, and so on. A pulse that seems to float on the surface of the skin and can be felt as soon as the therapist touches the wrist indicates that a cold is likely coming on.

These are subtle arts and developing the sensitivity to detect the slightest nuances takes years of practice. A novice student practitioner may at first only be able to feel the grossest signs whereas the trained professional will be able to decipher more of what the bioenergetic complex is saying. Some therapists have stated that it is only after 10 years of studying the pulse that they are finally starting to understand it.

The condition of the patient doesn't have to be determined through just these methods. The story of a person is told all over his or her body, and if therapists are trained to listen correctly, they will be able to determine a patient's condition through a number of other ways. The state of the muscles, the quality of the voice, the glow in the eyes, and the characteristics of the personality can all reveal a world of information. The face, too, can hold valuable clues.

The quality of people's voices, the way they breathe, the way they smell, and the way their bodies feel to the touch can all reveal valuable insight into their condition. Every imbalance is reflected in the body and will leave its marks. The level of the therapist will determine if those markings are read or go unnoticed. More than likely, experienced Second and Third Paradigm bioenergetic practitioners trained in the philosophy and practices of TCM will have the greatest likelihood of success in catching the more subtle signs and symptoms manifesting in a patient's pulses, tongue, and bioenergy system.

TUINA

The term *tuina*, translated to mean "lift and press," first appeared during the Ming Dynasty (1368–1644). Prior to this era, massage in ancient China had been known originally as *amma* and later as *anmo.* This distinction from the traditionally used terms, represented an evolutionary step in bodywork, a time when massage had become a fully fledged system of healing with its own comprehensive system of diagnosis and treatment.

Although tuina was frowned upon by the government during the Qing Dynasty (1644–1911), this healing art form flourished among the masses. After the People's Republic of China was established in 1949, the government initiated training programs to spread and develop tuina as a serious medical art. In the 1960s, tuina was developed to a degree where practitioners worked side by side with doctors in hospitals across the country. Today, tuina not only plays an active role in the Chinese medical community, it is also gaining recognition internationally.

Techniques

In **tuina**, there are many steps that need to be taken toward becoming a proficient therapist and many details that must be attended to. The physical application of tuina treatment is a demanding process and requires much practice to develop the skills, stamina, and strength necessary to perform each action correctly. In fact, for some chronic conditions to be relieved it may require every ounce of the practitioner's strength; therefore, it is of the utmost importance that the therapist be in good health.

The hands must be strong yet sensitive. The fingers must be nimble yet penetrating. Physically, practitioners must possess the fortitude to carry out techniques that require lifting, supporting, and twisting half the patient's body weight. The features and qualities of each technique must be learned in order to provide treatment most effectively.

Careful "listening" to the body before, during, and after the treatment is necessary to ensure that each technique being applied is appropriate for the moment. Otherwise, the technique must be changed immediately to fit the specific condition of the specific channel. One of tuina's major strengths is the arsenal of techniques that it can deploy toward a broad spectrum of ailments.

The quality of application of each tuina technique depends upon the condition of the patient being treated. Generally speaking, however, each stroke should be deep yet gentle, brisk yet rhythmic, and determined yet not aggravating. Although there are many names given to the array of techniques belonging to the tuina family of bodywork, they can be broken down into two basic categories: fundamental and subordinate. Fundamental techniques are the major strokes and maneuvers that are most often used during treatment. Subordinate techniques, tuina's minor collection of movements, are less frequently used.

The following briefly describes several of the most commonly used fundamental techniques.

Stroking, or light rubbing, is a simple motion applied with the entire palm and is often used as an introduction to treatment as well as a conclusion because of its ability to gradually build then descend softly. This maneuver can be applied either toward or away from the heart. Stroking toward the heart promotes the circulation of blood, qi, and fluids; boosts metabolism; reduces swelling; and calms the nerves. Stroking away from the heart relaxes the body, induces sleep, reduces numbness, and strengthens the channels.

Kneading is slow and soft at first, but this stroke builds in intensity to become deep and penetrating. Using the fingertips, this stroke can be applied to many parts of the body. The fingers provide support while the thumbs create a semi-circular forward motion. On larger parts of the body like the legs, hip, and lower back, the whole hand can be used to deliver a deep, broad pressure. While kneading the body, muscles can be pulled and squeezed with this motion. Kneading stimulates and strengthens the muscles and fascia. Kneading toward the heart promotes circulation, prevents muscle atrophy, and softens scars. Stroking away from the heart strengthens muscles and promotes their regeneration.

Twisting or wringing can be applied to long muscles like the calves and the biceps. The muscle is first lifted away from the bone with both hands. One hand pulls the muscle in one direction while the other hand pulls it in the opposite direction to create an "S" shape with the muscle.

The practice of *rubbing (or burning)* creates a penetrating heat that is absorbed into the many layers of tissue deep underneath the skin. It warms the channels; clears stagnation of qi, blood, and fluids; and reduces swelling. This stroke is performed directly on the skin in a straight line with even pressure throughout. Rubbing is focused on creating heat, not going for depth; therefore, this stroke should be mild with the pace falling around 120 strokes per minute. This maneuver can be performed with the fingers, pinky edge of the palms, or the whole hand, depending on the area of the body being worked.

The simple and powerful maneuver known as *pressing* is done with the thumbs or elbows, and can provide a very specific and penetrating pressure to release deep-seated conditions. This stroke can press directly into the points along the channels in order to diffuse qi and tension, but if greater circulation is desired, the movement can be applied with a forward, gliding motion.

Quick, rhythmic *percussion strokes* can be applied with just the fingers or the whole fist, with one hand or both at the same time. When using just the fingers, the fingers are fanned and relaxed. Contact is made using the pinky edges with quick, "karate-chop" motions of the hands. This can be either stimulating or sedating, depending upon the length of time this stroke is applied.

In other bodywork modalities, this stroke is also known as tapotement. A short burst of tapotement enlivens the nerves and wakes the body while a longer one will relax and sedate. Because this stroke is very effective on the nerves, this is an excellent technique for conditions like numbness and paralysis. Tapotement with the fists provides a deeper stimulation that penetrates to the core of dense tissues, while a lighter tapotement with the fingers just skims the surface and often serves as an ending stroke for treatment.

Vibrations can be done with just the fingers or the thick flesh at the base of the palm under the pinky finger. This technique can be stationary or can slowly progress forward to push and clear clogged channels. With the hand or fingers resting on the body, a tight, rapid shaking motion is applied. This motion, too, is tonic for the nerves and has benefits similar to tapotement. For muscle spasms and scars, this stroke is especially appropriate.

Circular strokes are well suited for tight or delicate spaces like the head and abdomen. This move can be done with the fingers, palms, or the whole hands. On the head, small semicircular motions of the fingers glide from the base of the skull, over the ears, through the thick cords of tension often found in the temples and ends near the borders of the forehead. Meanwhile the thumbs anchor into the northernmost point of the head and act as an axis from which the fingers swing. This stroke helps alleviate the pain or tension that often accumulates in the face, jaws, and even the shoulders.

Over the abdomen, sweeping strokes can be created with both hands or small, mini-circles can be used to trace over the path of the large intestines. These strokes benefit digestion, promote healthy bowel movements, improve menstruation, and flush out the energies that tend to stagnate in this area.

Stretches, rotations, and joint movements are also a regular part of tuina's repertoire of fundamental techniques. The head can be stretched forward, backward, side to side, twisted, and pulled. The arms can be pulled, stretched, and rotated in nearly every direction, as can the legs. The whole torso can even be flexed, tractioned, and rotated to free the spine and waist. These techniques serve to open and free the joints, areas where the greatest tendency lies for qi to become blocked and stagnated. These blockages can cause major imbalances in the overall bioenergetic system, which, if left untreated, can in turn manifest as serious physical conditions.

Principles of Tuina Practice

Before applying even a single stroke, the therapist must consider tuina's principles of practice. These principles were established to help the tuina therapist give a highly focused and effective treatment while providing the most ease and comfort to the patient.

1. Don't seek to treat pain—seek to treat the cause of pain. The cause of a headache may actually be in the neck or further down the arms. To treat just the area of pain would be to treat just the symptoms. While this would provide temporary relief, it wouldn't be a real solution.

2. The scope of each technique should gradually enlarge from a point to a line to an area.

3. The pace should reflect the pressure by starting slow then gradually becoming deeper and more rapid.

4. Treatment should progress from top to bottom, front to back, and from outside to inside.

5. Sensitive areas such as the insides of the arms and legs require a mild touch, while thicker areas on the outside of the arms and legs require a heavier hand.

6. The pace and pressure of each stroke should be calibrated according to the patient's condition.

7. The attitude of the practitioner should be warm and friendly but also serious and focused.

8. The patient should lie quietly for 5 to 10 minutes before the treatment begins. Tuina therapy does not begin until the patient is calm and quiet.

9. Only the area being worked should be exposed. All other areas should be covered and warm. The practitioner's attention should be absorbed into the area being worked and into the expressions of the patient's face. This is so that the practitioner is able to adapt the treatment at a moment's notice if the current approach is either aggravating or noneffective.

The Tuina Session

A tuina therapy session generally doesn't last more than an hour. Because each tuina treatment is specifically designed for the patient, treatment routines can vary dramatically in pressure, rhythm, pace, and direction. Although tuina is designed to be a more aggressive form of bodywork, the use of excessive force will damage the skin, injure the muscle, and may even break the bone. Therefore, the tuina therapist must be highly aware that while pushing the limit may be of benefit, crossing the line between just enough pressure and too much could be damaging. To ensure that the patient receives just the right touch, each stroke must be carefully calibrated to fit the needs and qualities of each patient.

When starting at the head, the thumbs are used to slowly wipe the forehead, beginning at the middle and pressing out to the sides over the temples. This stroke initiates from just above the eyebrows with each subsequent stroke starting just a little higher than the one before and ending at the hairline. A lighter version of this same stroke can be used to wipe directly over the eyes to reduce redness, swelling, and pain.

Vertical strokes starting at the center of the eyebrows and rising to meet the hairline can help clear blockages and stagnation in the head and face. Over the temples, circular strokes can be used to soften tension. The pace here is brisk and activating. Points on the head and face can benefit many conditions ranging from sinus congestion, headaches, blurry vision, and anxiety.[5] While many modalities ignore or simply gloss over the head and face, in TCM this is considered to be an important area where much tension is held and energy can be trapped.

Similar strokes are performed over the top and back of the head as well as around the ears. In just the head alone, a variety of strokes can be used, from simple straight stroking, to circular pressure, to vibration, tapotement, kneading, and pressing. This reflects a major strength of tuina. For every pain in the body, tuina offers precise solutions.

To work the back and waist, the patient is turned over onto the stomach. Issues here can be numerous, including muscle spasm, disc degeneration, and spinal herniation. Simple pushing strokes initiate the work, followed by kneading. Gradually, the depth and pressure of the strokes become more and more penetrating. All the strokes applied on the head and face can be carried over to the back, but the denser mass of tissues here allows for more powerful techniques to be employed. Heavy kneading with the palms, deep stripping with the thumbs, and penetrating pressure with the elbows help diffuse the stress, tension, and energy that often stagnates here (Figure 9-7). Rubbing can be

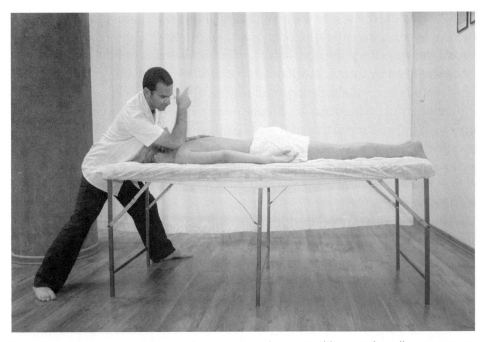

Figure 9-7 A woman receiving a tuina treatment by a practitioner using elbow pressure to help diffuse the client's stress, tension, and built-up energy. *Image copyright 2009, Salamanderman. Used under license from shutterstock.com.*

used alongside the spine to create an intense heat along the core of the back. To soften the thick buildup of tension and tissue regularly found in the lower back, a method called spine-pinching (where just the skin is lifted and twisted) can be utilized.

Turning the client back over, the abdomen can be worked to benefit all the internal organs in this area. This is one of the most vital areas of the body and dysfunction here can disrupt the functioning of every muscle and cell in the body. A unique feature of abdominal work is the use of a technique called whirling round-rubbing. Both hands are used to create a continuous circle of pressure that whirls around and around the abdomen. The hands flow one after another, tracing over the path of the large intestine again and again. The pressure is deep, but not aggressive and is adjusted as per the patient's tolerance. This is followed by an undulating motion of the hands, beginning just underneath the navel and rising up the body in waves. Simple strokes down the midline of the abdomen follow up along with kneading and vibration. A powerful palmar pressure can be applied at this point to break up intestinal adhesions, improve digestion, and benefit menstruation. A lifting motion on both sides of the waist further helps decrease tension and stagnation in the torso.

Working the chest opens the breathing, improves circulation throughout the whole body, frees the ribs, and releases repressed emotions. Palmar stroking all the way down the chest and to the abdomen, and kneading with the palm followed by thumb-work down the midline of the chest, disperses the tension and energy that can accumulate here. The thumbs can be used to comb through tension in between the ribs. Strokes starting at the top of the chest going down the midline of the body and flaring out underneath the ribcage help soothe emotions and clear tensions. Pummeling the chest further helps dissipate any tightness in that area. The whole upper torso can be stretched from side to side, flexed and extended, and twisted at the waist to complete treatment for the torso.

The arms can be treated with the patient sitting or lying on a table. Long, straight strokes begin at the wrist and glide up to the armpits. Kneading and compression up the arm helps relieve numbness, pain, or weakness. Since the channels in the arms include the Lung, Pericardium, Heart, Colon, Triple Warmer, and Small Intestine, these strokes also benefit conditions related to digestion, breathing, and heart functions. A rolling maneuver is used to soften the long muscles of the arms and muscles here can be twisted, pummeled, and pressed. The fingers can be adjusted ("cracked") with a tractioning motion that frees compression in the joints. Taking the whole arm, the shoulder, chest, neck, and back can be stretched in a variety of directions.

The legs are worked in much the same way as the arms, but the thicker tissue here may require more penetrating pressure. Channels in the legs include the Stomach, Spleen, Liver, Kidney, Gall Bladder, and Bladder. Because of this, conditions ranging from indigestion to headaches to urinary tract infections and premenstrual syndrome can be benefited by working the legs. Like the shoulders, the hip can be opened by stretching and rotating the legs.

AMMA THERAPEUTIC MASSAGE

The word *amma,* the oldest known word for massage, dates back approximately 5000 years to the period of the Yellow Emperor, Hwang Ti, and is translated as "push and pull." After the Han Dynasty of China (206 BCD–220 CE), Asian bodywork was known as *anmo,* translated as "press and rub." Then during the Ming Dynasty of China (1368–1644 CE) it became known as tuina, meaning to "lift and press." As this form of bodywork spread throughout the Orient, the original term amma was maintained by the Koreans, while anma was used by the Japanese.

The amma therapeutic massage of Tina Sohn, trademarked as AMMA Therapy®, is a newly evolved form of this ancient discipline. It has been taken to new levels of depth and precision by blending the energetic-based science of traditional Chinese medicine with newer, more material models of the human body. Western theories of anatomy and physiology have been closely analyzed side by side with traditional concepts of channels and energy. Because this hybrid modality approaches injuries and illnesses from both eastern and western perspectives, it is able to offer solutions that fit the modern lifestyle. This also allows practitioners of this modality to work comfortably alongside doctors, nurses, and other important members of the western modern health care establishment.

Tina Sohn, creator of amma therapeutic massage, was known as a healer of extraordinary abilities—a gift that was nurtured by her husband, Robert Sohn. She was what is known as a healing sensitive—someone who can literally "feel" the pain of others. Walking into a classroom she would often somehow feel that something was wrong with one of her students. Once with no prior knowledge of a student's condition, Mrs. Sohn was drawn to and pressed a point in the student's jaw, dissolving the pain of a tooth extraction that had been lingering for weeks.

In another situation, Mrs. Sohn came to the aid of a child in a hospital who had been coughing up blood for three months. Every known test had been performed, but the results revealed nothing that explained what was wrong. Mrs. Sohn, after only a moment of resting her hands on the child's head, revealed that the child's sinuses were bleeding. All the tests so far had only been conducted from the neck down due to the concern over the cough, but the blood was actually draining from higher up. After only a few amma sessions, some herbs, and dietary changes, the child recovered completely.[6]

Although a blessing to many, this gift could also be a curse. Her sensitivity to others was so great that Mrs. Sohn could become physically ill if she touched someone who was on powerful medications, steroids, or drugs. Although patients were screened, a few patients who had no idea what they were taking would still make it to her massage table and she would become sick—sometimes for days. But even after such instances, she returned day after day, year after year, continuing to treat the sick and teach her students her art.

Tina Sohn's training in the healing arts began early in her life when she was immersed into a world of acupuncture, herbs, philosophy, and martial arts. Her training began at the age of four when her grandmother would have Tina imitate amma techniques on her to help take away grandma's aches and pains. Often, Tina could "feel" someone's pain just by being near or touching them. Once, when Tina was a young child sitting in class, her teacher began to appear like a skeleton to her. Several months later he died from a disease from which he literally wasted away. Another time, Tina was in close proximity to a relative and she experienced pain in her kidneys. Then weeks later, he was diagnosed with kidney disease. For some time, Tina thought that she was the cause of these events and spent years trying to block her experiences and avoided getting close to people. However, with the help of Robert Sohn, her future husband, Tina was able to translate her rare abilities into a format that was teachable to others.[7]

Theory and Principles

The most obvious distinction of amma therapeutic massage from other formats with the same TCM background is the circular strokes that are applied to nearly every part of the body. As opposed to shiatsu's passive approach, amma is similar to tuina's more assertive style to influence and motivate the flow of qi in the body. Strokes are produced with the thumbs, fingers, palms, or fists and are always directed downward in order to ground the patient's energy.

A modality bearing close resemblance to its predecessors, amma utilizes the traditional methods of gathering information, including tongue and pulse diagnosis, and is based on the conventionally established meridian points and pathways. There are, however, some unique distinctions. In addition to the established points of acupuncture, Tina Sohn discovered extra points (located on and off the channels) that were found be highly beneficial. These points are called Tina Sohn Points (TS points), and have been tested on thousands of patients over the course of many years.

Also, the focus of amma therapeutic massage is on treating the tendino-muscle channels and cutaneous regions of the bioenergetic system, which are the superficial extensions of the 12 primary channels. Although they are located closer to the surface of the body, when manipulated competently their effects travel and have repercussions into the deepest layers of the bioenergetic system.

The Development of an Amma Therapist

Being able to effectively utilize the techniques and principles only achieves half of what a truly developed therapist can accomplish. Advancement to the highest degree only comes when there is a parallel development in the practitioner's internal world—requiring serious exploration of one's psychology.

The development of an amma therapist can be described in three levels. Each level is determined by the practitioner's body of experience, knowledge, and capabilities. The first level is that of a novice Asian bodywork therapist.

Aside from the strokes appearing different to the strokes of a basic massage and the focus of treatment being on the channels of energy system, there is little difference in the outcome, primarily general relaxation and stress reduction. It is in the second level, the level of the amma therapist, where energy's often complex dynamics are realistically understood and applied. The practitioner has come to a point in his or her training and practice where as a result of this deeper perspective, as an amma therapist he or she is able to treat more complex conditions and achieve more far-reaching results.

At the far end of the spectrum is the **healing sensitive**. The healing sensitive represents someone whose sensitivities have developed to the point of being able to read signs of physical, mental, and emotional distress with only the power of perception. Just as some are born great pianists and others must work night and day to become great, some are instilled with this level of sensitivity from birth while others have to earn it. This is a process that requires a unique fusion of dedication, knowledge, and compassion. The correct combination of these three elements can recalibrate our sensitivities to detect the subtle vibrations of illnesses, injuries, moods, and even thoughts. This direct "seeing" into the patient's condition provides a profound insight into what kind of treatment will be required, thus heavily impacting its results. Interestingly, these three levels parallel those of The Three Paradigms.

Physical, mental, and emotional fortitude are necessary qualities of achieving the features of a healing sensitive. Practitioners must have the physical endurance to treat the tenth patient of the day with the same energy, care, and skill as their first. They must have the intellectual prowess to understand the subtle ebbs and flows of energy and they must develop their emotional capacity to provide a level of care and compassion far beyond normal human concerns. Exploration of these subtle arts is bolstered through the practice of tai chi chuan, an internal martial art, which facilitates sensing, cultivating, and controlling energy. Amma therapeutic massage is as much about self-growth as it is about treating the patient.[8]

A General Treatment in Amma Therapeutic Massage

Amma therapeutic massage treatments are performed on a bodywork table and can last anywhere from 45 minutes to more than an hour, depending on the issue(s) being treated and the time needed to review recommendations, exercises, medical tests, and so on. During treatment, patients generally are wearing underwear and are fully draped at all times or they may choose to wear a hospital-type gown or loose clothing. Before the amma practitioner begins the treatment, a thorough review is taken of the patient's medical history;

medications; presenting complaints, signs, and symptoms; and the patient's dietary habits and exercise patterns. Usually this information can be obtained from a fairly detailed patient health history form, which needs to be completed in advance, and a brief interview during the first visit. If there is enough advance time for the appointment these forms may be sent to the patient's home where they can be filled out carefully, with much thought and detail.

After a complete assessment is made, a treatment plan is formulated. Since patients bring with them their own set of energetic imbalances, amma practitioners need to identify what they are through a series of diagnostic procedures including palpation and pulse and tongue diagnosis. As mentioned earlier, these assessment tools offer information about the condition of patients' organs, imbalances in their underlying energy system, and their overall constitution. Using palpation, amma professionals pay attention to areas of sensitivity or pain, as well as any discomfort related to specific motions or postures. Consideration is also given to structural deviations, spasms, and palpable masses and their possible effects on energy system blockages and imbalances. Of course, attention is also paid to skin temperature and skin changes.

Since amma therapeutic massage also uses an integrative approach to assessing patients, practitioners will also consider any other available, relevant information including test results such as blood, X-rays, MRIs, EKGs and so on. If necessary, therapists will research the medications their patients are taking and look for any serious side effects or complications from these medicines that may be playing a role in what their patients are presenting.

Full-body amma treatments may include the vigorous manipulation, often with the use of herbal liniments, of particular points, energy channels, and areas of the body utilizing specific circular hand techniques including circular thumb pressure; circular digital, palmar, ulnar, or palm-heel pressure; direct thumb or digital pressure; and a variety of other stroking and embracing hand techniques that require both great skill and strength to perform properly. For maximizing the effects of amma treatment, practitioners usually recommend specific exercises directed at a particular problem or forms of exercise like tai chi chuan, qi gong, or hatha yoga for developing and maintaining optimum health. Diets and detoxification regimens are also often a big part of the amma process along with appropriate herbs, vitamins and supplements.

When amma therapeutic massage professionals are practicing at Second or Third Paradigm levels, their work is often used to aid in the treatment of a wide range of more serious conditions. Some of these include but are not limited to: osteo- and rheumatoid arthritis, hypertension, diabetes, ulcers, colitis, respiratory and circulatory conditions, various cancers, and autoimmune and neuromuscular diseases. In addition, amma treatments for the full range of infant and childhood illness are also quite effective and beneficial.

ACUPRESSURE

From one view the origins of acupressure can be said to date as far back as a human being's instinctive impulse to rub or press a painful area of the body. To this day people still automatically do that. But the cultivation and evolution of this practice of applying finger pressure to various points or loci on the body has no greater history than with the Chinese where it has been used for more than 5000 years. Gradually through a combination of great intuition, as well as trial and error, the Chinese discovered that applying pressure on various points not only relieved pain in the local area of those points, but that it also brought relief and other benefits to parts of the body far from the points themselves. With further experimentation, including the use of pressure tools such as stones and arrows on the battlefields, the Chinese began to discover new point locations and recognized that their repeated manipulation not only alleviated pain but also positively influenced the functioning of the body's physiology, particularly the internal organs. Eventually, after years of observation, palpation and deep insights, the Chinese physicians mapped out the underlying complex energy system of channels and points which serves as the basis of traditional Chinese medicine and treatment in all forms of Asian bodywork and acupuncture.

The Chinese method of acupressure can also be viewed as a close relative of some of the lineages and variants of Japanese shiatsu particularly in the west, especially given the fact that China greatly influenced the development of the Japanese bioenergetic healing arts. For example, the more recent Tsubo Therapy work of Katsusuke Serizawa, a form of shiatsu therapy which is the subject of his 1976 book *Tsubo: Vital Points for Oriental Therapy* is viewed as a form of acupressure in the United States. It is not uncommon to find the terms shiatsu and acupressure being used interchangeably describing hybrid forms of Asian bodywork therapy. Today acupressure is also the foundation of other forms of bodywork, including the popular Jin Shin Do® Bodymind Acupressure® and some other forms of shiatsu.[9]

Acupressure can be essentially understood as point therapy. Its name, however, is misleading because "acu" means needle (as in acupuncture) and also "pressure" implies that pressure is a key element. The effectiveness of treatment, however, is not dependent upon the amount of force exerted and there are of course no needles involved in the practice of acupressure. In fact, acupressure is a system that utilizes gentle stimulation of the points. As opposed to physically "doing," the acupressure therapist is patiently attracting energy to a point through light touch. Points are held until a pulsation is felt under the fingers—an indication that qi is now flowing freely through the area. Through a specific sequence of pressing, rubbing, or lightly touching points, a wide variety of results can be achieved (Figure 9-8). Because subtle treatments are more effective when the body is in a state of relaxation, a typical acupressure session may often begin with the more vigorous manipulations of tuina.[10]

The underlying practice of acupressure, its theories, principles, assessment methods, and treatment planning, are directly in line with acupuncture and

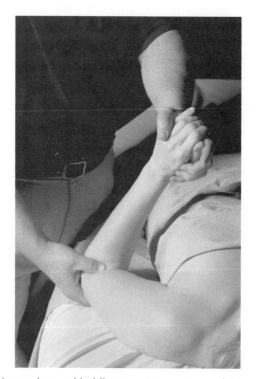

Figure 9-8 A therapist pressing and holding an acupressure point on his patient's elbow.

the use of TCM. This includes diet, herbs, exercise, and meditation, to achieve and maintain overall health, wellness, and balance. Because they are more closely connected through touch to the changing dynamics of the body's energies, acupressure therapists have the advantage of being able to immediately sense the activities of each point. These practitioners are able to make real-time modifications the moment change arises.

General Benefits of Tuina, Amma Therapeutic Massage, and Acupressure

- Relieves stress and tension
- Instills a sense of well-being and connectedness
- Improves digestion and circulation
- Promotes menstrual regularity and comfort
- Relieves head- and backaches and other musculoskeletal conditions
- Strengthens immune system
- Improves stamina
- Relieves post-traumatic stress
- Promotes healthy pregnancy
- Eases childbirth
- Improves reproductive system disorders
- Reduces high blood pressure
- Treats a broad range of conditions, depending upon the practitioner

Precautions

Tuina, amma, and acupressure can be applied with caution as long as the following conditions are avoided:

- Open cuts and sores
- Broken bones
- Rashes
- Bruises
- Phlebitis
- Pregnancy—certain points should not be pressed
- Patients receiving UV therapy. (After UV therapy ends patients must wait 7 to 10 days before receiving treatment)
- Infectious diseases like hepatitis

Contraindications of Tuina, Amma Therapeutic Massage, and Acupressure

Tuina, amma, or acupressure may either be ineffective or damaging to the following conditions:

- Acute fever and flu
- Malignant tumors
- Advanced internal organ disease (kidney failure, respiratory failure, nephritis)
- Very unstable blood pressure
- Poisoning (food, snake, insect, etc.)
- Acute inflammations (appendicitis, severe arthritis, peritonitis)

SHIATSU

While the literal translation of the word shiatsu (Japanese for "finger pressure") suggests simplicity, this basic definition belies a rich and sophisticated system of healing with roots that trace back to ancient China. Since its inception in Japan, shiatsu has evolved with its own unique theories, philosophies, and techniques. This evolution, however, was not a linear process. At one point, shiatsu was nothing more than the rote imitation of healing delivered by untrained body-rubbers. At another point it almost faced extinction due to the shifting tides created by the Second World War. However, the strength of this approach has survived its critical stages of development and has matured into a system with its own branches and offspring. Today, there are many different forms and styles of shiatsu—some that differ like night and day, and others that bear obvious resemblance to their forefathers.

The two main forms of shiatsu being practiced today are Namikoshi shiatsu (Nippon style) and Zen shiatsu. Although Tokujiro Namikoshi came to the United States first, it was the warm, meditative approach of Zen shiatsu that really grasped the attention of the American public. Namikoshi's style had been developed in a time of Japan's modernization following the Second World War and had been stripped clean of traditional Chinese medicine theories involving energy, the Five Elements, and channels, in order to present a "legitimate," scientific face to the world. American students however, wanted to explore more than just the physical realm. Tired of the clinical approach to life that had been building in the West, they sought a deeper understanding of themselves and the world around them.

It was around this time, in the late 1970s, that Zen shiatsu came into the picture. A former student and teacher at Namikoshi's school of shiatsu, Shizuto

Masunaga offered a style of shiatsu that re-integrated its original core of spirituality and energy. With his special interest in exploring the mental, emotional, and spiritual components of the human entity, he crafted a system that merged theories from western psychology, traditional Chinese medicine, a modern understanding of the body, and Zen Buddhism. By exploring the connections between the energetic theories of the East and the result-based science of the West, Masunaga created a bridge for students who wanted to cross the boundaries to explore the mysterious force of energy that the Japanese called ki (qi). Because Masunaga was able to root foreign concepts into conventional western understanding, Zen shiatsu had a wide appeal and has become one of the most popular forms of shiatsu in the United States today.

Following the deaths of Namikoshi and Masunaga, other forms of shiatsu have emerged, each with their own unique aspects. Macrobiotic shiatsu emphasizes living a life that is in harmony with the natural order of the world. Self-care and lifestyle changes including exercise, stretching, postural alignment, breathing, diet, and home remedies are a major component of this approach.[11] Five Elements shiatsu focuses on using the TCM theory of the Five Elements as its major diagnostic tool to understand and treat the layers of the bioenergy system of the body, including the energetic imbalances that often accumulate over a lifetime. Other styles include Ohashiatsu®, Integrative Eclectic shiatsu, acupressure shiatsu, and more—each offering a unique interpretation of either the scientific approach of Namikoshi shiatsu or the more energetic and spiritual approach of Zen shiatsu.

Zen Shiatsu

Although born into a family of shiatsu practitioners, it wasn't until later in his life that Masunaga took up the family trade. His first inspiration was psychology, and he even taught the subject at Namikoshi's school of shiatsu.[12] The story of Masunaga's efforts entail not only tying the spiritual essence back into shiatsu but also his significant contributions to its evolution by developing theories unique to his system.

Theories and Principles

Although the roots of Zen shiatsu dig deep into the heart of TCM, there are significant differences. A practitioner of TCM uses multiple approaches while a practitioner of Zen shiatsu focuses mostly on balancing the channels, also known as meridians or pathways. While points are still utilized, it is specifically the channels that Masunaga was drawn to. This may be the reason that Masunaga's personal experience of channel location diverged from the TCM standard.

Masunaga's channel extension system of 12 bilateral pathways unique to Zen shiatsu are similar to, but not the same as, those defined by TCM. Masunaga felt that the meridian system of TCM was not sufficient to address the fact that the energy of each channel permeates the entire body. So he developed what he felt was a more complete integrated map of the energy channel system (Figure 9-9). The biggest difference is in the use of the extensions of each primary channel, many of which follow the known auxiliary pathways of TCM. They each (all 12) travel through the arms, legs, and abdomen (hara), where they can be palpated and used in the process of assessment and diagnosis. (To get a comparison of the difference between Masunaga's channel system and that of TCM's refer back to Figure 5-7 in Chapter 5.)

Assessment

Masunaga defined the fluctuations of the body on a day-to-day, moment-to-moment basis in terms of **kyo** and **jitsu**. Kyo is the activation of some internal need or desire. Jitsu is the response to that need. Together they perform the actions of balancing and counterbalancing. In essence, the theory of kyo and jitsu is an expression of the fundamental TCM principle of yin and yang.[13] Kyo is yin. Jitsu is yang. Yang is the activating force that seeks. Yin is the grounding force that receives. In the body, kyo conditions reflect as weak, empty, and "needy." Jitsu conditions manifest as tight, painful, and full.

While TCM diagnosis takes into account both the history and current status of the patient, Zen shiatsu focuses on the immediate present. The key question in diagnosis is, "What is the current health of the patient and how is the energy distributed?" While diagnosis can reveal an elaborate picture of the body's story, only two factors are considered essential:

1. The most full, or jitsu, meridian
2. The most empty, or kyo, meridian.

While it is important to treat jitsu, it is even more important to treat that which initiated jitsu—kyo. Kyo must be energized and reinforced while jitsu must be diffused and dispersed. An interesting distinction between TCM and Zen shiatsu diagnosis is that TCM seeks the cause or root factors while Zen shiatsu expresses the cause as having only two roots: the two meridians acting as kyo and jitsu—yin and yang.[14]

HARA DIAGNOSIS   One of Zen shiatsu's most important ideas is that of the hara. The hara is a multilevel concept that is much more than just a point located deep in the lower abdomen a few inches below the navel. It is the

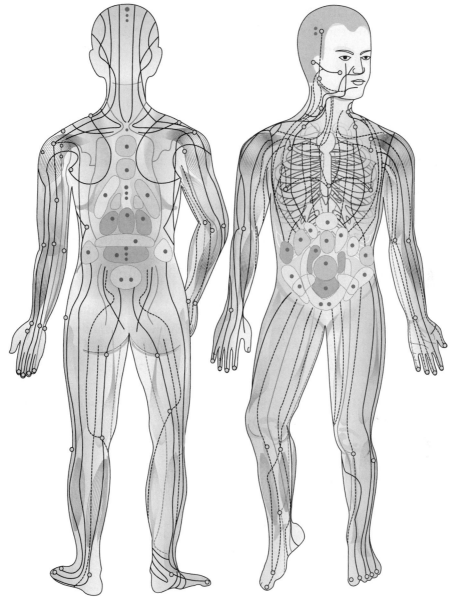

Figure 9-9 Masunaga's channel extension system of 12 bilateral pathways unique to Zen shiatsu. Each pathway (all 12) travels through the arms, legs, and abdomen (hara), where they can be palpated and used in the process of assessment and diagnosis.

physical center of gravity, the equivalent to the tan tien also known as the "field of elixir" in Traditional Chinese medicine. It is a person's energetic source of power and healing, and a psychological place of correct intention. It is considered the seat of one's life force and can be strong or weak, depending on the person's constitution. Just as examining the tongue or pulse can reveal the internal state of the body, palpation of the abdominal region through hara diagnosis can reveal a world of information about the nature of what the patient is experiencing.

Hara diagnosis, accomplished through abdominal palpation, is the primary assessment technique of Zen shiatsu and is often used in the prescribing of herbs and acupuncture. At one time a commonly practiced Chinese technique, abdominal palpation became important in the practice of Kampo, the Japanese version of the practice of Chinese medicine. Kampo took root around the beginning of the 18th century (Figure 9-10).[15]

Hara diagnosis consists of evaluating which energies are kyo and which energies are jitsu in order to determine the right course of action in treatment A jitsu pattern in the Liver can explain the stress or frustration that someone may be experiencing. A kyo pattern in the Spleen can shed a light on the patient's dampened levels of energy.[16] Evaluation of the hara is conducted with the slightest pressure of the fingertips—barely enough to indent the skin because here the practitioner is feeling for the organ's energy—not the organs themselves. Evaluation can be accomplished with either one hand or two (Figure 9-10). The one-handed sequence is a good way to get a feel for each individual's energies. Although the diagnosis is itself orchestrated with one hand, it is always connected to and working in concert with the mother hand. When assessing the upper portion of hara, the mother hand grounds at the Heart area. When evaluating the lower hara, the mother hand connects to the Spleen area over the navel. A more advanced technique is to operate with both hands. This is a more complex rhythm to follow and should only be practiced once the giver can locate the diagnostic areas with proficient accuracy.

The most important step in diagnosis is to approach it with a sense of peace and openness. This requires the giver to first take a moment to observe his or her own internal state. No matter what the giver sees within (anger, frustration, boredom, love, or compassion), this moment will allow the giver to contact and establish an inner presence that is connected to a grounded place and able to more objectively observe.

First the giver seeks to find the most jitsu energy. This is not a lingering or deliberating process. The sequence is given slowly but steadily, without

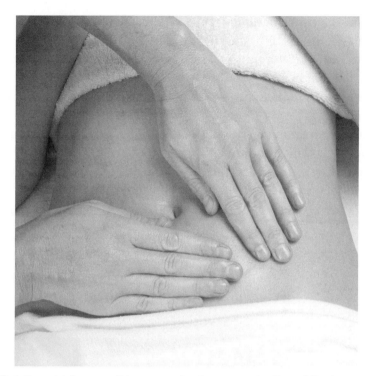

Figure 9-10 A Zen shiatsu practitioner conducting an evaluation of the hara. *Image copyright 2009, Jennifer Sharp. Used under license from shutterstock.com.*

pausing to think about what one is feeling. In this process, to think is to get in the way. This is a process that is achieved by feeling, not thinking. Jitsu patterns are invariably:

- Obvious
- Active
- Resilient
- Reactive

Although many have reported additional sensations of heat, tingling, pulsing, or a pushing away, these sensations can vary from receiver to receiver. If this process is approached with a quiet and grounded manner, the most jitsu energy will make itself known immediately. However, if after several attempts a conclusive diagnosis can't be reached, practitioners should perceive this as the perfect opportunity to exercise their sixth sense.

Finding the energy that is most kyo is difficult on its own because kyo has the fundamental properties of being hidden and withdrawn. However, once jitsu has been found, kyo can be tracked more easily. Placing one hand on the jitsu, the other hand carefully circles around the hara to listen for the area that connects, vibrates, or resonates with jitsu. Different practitioners have reported different sensations when this connection is felt. Some have reported it as a "blip" passing between the two areas. Others have described sensations of buzzing, kyo swelling, jitsu diminishing, or a sense of completion.

A similar evaluation can be conducted on the back. While this method is approached in a similar manner, the back reflects more chronic conditions and longstanding imbalances; therefore, the back diagnosis may not reflect the diagnosis of the hara. Because of this, only one of these methods should be employed.[17]

DIAGNOSING ENERGY   Visually observing the patterns and movements of ki in the body is said to be surprisingly easy provided the practitioner has at least a year's worth of training in both shiatsu and energetic exercises such as qi gong and tai chi chuan. When observing ki, three key questions are silently asked of the receiver:

1. "Is their ki up or down?"
2. "Is their ki strong or weak?"
3. "Is their ki flowing or blocked?"

When connected to the hara and observing with relaxed focus, the patterns of ki flow are said to become apparent. Looking at the ki allows the practitioner to form a plan of action tailored exactly to the receiver's needs. Reviewing the energy patterns after treatment can reveal the effectiveness of the treatment.[18]

Techniques

Zen shiatsu is the expression of the dynamic interplay between yin and yang. Yang represents movement and yin represents stillness. Applying pressure to the receiver's body is an act of yang while the calm, centered state in which the giver applies that pressure is yin. This concept is also expressed in the therapist's hands. One is used to support and listen while the other is used to move and take action.

The still hand—the mother hand—takes on the role of grounding the patient while the child hand, its active counterpart, has the function of activating the circulation of ki. Each hand will take its turn playing the role of mother or child as necessary; thus it is not important which hand takes which role. What is significant, however, is that the two are "in touch" and are working as one. This principle is applied to not only the hands, but to the use of elbows, knees, and feet as well.

Cooperation between the various parts of the therapist's body must also be reflected in the correct relationship between body and mind. This connection is imperative in order to properly express another core tenet of shiatsu—that of continuity. Each movement should flow from one to the next while contact is being consistently maintained with the client. This smooth flow of physical movement, however, must first be initiated in the mind. A conscious effort is necessary to continuously direct one's focus and intent towards creating fluidity of motion.

Even the roles of the shiatsu practitioner and the client are defined in a way that emphasizes the nature of their intertwined relationship. The therapist is called the giver and the client is known as the receiver. This is a dynamic that is only complete when the two come together in a balanced and harmonious way. From this perspective, the roles of both the therapist and the client are equally important. Without one, the other couldn't exist.[19]

While newer techniques have been developed to practice shiatsu on a massage table, it is most often practiced on the floor with a shiatsu mat, thick carpet, or a blanket. One of the unique aspects of working on the floor is that therapists have more "tools" at their disposal. While traditional massage therapists will often utilize only their hands, forearms, and elbows, a shiatsu practitioner can use the knees and even the feet. Because of this, shiatsu is a more whole-body experience for the giver. Even when pressure is applied with just the thumbs, the weight of the whole body can be used to lean into a point or channel. This not only gives the therapist a mechanical advantage, it also allows the practitioner to better "listen" to the client's body. Tensing the hands to push into the client's body will put up a wall between what the therapist is doing and what the client is feeling. By simply allowing the weight of the body to be transferred from the hands into the patient, the therapist can remain relaxed and receptive. This treatment style reflects Zen Buddhism's approach to spirituality—simple and direct. [20] With every stroke, pressure goes straight into the channels—there are no circles, no sweeping motions, and no deviation. The goal is crystal clear: to contact the ki in the most straightforward manner possible.

Shiatsu practitioners apply pressure along the body's energetic channels. Palming is often the first method utilized because of its nonabrasiveness. It provides a generalized pressure that is soothing to the body and prepares it for more penetrating work. Deep work right from the start can trigger a defensive tightening of the muscles, so palming provides an easy, noninvasive way to introduce touch to the body.

Once a layer of palming has been applied, the practitioner may choose to go deeper by using the thumbs. This provides a more focused pressure that can help release long-sustained blockages along a channel. Along with the thumbs, the fingers can be used when precise, delicate work is called for, like around the head and face.

A more vigorous alternative to the thumbs or fingers are the knuckles, which are well suited for working along the thick musculature found in the back. For the densest areas, the elbows, knees, or feet may be employed. Because the pressure can be intense, therapists will often palpate the area first with their hands before applying deeper pressure.

In addition to applying pressure to stimulate the channels, stretches and rotations of the head, neck, arms, and legs are frequently utilized. These joint movements are effective ways to activate the flow of blood and ki in the channels of the body.

PRINCIPLES OF PRACTICE

1. Relax: Tension interferes and distracts from being able to sense the receiver's ki. Relaxing allows the giver to be more in tune and connected with the receiver's energy.

2. Penetration, not pressure: The idea is not to simply apply pressure on the channels, but to penetrate into the receiver's energy system by relaxing into it and allowing it to open.

3. Stationary, perpendicular penetration: Being still allows time and opportunity to listen and assess the receiver's ki. Approaching the channel perpendicularly enables direct access into the receiver's energetic pathways.

4. Two-hand connectedness: Even while only one hand is being utilized to treat, the other hand should be part of every motion. Again, this is the principle of yin and yang in motion. While one hand actively engages the receiver's body, the other hand is quietly listening, grounding, and supporting.

5. Meridian continuity: Contact is made not only on the points, but throughout the entire channel.

6. Move from the hara: This means that the practitioner is using their body in the most connected, mechanically advantageous way while coming from a place of balance and centeredness. Being consistently connected to the hara throughout the treatment is the "epitome of good shiatsu."[21]

The Session

The session begins with the client fully dressed in loose and comfortable clothes and lying on the floor on a soft, padded mat or blanket for cushioning. The therapist kneels down by the head and quietly places his or her hands on the receiver's temples. This soothes the nerves and clients may feel a subtle release of tension as they start to let go of the stresses of the day. Intricate thumb and finger work traces the head and face around the eyes, cheeks, ears, and mouth. People are often shocked at the amount of tension that they hold there.

Specific points on the head and face help clear the sinuses, reduce jaw pain, improve vision, and calm the mind. To relax the neck, the head may be gently rolled from side to side to help stretch the thick sinews composing the muscles of the area. Turning the head to one side, the therapist can work on the exposed musculature of the neck to clear the many channels that run through this area.

The sequence of the giver's strokes is applied in the direction of each channel's flow of energy. Once the head is cleared, the giver places the hands on the receiver's shoulders near the chest and applies a slow, back and forth pressure that urges the shoulders to release down onto the mat. This is done in sync with the receiver's breath. As the chest opens, the shoulders begin to relax. This area, particularly centered around the solar plexus, has a strong connection to the emotions; therefore relaxing it can have dramatic effect. As pent-up feelings are released, the receiver will often experience positive changes in their state of mind.

Next, at the side of the body, the receiver's arm is brought out at a 45-degree angle from the body. The mother hand supports the client at the shoulder while the child hand applies a calming sequence of strokes down the arm along the Lung channel. This is an important area for those suffering from breathing problems or for when someone is sick because, from a TCM standpoint, the Lung energy plays a crucial role in supporting the immune system.

Arm rotations accompany the massage work, with one hand supporting the shoulder and the other taking a firm, but gentle hold of the wrist. The arm is moved in a wide arc that helps open the shoulders and chest while alleviating tensions that can cause headaches, neck, and back pain, and difficulty breathing.

Because of the greater emphasis that Asian bodywork places on the internal state of the body, a Zen shiatsu session will often incorporate abdominal or hara work. This is considered the most important aspect of the body because it is the source of one's major processes—digestion, detoxification, and reproduction. Clearing stagnation here can have a major influence on one's overall health and level of energy, emotional state, and, for women, menstruation. Some forms of shiatsu even specialize in treating the hara exclusively.

To loosen the tight grip that people often have in their hips, the legs can gently be rolled from side to side. This rocking motion invites the thick muscles of the hips to relax and let go. Relaxation is stimulated further down the leg and as the whole area begins to ease, the knees and feet fall out to the side. With the same methodical pace, the sequence of strokes continues down the leg, following each channel down to its end. Points are applied and held on channels of the legs to improve many conditions, including sluggishness, indigestion, stress, and anger.

Work on the back begins with the giver once again at the head of the recipient. Deep thumb strokes applied to the shoulders and in between the shoulder blades penetrate the tension that concentrates here. The thumb work is applied down the full length of the back on either side of the spine. The dense tissue here may require a more vigorous pressure, which can be supplied by the forearms or elbows.

Although this work treats mostly the Bladder channel, the main channel covering the back, key points along the inside path of this channel also benefit every other organ in the body. According to TCM, there is a group of special points along the Bladder channel where the ki of each major organ surfaces. Treatment of each of these points will tonify its associated organ and, when indicated, can be used as part of a specific treatment plan for a variety of imbalances.

The hips may require a deeper pressure as well since this is where the densest concentration of muscle tissue is found. For this purpose, the knees can be employed. By carefully placing the knees directly in the powerful muscles of the hips, the therapist can comfortably apply a broad but penetrating pressure. For those suffering low-back pain, this will often provide a welcome relief.

The legs are worked in the same fashion as the arms. The therapist may use a flat, palmar pressure to start here to ready the muscles for deeper work with the thumbs. The mother hand gently supports the receiver at the top of the hip while the child hand follows the path laid out by the channels down the legs.

A unique feature of Zen shiatsu is the side-lying position that is often utilized. Aside from providing a welcomed change of positioning, the side-lying position allows the giver easy access to areas that can be tricky to get to from the front- or back-lying positions. The channels that are accessed when the body is on its side can, among many things, be used to promote healthier digestion, detoxification, and emotional flexibility. Also, supporting the client from behind while in the side-lying position can give the client a warm sense of safety.

Throughout the course of treatment, movements are fluid, deep, but not aggressive. Stretches and rotations blend into the treatment as the receiver is pressed, pulled, lifted, and twisted. Working from the floor not only allows the therapist a wider range of movement options, it also offers clients a sense of freedom and security that's impossible to feel on a table.

Namikoshi Shiatsu

Namikoshi shiatsu (also known as Nippon style) was created by Tokujiro Namikoshi. Tokujiro, born November 3, 1905, first became involved with bodywork when he was only seven. After a long and grueling journey across Japan to relocate their home, Tokujiro's mother suddenly began complaining about knee pains. At first everyone thought it was just a result of the journey and assumed it would pass, but the pain grew worse, spreading to her ankles, shoulders, elbows, and wrists. With no doctor and no medicine, it was up to the children to make mother feel better.

Frequently she would say to Tokujiro that his hands felt the best. Encouraged by the praise, the young boy worked even more diligently. Although ignorant about anatomy, physiology, channels, and points, Tokujiro's little hands could tell the difference in the way tissue felt and modified his treatments accordingly. Eventually he discovered that the most effective method was to use pressure 80 percent of the time while rubbing only 20 percent. Young Tokujiro was eventually able to cure his mother completely—beginning a lifelong study in shiatsu.

In 1925, Tokujiro Namikoshi opened the Shiatsu Institute in Hokkaido and in 1940 he opened the Japan Shiatsu Institute. In 1955, after the end of the Second World War, the Japanese Health Ministry was directed by the United States to research the 300 or so unregulated therapies currently being practiced in Japan and approve only the ones that demonstrated effectiveness in clinical trials. Of those, shiatsu was the only one that received government approval.[22]

In 1957, Namikoshi's Shiatsu School was officially licensed by the Minister of Health and Welfare to become the first and only school in the country to provide specialist education for this field and in 1964, shiatsu finally received recognition as a distinct form of massage separate from other forms of bodywork. Today, Namikoshi shiatsu is the most popular form of shiatsu practiced in Japan, and schools and practitioners can be found worldwide.

Theories, Principles, and Treatment

Namikoshi shiatsu is a pressure point-based system that was founded on the modern western understanding of the body including anatomy, physiology, and pathology. Located on or over the muscles, nerves, blood vessels, lymph vessels, bones and endocrine glands, Namikoshi's pressure point system directly affects the nervous system, which in turn affects the internal physiological organ systems of the body. Nevertheless, many of Namikoshi's pressure points do correspond to acupressure points also found on the energy channels or meridians of Chinese acupuncture and commonly used in the other forms of shiatsu (Figure 9-11).

Whereas in Zen shiatsu the therapist liberally uses the various parts of the body, including the elbows, knees, and feet, Namikoshi shiatsu is a minimalist style that primarily utilizes the thumbs, as well as the fingers and palms. Working from the principle that everything is connected, the entire body is manipulated and every pressure point is treated during each session. The scope of the treatment is then narrowed to the areas of greatest need. Although certain conditions may require extra work directly in the area of pain, sometimes points on distant areas of the body provide the greatest relief. Assessment and treatment occur at the same time—feeling (palpating) as you treat and treating as you feel. This sense of immediacy is reminiscent of Namikoshi's treatment approach to his very first patient, his mother.[23]

THE SCIENCE OF NAMIKOSHI SHIATSU   By design, Namikoshi shiatsu affects nearly every physical system in the body, including the muscles, nerves, respiration, digestion, circulation, and immune function. As opposed to focusing on the energy system (ki), Namikoshi chose to derive a scientific explanation for his treatment's effectiveness. By viewing the body through modern eyes, he found that simple pressure into the body could also relieve congestion that occurred at the cellular level, sweeping out waste and biotoxins that often amassed at sites of pain and injury. This not only improved cellular functioning but also lengthened the cell's lifespan.

By varying the speed and quality of pressure, Namikoshi found that he could achieve different results. A quick succession of pressing and releasing was found to generate a small electrical charge in the cells that boosted their energy levels. When compressions were held for a longer period (3–5 seconds), it would stimulate portions of the brain that regulate a muscle's length during rest. The sustained pressure reprograms the brain's setting to increase the muscle's natural resting length, thus eliminating stress, tension, and spasms in the muscle.[24]

Unique to the Namikoshi style, three key reflexes in the body are stimulated because of their powerful healing properties. The cutaneovisceral reflex (cutaneo = skin, visceral = organ) can be triggered just by touching the skin. This touch then reverberates through the nerves to the organs and deeper

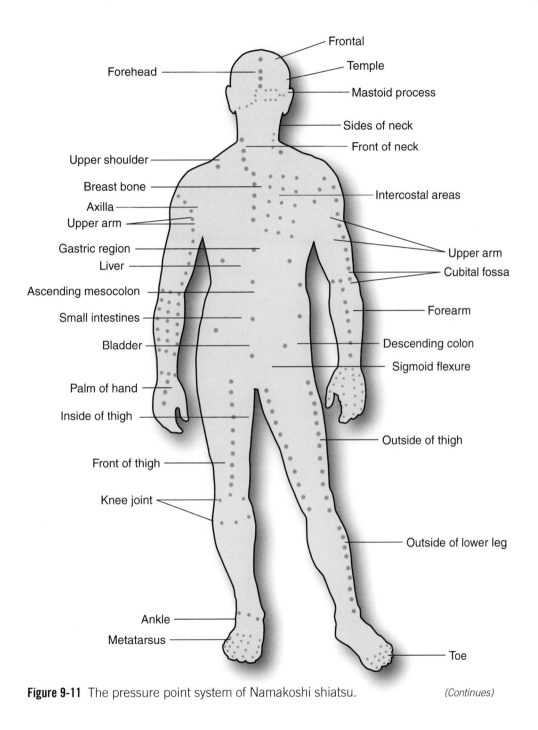

Figure 9-11 The pressure point system of Namakoshi shiatsu.   *(Continues)*

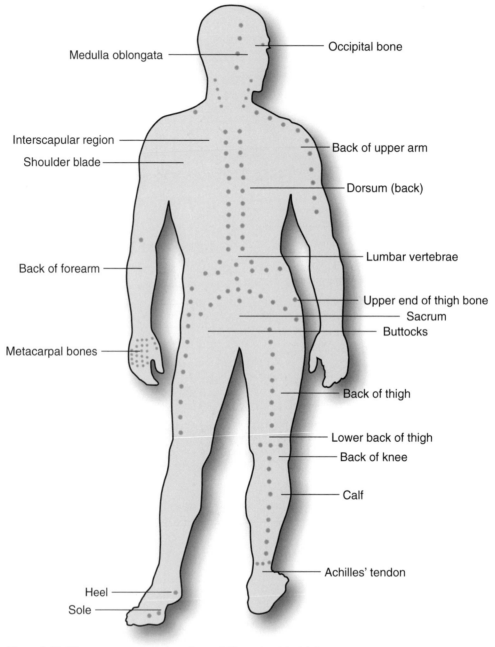

Figure 9-11 The pressure point system of Namakoshi shiatsu. (Continued)

tissues that are not directly accessible through palpation. The ocularcardiac reflex (ocular = eye, cardiac = heart) elicits a deep relaxation response from the body. The carotid sinus reflex prompts the brain to lower blood pressure. Carotid in Greek means "to plunge into sleep or stupor." It was named so because compression of these arteries can cause a loss of consciousness. When this reflex is stimulated appropriately, however, it creates a positive, healing effect.[25]

Although entrenched in modern theory and principles, Namikoshi still emphasized the importance of taking action to prevent illness and injury as opposed to waiting until something goes wrong. This style has been shown to have a wide array of positive effects on the body and can be used for simply improving general health or for resolving numerous specific conditions, including asthma, rheumatism, diabetes, and sexual dysfunction.

Five Element Shiatsu

Five Element shiatsu, a recent derivation of the more traditional forms of shiatsu, gets its name from its unique emphasis on using the theory of the Five Elements of TCM for much of its diagnosis and treatment. In addition, it also utilizes TCM theory as its theoretical basis, as do most all other forms of Asian bodywork therapy. Cindy Banker and Robbee Fian, two of the group of founders of the American Organization of Bodywork Therapies of Asia (AOBTA) worked to develop this style of Asian Bodywork in the early 1980's.

The basic method of Five Element shiatsu is to identify a pattern of energetic imbalance through use of various TCM assessment techniques including pulse and tongue diagnosis and the four examinations: 1) looking, 2) listening, 3) smelling and tasting, and 4) touching. Considerations of the patient's lifestyle and emotional and psychological states are also reviewed. Once all of this information is assimilated by the practitioner, an appropriate treatment plan specific to the patient's energy imbalance is developed and facilitated. Five Element practitioners employ a variety of standard forms of shiatsu treatment techniques to effectively accomplish their treatment goals. This includes acu-point pressure and manipulation of the channels and soft tissues of the body using the fingers, hands, elbows, forearms, knees, or feet to apply gentle pressure and stretching.

Another main focus of this form of shiatsu is to treat the person at the level of the spirit. Practitioners of Five Element shiatsu regard this as the highest form of healing because it focuses on the absolute core of an individual—that aspect of a person that connects to the underlying universe. This is a multilevel process that involves filtering through the many layers of imbalance that people have often developed over a lifetime. The dynamics of the body's energy system are analyzed according to the interplay of the Five Elements as depicted in the Chinese pentagram (see Figure 9-2).

Five Element Theory holds that from birth, each one of us resonates most with one particular element. This is considered to be a person's constitutional factor. The constitutional factor describes a person's physical make-up, emotional tendencies, and personality traits. For example, an earth element constitutional factor indicates a grounded nature with great aptitude for fostering trust, creating strong relationships, and caring for others. When those with an earth constitutional factor become imbalanced, however, they can lose their warmth and become apathetic towards even those that are close to them. By nurturing and treating the strength of the constitutional factor, Five Element practitioners seek to bring balance at the root level.

In the end, Five Element shiatsu focuses on helping the recipient address the most complete picture possible, including diet, lifestyle, and emotional wellbeing. Education and collaboration between practitioner and patient enables the patient to learn how to create his or her future health.[26]

Macrobiotic Shiatsu

Like so many of the other pioneers of different forms of massage and bodywork therapy, it was illness that became the catalyst for Shizuko Yamamoto, founder of the International Macrobiotic Shiatsu Society, that sparked her interest to search for new ways to improve her emotional and physical states. This search ultimately led her to several Japanese master practitioners. Her main teacher was George Ohsawa, credited for bringing **macrobiotics** to the West and considered by many to be the father of modern macrobiotics. He was the one who asked Shizuko to come to the West and continue her work there. She also studied with Morihei Ueshiba, the founder of aikido, and Masahiro Oki, an originator of a unique form of yoga.

Macrobiotic shiatsu, developed by Shizuko Yamamoto, places heavy emphasis on simple changes in lifestyle that can have dramatic impacts on one's health and wellbeing. Since the foods that we eat are the raw materials that literally become our cells, bones, skin, and blood, diet is a primary focus of this approach. *Macro* is Greek for "great" and *bios* means "life." Macrobiotics, then, is a way of life that seeks to coordinate and harmonize with the natural order of the world.[27]

Macrobiotics views food as containing a living energy (or ki) that impacts the ki of the individual when eaten. An easy way to determine the properties of specific foods is to consider their behavior. Vegetables that root into the ground encourage ki to move downward in the body. Food like onions and garlic that grow outward work to draw ki to the surface of the body. Different methods of food preparation also impact the effects of foods. Stewing draws ki downward, while steaming creates an upward affect, and pressure cooking pushes ki deep into the body.

The macrobiotic diet consists almost entirely of whole, living foods. Grains, beans, and seeds will sprout if left in water. Fruits and vegetables are alive and continue to ripen. Foods like biscuits, rice cakes, and pasta, on the other hand, are considered dead foods because of their low ki content. This approach recommends that the basis of our nutrition should be whole cereal grains (40–60%), followed by vegetables (25–35%), then beans (10–15%), soups (5%), and sea vegetables (5%).

Techniques of Macrobiotic shiatsu are Zen shiatsu inspired, drawing on their uninhibited style of utilizing the hands, knees, elbows, and feet. In addition, Reiki-like palm healing can be conducted in which the practitioner visualizes sending ki deep into the receiver's body.[28]

General Benefits of Zen, Namikoshi, Five Elements and Macrobiotic Shiatsu

- Relieves stress and tension
- Instills a sense of well-being and connectedness
- Improves digestion
- Promotes menstrual regularity and comfort
- Relieves headaches
- Relieves back pain
- Improves frozen shoulder
- Relieves sciatica
- Relieves sports injuries
- Improves joint mobility
- Strengthens immune system
- Improves stamina
- Relieves post-traumatic stress
- Promotes healthy pregnancy
- Eases childbirth
- Reduces blood pressure

Precautions of Zen, Namikoshi, Five Elements and Macrobiotic Shiatsu

Shiatsu can be applied with caution as long as the following conditions are avoided:

- Open cuts and sores
- Broken bones
- Rashes
- Bruises
- Phlebitis
- Pregnancy—certain points should not be pressed

Contraindications of Zen, Namikoshi, Five Elements and Macrobiotic Shiatsu

Shiatsu may either be ineffective or damaging to the following conditions:

- Acute fevers and flu
- Malignant tumors
- Advanced internal organ disease (kidney failure, respiratory failure, nephritis)
- Very unstable blood pressure
- Poisoning (food, snake, insect, etc.)
- Acute inflammations (appendicitis, severe arthritis, peritonitis)

Training of a Practitioner

Training of an Asian Bodywork Therapy Practitioner (Tuina, Amma Therapeutic Massage, Acupressure, Zen Shiatsu, Namikoshi Shiatsu, Five Element Shiatsu, and Macrobiotic Shiatsu)

Training in these varied forms of Asian Bodywork takes place on many levels and can range from a 12-hour weekend workshop designed for home practice and self-care, to part of a professional licensing program requiring more than 1000 hours of schooling. In some cases, an associate's degree is even required. Much depends on the state and the school where it is being offered. In most jurisdictions, the practice of any form of Asian bodywork therapy will legally fall under the license to practice massage therapy. As a result, massage and bodywork therapy students will usually study Asian bodywork forms such as shiatsu or tuina in a specialty track as part of a larger, more comprehensive state licensure-qualifying massage therapy and bodywork program. The hours in these programs will be devoted to the study and practice of the theories and techniques of each modality. Usually, students also receive professionally supervised clinical experience where they practice on the public. Generally speaking, what particular forms of Asian bodywork are taught at different schools throughout the country is mostly dependent upon the instructors living around the institution's local area.

There are also numerous stand-alone Asian bodywork schools across the country that offer various forms of Asian bodywork programs that are approved by the AOBTA (American Organization for Bodywork Therapies of Asia). Although these programs require a minimum of 500 hours of training, they often run much longer. In addition, many western-based massage therapy schools also offer full, but separate, 500-hour or more Asian bodywork therapy programs, producing an East-meets-West theme to the school.

These longer programs, which entail more rigorous practical hands-on training, must also include study of western anatomy and physiology as well as TCM theory, principles, and diagnosis, treatment of specific conditions, physical arts (such as qi gong and tai chi chuan), and student clinic.

Graduates of these programs, particularly those approved by the AOBTA, can take the Asian Bodywork Therapy exam of the National Certification Commission for Acupuncture and Oriental Medicine, in order to be designated Diplomats in Asian Bodywork Therapy (Dipl. A.B.T.). If the particular program and graduates meet certain other educational and additional requirements, they can also sit for the National Certification Examination for Therapeutic Massage and Bodywork (NCBTMB) and depending on which state they live in, will actually have to either pass it or the examination developed by the Federation of State Massage Therapy Boards known as the Massage & Bodywork Licensing Examination (MBLEx), for a license to practice.

JIN SHIN DO®: BODYMIND ACUPRESSURE®

The acupressure technique of Jin Shin Do® is one that has been bred and cultured from a style of Japanese bodywork called Jin Shin Jyutsu. Jin Shin Jyutsu was developed by Jiro Murai during the early 1930s through the 1960s. It is said that he became deathly ill in his early twenties due to his excessive style of living. Although his father and uncle were doctors, neither knew how to help. Accepting his fate, Jiro Murai insisted that he be taken to the top of a mountain where he could quietly meet his death.

While awaiting the end of his life, Murai recalled the hand positions that he had seen again and again on the meditating statues of Buddha found all throughout Japan. He experimented with these positions while awaiting his end, but instead of passing quietly into the night, something strange occurred. He began to feel hot, as if "rivers of fire" were running through his entire body.

Without food or water, he had become very sensitive and was able to feel currents of energy flowing through him. Eventually he was even able to control them. His later drawings would show that the patterns of energy flow that he experienced were almost identical to the traditional channels of acupuncture. When it was all over, Jiro Murai fell to his knees in gratitude—completely healed. He vowed to take what he had learned to the rest of mankind and from then on traveled throughout Japan teaching others simple ways to control their own ki through acupressure and meditation.

Jin Shin Jyutsu was brought to United States by Mary Burmeister, a Japanese American born in Seattle who had traveled to her homeland to learn Japanese. There, a chance encounter brought her into contact with Jiro Murai, whose first words to her were, "How would you like to study with me to take a gift from Japan to America?" For the next 5 years, Mary trained under Jiro's tutelage and became the vessel that would take Murai's work to the West. However, for 17 years this knowledge brewed inside of Mary until she felt she was ready to share this rare gift.[29] It was through Mary Burmeister's teaching that Iona Teeguarden was introduced to the healing art of Jin Shin Jyutsu.

After years of scholarly research, spiritual guidance, and clinical experience, Iona Teeguarden developed and branched into her own style of bodywork called Jin Shin Do.

Literally translated, Jin Shin Do means, "The Way of the Compassionate Spirit." Jin refers to the compassion that is necessary not only in healing others but also in healing ourselves. Without compassion, we cannot resist the forces of criticism, doubt, and insecurity that we project onto ourselves and others alike. Compassion is the first requirement of a Jin Shin Do practitioner.

Shin refers to the human spirit—the aspect of us that is eternal. Shin is the "organ" through which we experience the emotions of joy and love. Like a window, shin can be clear and bright or it can be dark, and cloudy. Shin allows us to touch higher levels in ourselves where we can understand our part in the greater world. When shin becomes blind to the natural order, we lose sense of who we are or what this life is all about. Our personal outlook becomes skewed and distorted.

Do refers to the Tao or "the Way." At its utmost, Tao refers to everything existing and nonexisting. It refers to the path of the entire universe, but at the same time it refers to our own personal path as well. For humans, it is the connection between us and the world around us that is important. Helping to establish this connection is the primary motivation of Jin Shin Do.

The principles of Jin Shin Do are principles that can be applied to anyone's life. More than just a path to physical healing, Jin Shin Do is ultimately a way of living and interacting with one's world. Its aim goes beyond helping the body to feel better by seeking to achieve balance in the entire structure of one's existence. Although the techniques, theories, and principles of Jin Shin Do are based on the complex and highly evolved roots of traditional Chinese medicine, it is still simple enough to be learned and used by nearly anyone.

The deep level of relaxation and rejuvenation that Jin Shin Do seeks is not only meant to benefit the body and mind of the receiver, it is also a means for practitioners of re-connecting to their higher selves through a process of letting go and allowing the spiritual connection to manifest by simply clearing the path. Like shiatsu, its focus is not only to benefit the receiver, but the giver as well. Through healing, one becomes healed. By giving, we receive, and by seeking to understand others, we understand ourselves.

Theory and Principles

Although its roots thread all the way back to the beginnings of Chinese medicine (some 5000 years ago), Jin Shin Do is a practice that has been refined for the New Age. The core of Iona Teeguarden's Jin Shin Do is formed mostly from a synthesis of traditional Japanese acupressure techniques, and classical Chinese acupuncture theory. Iona has also integrated psychological theories from the West to create a form of bodywork that represents the point where eastern and western theories and practices meet. The practice of Jin Shin Do also includes principles and methods of Taoist philosophy, such as breath work, meditation, and exercise to create a sophisticated system of healing that is able to positively affect a person on a number of levels.

Its approach, staying true to eastern philosophy, aims to maintain balance and well-being rather than trying to treat anything. This is a subtle but important distinction. Its motive isn't necessarily to "do" anything—rather it simply seeks to allow the individual self to connect with the energies of the larger, Universal Self. This idea of flowing with the Tao is such an important factor in Jin Shin Do that it could easily have been named Taoist acupressure.

Because traditional oriental philosophy sees the human entity as a continuous spectrum that is composed of body, mind, and spirit, any point can be accessed to create changes throughout the whole being. Jin Shin Do seeks to capitalize on this by utilizing a multifaceted approach that seeks to affect change on a number of levels at once. Bodywork re-balances the body's energies, breathing techniques open the body's vital centers, meditations are taught to calm the mind, self-reflection is encouraged to draw one's attention inward, and emotional release balances and clears unresolved armoring. Armoring is a person's way of unconsciously and psychologically protecting and defending him or herself that results in holding 'armor-like' deep tensions in the body's muscles. This in turn creates blockages and imbalances in the underlying energy system which can cause illness. Dietary changes, herbal supplements, and exercise are also used to reinforce the treatment. Because the techniques of Jin Shin Do weave deftly between the physical and energetic realms, the scope of a Jin Shin Do treatment can vary from dealing with neck and back pain, to deepening the breath, to clearing the mind and/or rebalancing the emotions.

The Bodymind Approach

Iona's work with the emotional component of an issue stemmed from her early years while being treated for chronic digestive problems. By exploring the thoughts and emotions that were so often intertwined with her pain, Iona discovered that she could profoundly enhance her own healing process. Gradually she learned to encourage clients to be open to feelings and images that may arise during their sessions. Through a process called body focusing technique, clients are encouraged to bring their awareness to areas being worked and feel what kind of tension, thoughts, or feelings may be lingering. Rather than repressing feelings, this process helps to explore and understand what's really going on so that achieving a more complete sense of healing becomes possible.

Through her work, Iona realized that emotions can morph into their opposites or create a segue into other emotions. Anger turned inward can manifest as guilt, but its outer face may present as resentment. Fear, on the inside, can become timidity, but turned outward it can become mistrust and suspicion. These emotion-to-emotion relationships have been explored and synthesized into the concept of the emotional kaleidoscope, which explores the interrelationship between one hundred different feelings and emotions. Based on the principle of Five Elements, each emotional spectrum is correlated to specific organ meridians and portrays how an emotion can sway to its extreme and which emotions are synergistic.[30]

Since there is such an intentional and strong emphasis on dealing with and balancing the emotional/psychological nature as part of treatment, Jin Shin Do® Bodymind Acupressure® could have easily been placed into the soma-to-psychic group of modalities. Modalities whose treatments are specifically intended to impact the body-mind connection to affect changes at the psychological level as well as the physical. However, since it is so deeply rooted in traditional Chinese medicine principles, and ultimately most all of the changes it seeks are through the effects of balancing the energy system, it has been grouped here within the bioenergetic level.

Channels & Points

Jin Shin Do® works with a system of eight channels that connect, nourish, and maintain the human organism. They are called the Strange Flows (also known as the extraordinary meridians or pathways) due to their unique characteristics.

Unlike the traditional 12 primary organ channels (the lung channel, stomach channel, heart channel, etc.) that are often emphasized and used in other forms of Asian bodywork, the Strange Flows have no points of their own (except for two, the Conception Vessel and the Governing Vessel). Instead, Jin Shin Do utilizes the points at which the primary organ channels and the Strange Flow channels intersect. Also unique to the Strange Flow channels is that they are not continuously transporting qi (again, with exception of the Conceptional Vessel and the Governing Vessel). In fact, these channels only engage when there is an imbalance that requires adjustment.

It's similar to a traffic jam. If the highway is blocked, traffic filters out through the side roads. The points utilized in Jin Shin Do act like the on and off ramps to the highway that help to control, balance, and neutralize excesses and deficiencies. Another name for this group of channels is the "Psychic Channels." This is because Strange Flows are not only strongly affected by touch and manipulation, but by the mind as well through meditation.

The points utilized in Jin Shin Do are the exact same points utilized in acupuncture and of course all the other forms of Asian bodywork that use the 12 primary channels and their points as the foundation of treating and balancing the energy system. However, the numbering structure has been altered to create a format that is more in line with the Jin Shin Do style. They are numbered going down the front of the body, up the back, down the outside of the arms and back up through the insides. Although Jin Shin Do acknowledges and has the ability to utilize all the points, there are 55 primary points that are emphasized.[31]

Techniques

The various techniques of Jin Shin Do are all meant to help achieve a sense of balance and stillness in our lives so that we can start to better see and experience the world. Often we are too mired in mental and emotional disturbances that cause us to react in fixed, rigid, and often unhealthy patterns. It is only when we step back that we can truly appreciate the fullness of a situation, and it is being in this place that allows us to act spontaneously and joyfully.

Often, it is not what is happening to us that causes grief, negativity, and unhappiness, but rather a result of the way we perceive the events unfolding. It's as if we are viewing the world through filters that only allow us to see and experience the things that each filter is set to receive. Our filters can be fear, anger, worry, happiness, and so on. Just like when we are wearing rose-colored glasses, everything we see is tinted rose and thereby altered in some fundamental way. After a short while we no longer even notice that all that we see is tinted and therefore in reality being misperceived because it looks so normal. Misperceiving the events and experiences of our lives through these different filters can psychologically stress us in a variety of ways and become reflected in our postures, attitudes, and behaviors. Our experience of these physical and psychological tensions reinforces the wrong perspective and continues this draining and painful vicious cycle.[32]

Hara Breathing

Throughout the ages, various techniques have been developed to strengthen the connection to the hara for both health and spiritual benefits. The hara breathing meditation taught in Jin Shin Do is a simple method that only requires that you find a comfortable, relaxing position whether you're standing, sitting, or lying down (Figure 9-12). The hands can be pressed together in a position of prayer, folded over the chest, or with the right hand over the left directly over the area of the hara.

All it takes for this simple yet powerful process to be initiated is deep, relaxed breathing, filling the lungs to their fullest capacity and exhaling completely while keeping the attention focused on the hara. Phrases like "The Source of Vitality" or the "Field of Healing" can be pondered to root the mind into the process of connecting to the hara. Since the hara is considered one's physical, energetic and psychological center of gravity, thinking about and meditating on this "space" will also help the process of realigning the body's energies.[33]

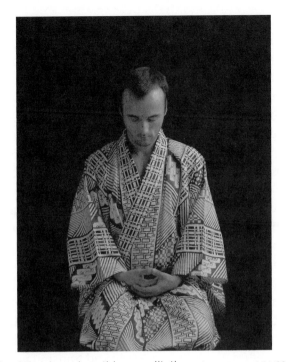

Figure 9-12 Man in sitting hara-breathing meditation. *Image copyright 2009, Tomasz Wieja. Used under license from shutterstock.com.*

This simple, basic pattern can be practiced to begin the process of opening and connecting to the hara:

1. Inhale through the nose for 5 seconds. Try to bring the breath all the way down below the navel while visualizing the breath descending to fill the hara. Visualization is a key element in this process and the strength of one's visualization will greatly affect the outcome of one's practice.
2. Hold the breath in the hara for 5 seconds. As the breath fills the lower belly, the hara will naturally fill with ki. Although the belly will expand during this practice, it will strengthen and tonify the abdominal muscles.
3. Exhale through the mouth for 5 seconds while contracting the abdomen and squeezing the navel towards the spine to empty the air before inhaling again.

The breathing should be so slow and gentle that if a feather was in front of your face it would barely move. Placing the hands over the area of the hara can help one get a better sense of where the breath may be blocked or if the belly is still holding rigidly.

Channeling Ki

Just as an acupuncturist uses needles to tap into the ki of the patient, the Jin Shin Do practitioner uses the hands to move and channel the ki during treatment. Here the principle of the Tao is again reflected. The process of channeling ki by utilizing one's own vital energy can be a draining experience because our own individual supply is a finite reservoir. A much more effective means is to draw from the great ocean of ki that we are immersed in every second of our life. Practitioners who have successfully learned to access this limitless supply can actually feel invigorated after performing a treatment because they too are absorbing energy even as they pass it on to the receiver. Although such ideas in the modern world may not be very mainstream, it is said that every one of us has the ability to channel energy. Some people are attuned to this process naturally, but like any skill it is something that can also be developed with practice.

In Jin Shin Do, this ability is developed through the meditation and creative visualization used to develop the hara. This stems from Taoist practices used to achieve "radiant health." Tapping into the power of the hara allows all the body's energies to become invigorated with new vitality. Achieving this is the first stage in learning how to direct ki. The stronger or more developed the hara, the greater the practitioner's ability to control and transmit energy.

This practice requires active visualization. As you inhale, feel the ki building in the hara. Then as you exhale, visualize the energy rising up the middle of the body to the heart. At this point concentrate the mind to push the energy out to the shoulders, spill down the arms, and pour all the way down into the hands. In a Jin Shin Do session, this is often done at the beginning and several times during the treatment.

Assessment

The first stage of assessment in Jin Shin Do is to determine whether a person is more yin or more yang. Someone who tends to be passive is considered yin and someone who is more aggressive is considered yang. In the body, cramped muscles, high blood pressure, insomnia, redness, and heat are all considered signs of yang. On the other hand, flaccid muscles, low blood pressure, fatigue, paleness, and cold is considered yin.

In the personality, yang may manifest with brisk actions, restlessness, strong voice, decisiveness, quick thinking, and talkativeness. Yin may present as slow movement, weak voice, drooping posture, and indecisiveness. Determining whether a client is yin or yang will completely change the direction and application of the treatment. Although those who are yang may have plenty of energy, it is often locked up in tension; therefore the energy becomes inaccessible and stagnates. They have an overabundance of energy in some areas while other areas are lacking. The focus of this treatment will be to release blockages and create a smoothly flowing stream of energy throughout the entire body. To alleviate this type of a condition, a firmer pressure is needed. In addition, breathing techniques for yang patients are designed to relax the body and release blocked areas that may have been established.

Yin personalities have the exact opposite problem. Their ki is too weak; therefore even small tasks may be a great effort for them. Their energy must be nourished and replenished. With yin types, a gentler pressure needs to be used and more attention must be paid towards channeling energy. Breathing techniques here are applied towards revitalizing the ki and exercises are taught for developing physical strength.

Original Constitution

A practitioner of traditional Chinese medicine must always seek to understand the nature of their patients in order to effectively treat them according to who they are as physical, mental, emotional, and spiritual entities. There are many methods of observation that can give insight into what is called the **original constitution**. This is the condition and attributes that a person is born with and remains relatively fixed and unchanging throughout the lifetime. This concept is similar to what is known as pre-heaven essence or pre-natal qi in traditional Chinese medicine.

One method of assessing a patient's original constitution is by examining the bony structure of the body. The physical form is a mirror of our psychological life and studying the skeletal structure, especially in the head and face, can garner valuable clues into the mental and emotional make-up of a person. Although there are 6 basic categories of facial shapes used in Jin Shin Do, in actuality there are myriad variations and many will be a combination of the 6 mentioned below.

1. Triangular—pointing up

   The triangular shape is a very yang sign. Generally this type of person is physically strong and is strong-willed.

2. Round

   The round face is also considered yang and has similar qualities, depending on the width of the jaw.

3. Rectangle/Square

   The rectangle or square-shaped face is the most yang. This type tends to be the most assertive and often has a highly developed skill for practical thinking.

4. Oval

The oval face represents the most balanced original constitution with neither yin nor yang playing a dominant role. Those with an oval face are neither fixed in one or the other; they tend to have more flexible lifestyles and attitudes.

5. Triangular—pointing down.

The triangular shaped face that is pointing down represents a more yin constitution and tends to be more cerebral and artistic. Because of this, those with a triangular face often rely on their well-developed powers of thinking and intuition to solve problems.

6. Long and Narrow

The long and narrow face represents the most yin constitution with attributes similar to the previous type, but with a greater need to develop the physical side.

Acquired Constitution

Acquired constitution reflects what we've done with what we've been given. This may parallel our original constitution or it can fluctuate greatly. Rather than considering the bony structure, determining the acquired constitution requires looking at the soft tissues of the body because muscle and sinew are much more responsive to lifestyle and environmental factors.

The first place that a Jin Shin Do Practitioner will often look for signs of acquired constitution is in the eyes. A strong spirit will be indicated in clear, bright, animated eyes. Cloudy, dull, and lackluster eyes on the other hand represent a spirit that is weak. The overall condition of the body is said to reflect in the positioning of the iris (the colored part of the eyes). An iris that is centered evenly on the top and bottom represents a balanced state.

An iris that rises upwards to reveal the whites of the eyes below indicates a yin state. Here, there is not enough energy and nourishment to sustain the body. People whose eyes are manifesting this condition are commonly more prone to accidents and depression. If the opposite scenario presents with the whites showing above the iris, this indicates a yang state. There may be an excess of energy that is not being used and may lead to hyperactivity or irritability. This can also indicate anger or lack of control. The level of the body's reserve energy is reflected in the skin underneath the eyes. If someone is experiencing physical or emotional fatigue, this area may be dark, lined, or swollen.

These are just some of the features that can provide a telling portrait of a person's life—who they are, how they've lived, and what they need. Jin Shin Do also utilizes basic principles of Chinese pulse diagnosis to determine the yin-yang condition of a patient.

The Session

The most common length of time for a Jin Shin Do session is one hour. However, this can be varied as needed. The client often begins fully clothed, lying on his or her back on a massage table. Hands and arms can either be positioned at the sides or over the hara with the right hand over the left.

The way of Jin Shin Do is a simple one. It involves merely holding a series of two points, not to create change, but to allow a release. Because the Jin Shin Do practitioner doesn't try to interject his or her own agenda, there is a sense of purity that is preserved. This reflects great faith in the founding principles of the Tao.

In Jin Shin Do, the finger pressure and technique remain relatively constant. The idea is to find the midpoint between too much and too little. When poised at the perfect balance, the greatest potential for healing exists. In Jin Shin Do terms, this provides the greatest potential to be connected with the Tao.

A complementary principle that Jin Shin Do incorporates into its treatment protocol is that of wei-wu-wei. This is the way of doing only when things need to be done. More than the physical act of doing minimally, this is the attitude or mindset that one should seek to come from. The inner state of peace and grace should be cultivated at all times unless it becomes imperative to make a shift. All things should be done from this place.

When applying this theory towards the goals and techniques of Jin Shin Do, it translates into manipulating only the points that are necessary. Jin Shin Do is an efficient system and doing any more than the necessary is considered excessive. The points are meant to regulate the body's energies—filling deficiencies and siphoning off excesses. Achieving this doesn't require the use of all the points—just a few select ones.

Points applied are pressed in pairs that complement one another. Sometimes both hands will be near the same area. At other times distal points will be used where the practitioner has one hand near the epicenter of the problem and the other hand at a point connected to it further down the arm or leg. Pressure applied builds gradually, meeting each layer of resistance and suggesting a release. Depth only goes until the point where contact is made with the body's ki. Just the right touch is needed. Points can be held anywhere from 30 seconds to two minutes, depending upon the level of armoring or resistance that is encountered.

There are three signs to look for when gauging the length of holding for each point:

1. Softening of the muscles around the point
2. Decreased or released soreness or sensitivity of the point
3. Feeling ki flowing through the point. This will feel like a strong, even pulse.

The last few moments of a session are considered delicate because it's the time when patients are the most open and vulnerable. This is when their defenses are down and they are the most willing to allow change to take place. The end of a session is also considered the most spiritual part of the treatment. At this point, the therapist must synchronize with the patient's state and soften his or her touch to transition from a more physical treatment to a more energetic one.

Because the body is in a greater state of sensitivity and receptivity, subtle techniques like visualizing ki flowing smoothly through the body and meditating on love, compassion, acceptance, and understanding on behalf of the patient can have a great impact. To close, a few points including the third-eye point between the eyebrows and the point above the heart center are held. This final balancing step grounds the patient—sealing the session.[34]

Benefits

The following are some of the conditions that Jin Shin Do can help to relieve:

- Muscular pain and tension
- Stress and emotion problems
- Head- and backaches
- Anxiety and depression
- Repression and frustration
- Fatigue
- Insomnia
- Menstrual/menopausal discomfort
- Digestive distress
- Sinus pain and allergies.

Precautions

The gentle nature of Jin Shin Do allows it to be used safely in many situations where other, more vigorous forms of massage therapy and bodywork may not be appropriate. However, there are still some precautions. Treatment can proceed with caution as long the following conditions are not aggravated:

- Open cuts and sores
- Rashes
- Contagious skin diseases
- Extensive bruising
- Phlebitis
- Broken blood vessels
- Pregnancy—some points should not be pressed

Training of a Jin Shin Do® Practitioner

Although most Jin Shin Do practitioners have completed at least a high school level of education, this is not an absolute requirement. Also, because of the level of maturity necessary to appropriately understand and deal with the emotional difficulties of clients, most Jin Shin Do practitioners are at least 18 years of age but generally older. Becoming a registered Jin Shin Do practitioner requires taking a series of educational theory and practice modules, logging experience hours, private sessions with authorized teachers, and practical examinations. Teacher training is much more extensive and includes beginning, intermediate and advanced coursework and training. All the exact details can be found on the Jin Shin Do® Bodymind Acupressure® website at http://www.jinshindo. org/requirement.htm.[35]

THAI MASSAGE

The legend of the statue of the Golden Buddha now resting in Bangkok reveals an intimate picture of Thai massage therapy. It was said that during the relocation of a giant clay statue of Buddha, the statue was dropped and cracked. At first the monks were horrified, but then they noticed something bright and shimmering just beneath the surface. The monks chiseled away the rest of the clay and discovered, to their amazement, that the entire statue was made of solid gold. It is thought that the statue was camouflaged during the Burmese invasion in 1776 to conceal the great treasure underneath.

While the truthfulness of this story remains uncertain, it speaks of the deepest aim of Thai massage therapy. The story of the golden Buddha reveals that there is an inner beauty inside each of us waiting to be discovered and it is this golden essence that Thai massage seeks to uncover.

In India, approximately 2500 years ago during the time of the Buddha, a group of students studying medicine were given a final assignment before they could graduate. They were asked to go out into nature and bring back something that had no medicinal value. Each of the students returned and presented what they had found: a rock, a dead fish, a poisonous plant, and a skull. One student, however, returned empty handed. "Sir," young Jivaka exclaimed to his teacher, "I cannot find anything that is not of medicinal value." In Jivaka's eyes, everything he had encountered had the potential to heal when used appropriately. Jivaka was the only student to pass the test and he went on to become a great healer and personal physician to the Buddha. Jivaka was said to have used massage, stretching (yoga-like) techniques, herbs and other remedies to treat sickness among the nuns and monks who were traveling with the Buddha throughout Southeast Asia, including Thailand (originally known as Siam), in an effort to spread Buddhism and this medical system. Although the exact dates of their travels are disputed, historians believe it most likely occurred in the second century, BC. It was Jivaka's teachings that later became the foundation of Thai massage. He is known as the "father of Thai medicine" throughout Thailand and homage is given to him by all serious practitioners.

In the third century BC, the famous Hindu emperor warrior Ashoka renounced violence to walk the peaceful path of Buddha, opening the gateway for Buddhism to spread even more throughout East Asia and carrying with it the teachings of Ayurvedic medicine. This was the system of healing that was later to merge with the form of massage that had evolved in Thailand up until that time. Thai Medicine consisted of four limbs—spiritual practices, nutritional guidelines, herbal medicine and massage known as Nuad Bo-Rarn ('ancient massage') or Thai massage as it is now known in the west. The fact that they called it ancient massage was a sure indication that it was considered sacred and had been handed down throughout the generations. Typical of indigenous peoples, the Thai continued to develop their own form of massage by assimilating Buddhism, Yoga, Ayurveda, and traditional Chinese medicine which had also spread throughout Asia. The Thai people held their medical system with the same reverence and veneration as their spiritual system. While most of the literature of this ancient healing art was destroyed in 1767 by the Burmese invasion of Thailand, there are detailed carvings and artwork at the famous Wat Pho temple located in Bangkok that have preserved some of the teachings and demonstrate how this system was used by the Thai people.[36]

Ayurvedic medicine is also the foundation for the ancient practice of yoga and the familial resemblance between Thai massage and yoga is immediately apparent. Whereas other forms of bodywork utilize massage techniques as its primary method of treatment, Thai massage utilizes yoga-like stretches as the major means to achieving the ends. For this reason, Thai massage has been playfully dubbed as "yoga for lazy people" and is also known as Thai yoga therapy.

Theories and Principles

Literally translated, Ayurveda means the science of life (*ayur* = "life," *veda* = "science"). Based upon India's holy books, the Vedas, the theories and principles of Ayurvedic medicine are said to have been revealed to India's great seers during a period of intense meditation. As if they were able to look at the entire world through a microscope, they saw that everything in existence was composed of five elemental forces similar to those of Chinese medicine.

Earth in nature provides structure to all things living and nonliving. In the body it is represented by the physical form of bones, tissues, and cells.

Water is the element of emotion, vitality, and life. In nature, water evaporates into fine mist to become clouds. Clouds become heavy and return to the earth in liquid form. Water again evaporates into the sky. This cycle is reflected in the body through the circulation of its vital liquids—blood, lymph, and fluids.

Fire is the sign of transformation. In the sky, fire is the king of creation. This element can melt solid objects and dissolve liquid into vapor. In the body, fire converts raw foods into substance that can be absorbed by the system and then transformed into energy.

Air represents our ability to expand, move, and change. It is a force that blows above, below, in between and around objects in its path. Its infinite capacity to expand represents the qualities of creativity and adaptability. In the body, the respiratory and nervous systems are within air's domain.

Ether, the most subtle force of all, provides the backdrop on which all the other elements exist. It gives definition to each form by maintaining space between objects, but at the same time it is a force that connects and adheres all things into one integrated endless unit. The earth is shrouded in ozone and atmosphere, protecting the planet and preserving its unique identity from the millions of other planetary bodies in space, but at the same time the invisible layers of particles finer than gas connect earth to sky, sky to space, and space to every other thing in existence. Although all-pervading, ether is an elusive force that exists in between spaces. In the body, it exists within the spaces of the pelvis, abdomen, mouth, ears, and nose. Ether also represents the vibrations of the invisible world, governing the sense of sound, intuition, and consciousness.

Tri Doshas

Combinations of these Five Elements join to form three vital forces known in Sanskrit, the most ancient language of India, as the tri doshas. Vata, pitta, and kapha describe three distinct combinations of the five elemental forms. The dosha of vata is formed by the fusion of air and ether. Vata represents the quality of movement. This not only refers to the actions of the arms and legs, but also the movement of blood, air, food, thought, and emotions. While vata has to do with that which passes through the body, pitta represents that which is absorbed. Pitta, the amalgamation of fire and water, is responsible for the digestion and assimilation of foods, ideas, and emotions that nourish our body, intellect, and perception. Kapha is created through the interplay of earth and water and provides a stable yet mobile structure while giving shape to bones, muscles, and organs. This dosha is responsible for feelings of being grounded, content, and compassionate.

The element of air that dominates the vata type of person is reflected in their thin structures, long, angular features, and thin lips. Creative and artistic, vata types are equipped with soaring imaginations. However, their minds can become as restless as the wind, constantly flowing from one project to another. The element of ether in this dosha allows the vata type to be sensitive to others, but this same quality can also make them anxious or skittish.

The fire contained in the pitta dosha is reflected in the passion and ambition of people of this type. They often have medium frames, piercing eyes, freckles, and fiery hair. With their aggressive and competitive nature mingled with their clear and focused mind, success comes easy to the pitta type. This tendency, however, can lead them to becoming workaholics and to burnout.

The water element of the kapha type of person is reflected in their soft features and moist skin while the earth element contributes to their large frame and solid build. Slow movers with a grounded disposition, kapha types are generally easy going, reliable, and patient. However, they tend towards becoming sluggish, lazy, and over-sentimental when out of balance.

The Principles of the Tri Doshas Applied to Thai Massage

Each dosha type requires a specific approach during Thai massage treatment. Vata types require a soft, calming approach to ground their high-flying minds. Too much pressure and stimulation can overwhelm the sensitive vatas, so the aim is to soften and sedate their overactive tendencies by using a mild, even-tempered approach. The pitta type on the other hand requires a more vigorous treatment approach to diffuse pent up energy and aggression. If pressure is too light, the fiery pitta may become even more aggravated. Here, firm pressure with a steady, flowing pace is required to harmonize the pitta type. The thick skin of the kapha type requires the most intense pressure of all because their dense bodies and slow nervous systems insist upon a heavy force in order to be activated. Although a soft and gentle approach may appeal to their fondness for rest and relaxation, this would only serve to plunge them deeper into slumber; therefore a 'heavy-handed' approach is necessary to penetrate through the layers of tension that can accumulate on their thick frames.

Energy Lines

According to Ayurvedic theory, there are 72,000 lines of energy running through the course of the body. Of these, Thai massage focuses on just 10 key lines known as the sip sen. Vital points along the sip sen are known as marma points. Unlike the points on the pathways of traditional Chinese medicine used in other Asian bodywork forms, marma points can range from the size of a penny to the size of a plate. Seven of the major marmas are located along the midline of the body and are popularly known as the chakras (Figure 9-13). Literally translated from Sanskrit, marma means "hidden" or "secret."

Techniques

The first and foremost element of every Thai massage is *mindfulness*. This is a preparatory phase that places the Thai massage therapist in the correct state of being for treatment. It heightens the sensitivities, sharpens focus, and encourages good body alignment. Many of the movements require repeated lifting of sometimes heavy limbs, which can be quite a rigorous ordeal for a therapist's back if he or she is not conscientious in applying correct technique. Also, because Thai massage utilizes positions that intertwine the bodies of giver and receiver, mindfulness helps prevent the practitioner from winding up in awkward, injurious, or even suggestive positions.

The second element of Thai massage is *rhythmic rocking*. Each stroke begins not from the hands, but from the meditative rocking of the therapist's body, which sets the tone and pace for the entire session. While sitting or kneeling, the arms are held straight, the spine is tall and erect and the body is allowed to sway like bamboo in the wind. The practitioner can go side-to-side, back and forth, or in circles like a whirlpool. Rhythmic rocking provides an energy-efficient method of applying pressure to the receiver because the therapist's whole body is involved in each movement. It also gives the therapist bigger "ears" because instead of just the hands, the entire body is now a listening device that helps pick up on the subtle distinctions of each individual client.

The third component of this modality is the *stance*. Working effectively from the floor requires a completely different utilization of the body than working on a table. Although working at ground level allows the practitioner to generate greater force and provides more options for movement, it also brings a greater risk of injury for the therapist and client. The various stances that are

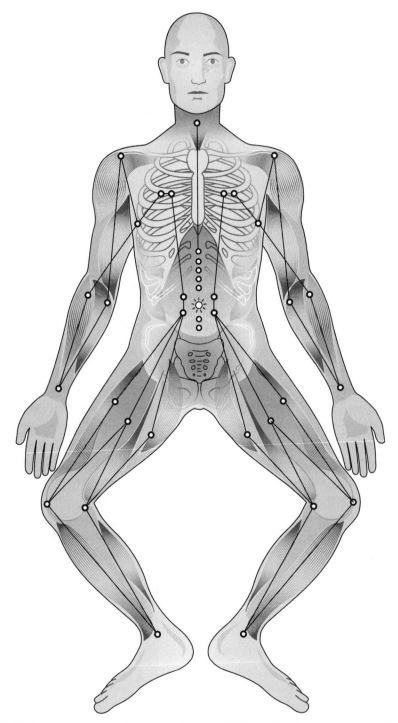

Figure 9-13 A chart based on the original drawings of the sip sen or energy pathways that are the focus of much of the treatment in Thai massage.

used in Thai massage have been developed to manage just this issue—some which are directly derived from yoga and tai chi.

Massage and stretching techniques are actually the final components of Thai massage. It is only when the previous three components are engaged that these can fully become effective. The hand techniques of Thai massage mirror that of shiatsu, with thumb and palmar pressure being used to generate mild pressure while the forearms, elbows, knees, and feet are utilized for when stronger pressure is needed. When stretches are applied, the therapist utilizes his or her entire body (Figure 9-14). Using only the hands and arms for this work not only creates excessive wear and tear on the therapist, it is not nearly as effective at creating the deep stretches that are the hallmark of Thai massage.

The Breath

In Ayurvedic medicine, people's relationship to the world can be explained by studying the qualities of how they breathe. Those who breathe deeply and fully are exhibiting signs that they are at ease with their current position in life. The fullness of their inhalation shows that they are able to take all that they need from their environment and the completeness of their exhalation is a sign that they give back just as much as they take, resulting in a balanced state. Rapid

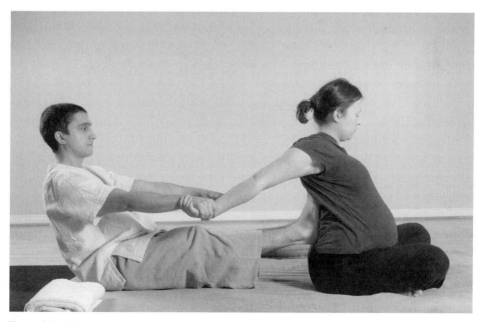

Figure 9-14 Thai massage being performed on the back of a pregnant woman. *Image copyright 2009, Yanik Chauvin. Used under license from shutterstock.com.*

breathers who take in short, staccato breaths reveal stress and apprehension in the ways they meet life. They may experience a general feeling of insufficiency, so they take what they need in quick gasps before it is gone. Slow breathers who take in only a small quantity of air reveal weariness and a lack of motivation—they literally aren't receiving enough inspiration in their lives and this is often reflected as a feeling of absence.

Breathing techniques known as pranayama (*prana* = "energy," *yama* = "control") have been developed to combat these disorderly patterns of breathing. (Note that Hindu word prana is the same as the Chinese word chi and the Japanese word ki for energy) Methods like mindful breathing or synchronized breathing are general approaches that can be used with anyone while others, like the cooling breath, are designed specifically for the fiery pitta clients.

The Session

With the patient comfortably seated and the therapist positioned behind, a moment is taken in contemplative silence to allow both giver and receiver an opportunity to become present to the moment. Often, therapists will have their hands pressed together at their chest during this preparation. Slowly the hands descend to the top of the receiver's shoulders and the rocking rhythm begins. Initial contact is soft, quiet, and inquiring. Like a weight at the end of a string, the therapist's hands hang straight down from the shoulders—not locked or closed, but relaxed and poised. Back and forth, left to right, and back to left again, the therapist's hands softly plunge into mounds of tension often trapped high in the shoulders. The neck and arms relax and fall limp to the sides as their tension evaporates.

With a firm, but yielding grip, the therapist takes the receiver's arm high to the sky. The whole front body stretches wide open, including the abdomen, chest, and shoulders. The more the relaxation settles in, the heavier the recipient seems to become. This is why good body mechanics is so important. At some points the giver is responsible for almost the entire weight of the receiver.

The receiver's hands are then placed behind the head with the elbows flaring out to the sides like handle bars, which can be taken by the giver to bend, twist, and turn the receiver's torso. Then, placing the receiver's legs straight out in front, the upper torso can be guided forward for a deep stretch of the legs and back. Here the therapist applies a firm series of palmar pressure along both sides of the spine, deepening the stretch and softening the muscles of the back.

With the client lying down, the chest, shoulders, arms, and legs can be worked in a fashion similar to shiatsu. The arms and legs can be rotated in their sockets, pulled across the body, and stretched away from the torso. Lying on the floor provides a sense of security unattainable on a table. Subconscious fears of falling off do not arise and the body melts in to the ground.

A proper Thai massage session requires 90 minutes and can sometimes take two hours. Like in a yoga class, the session ends in savasana, the corpse pose, with the client resting on his or her back. Here the marma points and muscles of the face are massaged, sometimes with a few drops of essential oils blended specifically according to the client's dosha. Afterwards, contact is broken gingerly and the session ends as it began—with a moment of silence.[37]

General Benefits

- Relieves physical stress and tension
- Rejuvenates the heart and mind
- Instills a sense of wellbeing and connectedness
- Improves energy, digestion, and immunity
- Increased flexibility and emotional openness
- Refreshes the spirit
- Provides a sense of deep relaxation

Precautions

As long as precautions are taken and the following conditions are avoided, Thai massage can still be applied without injury or damage:

- Open cuts and sores
- Broken bones
- Rashes
- Bruises
- Phlebitis
- Pregnancy—certain points and positions should not be used

Contraindications

Thai massage may either be ineffective or damaging to the following conditions:

- Acute fevers and flu
- Malignant tumors

- Advanced internal organ disease (kidney failure, respiratory failure, nephritis)
- Very unstable blood pressure
- Poisoning (food, snake, insect, etc.)
- Acute inflammations (appendicitis, severe arthritis, peritonitis)

Training of a Thai Massage Practitioner

The popularity of Thai massage has grown rapidly in the past couple of decades, and so have the variety of training options available to the public. Three-hour "taster" workshops are offered in which a short full-body massage is taught. Fifteen-hour courses are also available for massage therapists who simply want to incorporate features of the Thai modality into their treatments. For those who want the full experience, however, more intensive courses and programs are available and can run up to several hundred hours of training.

Many schools of massage therapy across the United States offer Thai massage as an elective specialty track that enrolled students can choose to take within a larger state licensure qualifying diploma or certificate program. These schools also offer shorter versions as part of the continuing education offerings they run for graduates and other practicing massage professionals.

Excellent training opportunities are also offered in Thailand, where beginner students, massage therapists, massage therapy instructors, and yoga instructors travel to Asia and immerse themselves in the study and practice of traditional Thai massage.

No matter what level of training is sought, in this country the laws that guide the education, training, and practice of massage therapy and bodywork vary from state to state. It is important to check the local and state regulations and learn what is legally required before deciding where to train and, of course, before ever practicing on the public.

SUMMARY

This chapter introduces the bioenergetic level of massage therapy and bodywork, which includes modalities with the intent to primarily treat the underlying and enlivening layer of the body commonly referred to as the energy body. Although this is accomplished through a rigorous manipulation of the soft tissue, the specific intention and focus is to create changes at the energetic level, including the meridians and acupuncture points, in order to balance and heal the physical body. The chapter provides an understanding of how the modalities of Tuina, Amma Therapeutic Massage, Acupressure, Zen Shiatsu, Namikoshi Shiatsu, Five Element Shiatsu, Macrobiotic Shiatsu, Jin Shin Do®, and Thai Massage each fit into the bioenergetic level of massage including how they differ, and how they are similar to each other. A basic overview of the history, the theory and principles, process of assessment, as well as a description of the techniques involved, are presented for each of these modalities of the bioenergetic approach. This chapter also acquaints the reader with what the general experience of undergoing a treatment session is like and identifies who are the best candidates to seek this form of treatment and what conditions are most benefited. Also presented is a list for each of these modalities of their general benefits, contraindications and/or precautions. A brief discussion about training, licensing, certifications, and requirements is also included.

CHAPTER REFERENCES

1. Sohn, T., & Sohn R. (1996). *Amma therapy*. Rochester, VT: Healing Arts Press.
2. Lundberg, P. (2003). *Book of shiatsu*. NYC: Fireside.
3. Lundberg, P. (2003). *Book of shiatsu*. NYC: Fireside.
4. Sohn, T., & Sohn, R. (1996). *Amma therapy*. Rochester, VT: Healing Arts Press.
5. Changye, L. (1992). *Concise tuina therapy*. Jinan, China: Shendong Science & Technology Press.
6. Sohn, T., & Sohn R. (1996). *Amma therapy*. Rochester, VT: Healing Arts Press.
7. Sohn, T., & Sohn R. (1996). *Amma therapy*. Rochester, VT: Healing Arts Press.
8. Sohn, T., & Sohn R. (1996). *Amma therapy*. Rochester, VT: Healing Arts Press.
9. *About acupressure shiatsu*. (2006). Retrieved April 8, 2007, from http://www.acupressuretherapy.com/acupressure.html
10. Henderson, J. (2007). *What is Shiatsu?* Retrieved March 31, 2007, from http://www.balanceflow.com/BAacupressure.htm
11. *ABT styles*. (2007). Retrieved March 31, 2007, from http://www.aobta.org/about-forms.html?start=1
12. Henderson, J. (2007). *What is shiatsu?* Retrieved March 31, 2007, from http://www.balanceflow.com/BAshiatsu.htm
13. Lundberg, P. (2003). *Book of shiatsu*. NYC: Fireside.
14. Cooke, C. B. (1998). *Shiatsu theory and practice*. Edinburgh: Churchill Livingstone.
15. Dharmananda, S., Ph.D. (2007). Zen Shiatsu: The legacy of Shizuto Masunaga. Retrieved March 31, 2007, from http://www.itmonline.org/arts/shiatsu.htm
16. Lundberg, P. (2003). *Book of shiatsu*. NYC: Fireside.
17. Cooke, C. B. (1998). *Shiatsu theory and practice*. Edinburgh: Churchill Livingstone.
18. Cooke, C. B. (1998). *Shiatsu theory and practice*. Edinburgh: Churchill Livingstone.
19. Lundberg, P. (2003). *Book of shiatsu*. NYC: Fireside.

20. Kirk, L. (2007). *History of shiatsu*. Retreived March 30, 2007, from http://www.shiatsutherapy.ca/shiatsuhistory.htm

21. Lundberg, P. (2003). *Book of shiatsu*. NYC: Fireside.

22. *The history of Namikoshi shiatsu therapy*. (2003). Retrieved April 2, 2007, from http://www.namikoshi-shiatsu.com.au/

23. *What is Namikoshi shiatsu?* (2003). Retrieved April 2, 2007, from http://www.namikoshi-shiatsu.com.au/about.html

24. *What is Namikoshi shiatsu?* (2003). Retrieved April 2, 2007, from http://www.namikoshi-shiatsu.com.au/about.html

25. *The history of Namikoshi shiatsu therapy*. (2003). Retrieved April 2, 2007, from http://www.namikoshi-shiatsu.com.au/

26. Banker, C. (2006). *What is 5 element shiatsu?* Retrieved April 4, 2007, from http://www.cindybanker.com/five.html

27. *ABT styles*. (2007). Retrieved March 31, 2007, from http://www.aobta.org/about-forms.html?start=1

28. *Macrobiotic shiatsu*. (2006). Retrieved April 4, 2007, from http://www.chienergy.co.uk/freeinformation_sh.htm#macrobioticshiatsu

29. *What is JSJ about Mary*. (2005). Retreived February 10, 2007, from http://jsjinc.net/mary.php

30. Teeguarden, I. (1999). *Acupressure way of health: Jin Shin Do*. Tokyo, Japan: Japan Publications

31. *The development of Jin Shin Do bodymind acupressure*. (2006). Retrieved February 7, 2007, from http://www.jinshindo.org/development.htm

32. Teeguarden, I. (1999). *Acupressure way of health: Jin Shin Do*. Tokyo, Japan: Japan Publications.

33. Teeguarden, I. (1999). *Acupressure way of health: Jin Shin Do*. Tokyo, Japan: Japan Publications.

34. Teeguarden, I. (2002). *A complete guide to acupressure: Jin Shin Do*. Tokyo, Japan: Japan Publications.

35. *Requriements*. (2006). Retrieved February 7, 2007, from http://www.jinshindo.org/requirement.htm

36. Gold, R., *Thai Massage: A Traditional Medical Technique* (1998) United Kingdom: Churchill Livingston

37. Chow, K. T., & Moody, E. (2006). *Thai yoga therapy for your body type*. Rochester: Healing Arts Press.

10

CHAPTER

The Energetic Layer of the Massage Therapy and Bodywork Continuum

CHAPTER GOALS

1. Develop an understanding of how the modalities of Therapeutic Touch, Reiki, and Polarity Therapy fit into the energetic approach of massage.

2. Recognize the significance of these modalities, how they differ, and how they are similar to each other.

3. Develop a basic understanding of the theory and principles of each of the modalities.

4. Develop a basic understanding of the process of assessment used in each of the modalities.

5. Develop a basic understanding of the techniques involved in each of the modalities.

6. Become acquainted with the general experience of a session in each of the modalities.

7. Identify who should seek this form of treatment and what conditions are most benefited by each of the modalities.

8. Become aware of contraindications and precautions related to each of the modalities.

9. Become knowledgeable about the training, licensing, certifications, and requirements that one needs in order to practice within each of the modalities.

INTRODUCTION TO THE ENERGETIC LAYER OF MASSAGE THERAPY AND BODYWORK

Almost every culture has recognized the existence of an all-pervading underlying force that enlivens and integrates the world. In India this force is known as prana. In Hebrew it is called ruach. Followers of Islam call it baraka and in the Orient it is known as qi or ki.[1] This energy is often described as the breath of life because it is considered the vital essence that animates and gives life to the physical form (Figure 10-1). When this energy is full and balanced in an individual it provides radiance and vitality. When lacking and imbalanced it leaves one cold and weak. It is a very rarefied form of matter, but at the same time it is still a physical substance. It can be palpated, it can be moved, and it can even be controlled. Some gifted healers claim that they can see this energy field called an aura. The manipulation and control of this energy for the purpose of healing is the focus of this chapter.

To those unversed and unfamiliar with energetic bodywork, these modalities seem like an otherworldly science. Even those who have seen or felt the benefits of energetic bodywork firsthand may not comprehend it and may view

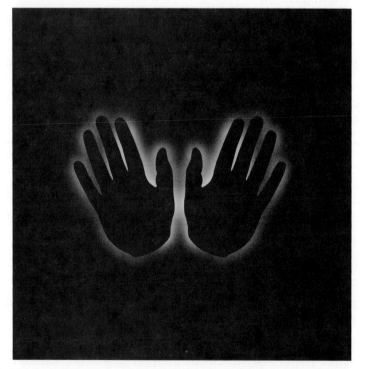

Figure 10-1 A pair of healing hands showing the energetic aura emanating from them. *Image copyright 2009, Tara Urbach. Used under license from shutterstock.com.*

it as a mysterious and complex phenomenon. Practitioners of this approach, however, often claim their work to be a simple act based on nothing more than the natural laws of the everyday universe.

At the core of **energetic bodywork** is the belief that the totality of the universe is an expression of energy and is connected in a vast, underlying network that nourishes and affects every particle of life. Some of these connections are visible like the network of blood vessels within the human body or the rivers that connect the waterways of the world. Others are more elusive and can only be felt, like the emotional ties that bind people to one another. Invisible as they may be, they still form potent bonds that can be harder to break than steel.

These underlying vital pathways that link and feed everything are seen as absolutely necessary for existence. Just as an arm or a leg would weaken and die without a supply of blood and oxygen, so too would our life end if this energy didn't circulate within us. In this way the human entity can be seen as baby nestled in the womb of an energetic universe, being continuously fed through invisible cords of energy. If this connection is severed, the body is no longer able to receive nourishment and its ability to sustain life ceases. The strength of this connection determines our health and well-being on all levels—physical, mental, and emotional. When this connection is strong, the body is full of health and vitality. When it is weak, the amount of vital energy received by the body diminishes, upsetting the individual's physical and psychological health.

Interestingly, the practice of energetic bodywork almost invariably produces a profound change in an individual's concept of life. In fact, this change is ultimately a prerequisite for the competent practice of energy work. The study of energy in the United States is not an education that is readily served in school or as part of one's normal education. Because of this, coming to terms with that which is invisible often requires bending oneself to a new set of rules and ideas that may be completely foreign to one's established foundation. Even just accepting the concept of energy requires a radical shift in understanding life and oneself because it also means accepting that we are not isolated entities from the world around us. The realization that one's words, actions, and very being affects everyone and everything can stretch the edges of one's conscience so that a greater sense of responsibility for the world around is felt.

However, once this idea is embraced it can be deeply comforting to feel the limits of the self stretching endlessly—especially for those whose life is coming to an end. With this shift in perspective, death can become an acceptable, embraceable act that is to be faced with peace and understanding. It is no longer seen as the loss of everything, but simply another passing—a transition from one form to another without any real loss at all. So while energy work provides a mode of dealing with pain in the physical body, it also provides a means for dealing with pain on deeper levels where medicine and surgery cannot reach.

Each modality in the following chapter adapts the same universal principles in slightly different ways. Although there exist many additional forms of energetic bodywork, the three discussed in this chapter are by far the most practiced and well known. Therapeutic Touch (TT), often referred to as Non-contact Therapeutic Touch (NCTT), is an approach seemingly made for the masses. Its practice is simple and intuitive, yet despite its ease of use it can still be a powerful healing apparatus. Reiki is a more complex form with special symbols and mantras that channel particular variations of the universal energy to create specific effects. Although not as accessible to the novice as it is to the experienced practitioner, anyone is said to be able to channel Reiki energy.

The most complex of the three methods of energetic bodywork covered here is Polarity Therapy. In truth, **Polarity Therapy** spans the entire breadth of bodywork. Upon first look it is somatic, somato-psychic, bioenergetic, and energetic all raveled into one. However, at its core it is primarily an energetic healing art that includes manipulations, light stretching, and light contact, as well as hand movements off the body to move, and balance the energy.

THERAPEUTIC TOUCH

Developed in the early 1970s by Dora Kunz and longtime colleague and student Delores Krieger, Ph.D., RN, Therapeutic Touch is a simple and direct form of energetic bodywork that seeks to balance the human energy by projecting and moving it with the hands. The practice of Therapeutic Touch, much like those of the traditional forms of Chinese massage therapy, is predicated upon the underlying assumption that human beings are complex energy fields (Figure 10-2). (As discussed in Chapter 9 on bioenergetic forms of massage therapy and bodywork, the Chinese took the concepts of energy to a much deeper and more complex level, evolving their whole system of traditional Chinese medicine (TCM) out of it.) The other major operational principle of Therapeutic Touch is that there is a natural potential in human beings to be able to enhance and advance the healing of others.

Dora Kunz, a past president of the Theosophical Society of America, was known as a healer of striking sensitivities and it was her early work that was formulated into the Therapeutic Touch of today. Her heightened sense of perception allowed her to identify subtle nuances in the human energy field that couldn't be detected by conventional medical means. Because of this she

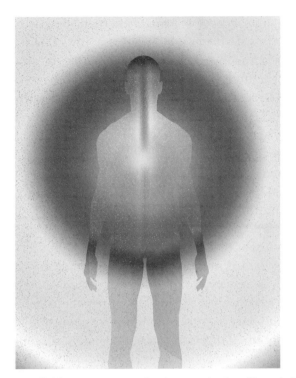

Figure 10-2 The energy field encompasses the human body, although it may appear to us that it is inside the body, much like water in a bottle. However, the correct understanding is that the body lies within an invisible energy field that surrounds, permeates, and enlivens it. *Image copyright 2009, Bruce Rolff. Used under license from shutterstock.com.*

developed a special relationship with doctors and scientists, who referred their unusual and perplexing cases to her for diagnosis and treatment.

Therapeutic Touch was officially developed and conceived with Delores Krieger, a longtime professor and nursing educator from New York University, at Pumpkin Hollow Farm, one of the Theosophical Society's spiritual retreat centers where patients were sent by their physicians. Soon the farmhouse and cabins filled with patients waiting to be treated and students wishing to learn.

Although Dora Kunz passed in 1999, Therapeutic Touch is still being carried on by her successors. Today, however, it is not only taught at Pumpkin Hollow, but also worldwide, and is practiced as an alternative therapy in hospitals and other health care facilities.[2]

Theory and Principles

Therapeutic Touch is one of the simplest forms of energetic bodywork and functions almost entirely on the basis of intention. This simplicity, however, does not imply a weakness. Its intuitive and straightforward manner allows it to be a highly accessible form of energetic bodywork that can be just as powerful as any other form of energetic healing. The term "Therapeutic Touch" is actually a misnomer, because its practice doesn't actually require physical contact, hence its alternative name Non-contact Therapeutic Touch (NCTT). The focus of treatment is on the underlying human energy field rather than the physical body itself, so the hands don't actually touch the other person.

Like Reiki, Therapeutic Touch utilizes the energetic system of the chakras. There are seven major chakras or vortices of energy in the body and two minor ones in the hands. It is through the chakras of the hands that the healer is able to direct energy into the receiver. Unlike Reiki, however, practitioners of Therapeutic Touch do not see their work as only producing positive effects. Therapeutic Touch sees energy work just like any other form of therapy that can be damaging if used inappropriately. Too much treatment can lead to what is known as "energy overload" and can worsen a condition. Or, treating without knowing exactly what's going on in the patient's energy field or without knowing exactly why a certain technique is being applied is seen as irresponsible intervention. If this is the case, the patient should seek out another practitioner.

Two of the major areas where the effects of Therapeutic Touch have most notably made their mark is in dealing with illnesses involving psychological stress and in terminal cases to ease the passing from life to death. Because psychological stress is seen as a huge component of illnesses these days (over 70 percent of all diseases are said to be linked to psychological stress), Therapeutic Touch can assist in a variety of conditions. In the case of the dying, Therapeutic Touch has been found to ease the burden of a patient's final transition. In a time of confusion, pain, and fear, Therapeutic Touch can ease the suffering and help bring about a state of calm, peace, and acceptance so that patients can enter into their final stage with grace, understanding, and even gratitude.

Skepticism

Interestingly, Therapeutic Touch has found a special home in the nursing profession. Usually, practices that are deemed fringe sciences do not mingle with the established medical system. However, Therapeutic Touch's acceptance by the nurses in the United States and Canada has put it right alongside modern medical practices—thus putting Therapeutic Touch under the scientific spotlight. Skeptics of Therapeutic Touch proclaim that it is nothing more than "faith healing" or the placebo effect in action.

As opposed to battling the argument that the power of suggestion is what's really at work in energetic healing, practitioners of Therapeutic Touch embrace it by trying to instill the patient with a strong sense of belief that treatment will be effective. "Placebo" is viewed as just another word for self-healing and is recognized as a powerful motivator for healing. It is this same power that is in effect when a doctor walks into the room of an ill patient. Sometimes just being in the presence of someone who knows how to deal with your pain provides that immeasurable something that jump-starts the healing process. Furthermore, proponents of Therapeutic Touch claim that some of the most profound responses to this modality have occurred in those who are thought to be incapable of responding to suggestion, such as **coma** patients, heavily anesthetized post-operative patients, and premature babies.[3]

Assessment

Assessment of the energy field is required to determine the nature of the energetic imbalance and is done with the receiver either comfortably seated or lying down. Starting at the head, the therapist hovers his or her hands 2 to 3 inches from the midline of the receiver's body and sweeps them out in opposite directions to the sides. The hands are then brought back to center, this time a few inches lower, and the same sweeping motion is applied again. This continues until the entire body is covered head to toe and front to back. At each level the therapist is looking for signs of irregularity or deviation from the normal pattern of healthy movement in the energy field. Ideally, the energy field should feel smooth, integrated, symmetrical, and free flowing. Turbulence, dips, or bulges in the energy field indicate that there is an imbalance. Areas where disturbances are felt in the energy field are called cues and can come in five main forms:

1. Temperature differences: Certain areas over the body may feel hot or cold compared to other areas of the energy field.
2. Magnetism: Some areas may feel like they are drawing in while other areas feel as if they are repelling and pushing out.
3. Tingling, pins and needles, little bubbles bursting, or slight electrical shocks.
4. Rhythmic pulses.
5. Intuitive insights: The therapist may experience a sudden flash of thought or vision when going over certain parts of the energy field.

Along with the various sensations that may arise, the therapist is also looking for differences and asymmetries in the recipient's energy field.

During this process it is important that the giver retain a sense of openness. Anything they feel should be accepted without judgment. The clues may come as subtle hunches, vague notions, or even strong impressions. During the initial assessment it is important to acknowledge these sensations but not to linger. The practitioner must get a sense of the recipient as a whole before poring over the details.

Techniques

There are three major components of treatment: rebalancing, modulation, and unruffling. The goal of **rebalancing** is to create symmetry and equilibrium in the receiver's field of energy. This is where the rule of opposites comes into play. For each type of energetic disturbance, an exact and opposite energy is created to counter the imbalance. If practitioners sense heat in the energy field, they seek to bring balance by supplying the opposite—cold. Here practitioners mentally replicate the feeling of cold by concentrating on a time when they felt cold and then project this thought into their recipient's energy field, thus calming and reducing the heat and bringing about balance. In the same manner, excesses are drained, insufficiencies are filled, tensions are softened, and irregularities are smoothed out.

The process of **modulation** has to do with modifying the recipient's existing energy. Rather than pumping energy in or out as done in rebalancing, here the therapist is concerned with enhancing or adjusting the levels of energy already in the recipient's field. This is done by visualizing and projecting specific colors. Like sound, colors are a specific wavelength of energy and just as different sounds can convey different emotions, so too can different colors yield different effects.

A clear royal blue like the color of ocean waves has been shown to soothe and pacify and can be used to resolve panic, fear, and hypertension. Vibrant yellow like the sun's rays has been found to have a stimulating effect and can be used to combat sluggishness, depression, and lack of motivation. Green has a neutral but energizing effect and is useful for providing balance and stability. The effectiveness of this technique has to do with the therapist's ability to realistically create an experience of that color. To do this, practitioners can allow their entire senses to be filled with the feelings of running through an endless green pasture, being bathed in sunlight, or being gently lapped in cooling ocean waves.

Turbulent energetic vibrations are often related to psychological stress such as fear, nervousness, or anxiety. The texture of this type of energy may feel rough, tangled, agitated, and disorganized. **Unruffling** is the clearing of these disruptive energies by pushing them out and away from the receiver's field. In this technique the hands "wipe" down the body to comb through energetic knots and tangles to create a smooth, synchronous flow of energy. This process reestablishes harmony in the field and produces a calm emotional composure.[4]

The Session

Every treatment begins with a short centering in order to break away from the day's distractions. This is the therapists' time to prepare their senses for the session. Picking up on energetic cues requires much more deftness of perception than "normal" dealings with the outside world; therefore, therapists must recalibrate their sensitivity to feel and handle the subtle vibrations of energy. Therapeutic Touch practitioners must be able to extract their awareness from external distractions and quiet their own internal noise so that it doesn't interfere with the treatment. This is also the time to put aside personal thoughts and emotions in order to open oneself to another's voice. Once the internal chattering ceases, new and previously hidden qualities can be noticed.

After centering, a whole-body assessment of the receiver's energy field is conducted. In this phase, therapists seek out imbalances and irregularities in the flow of energy. Often patients won't be aware of the energetic disturbances in their own field, but usually they'll feel the effects of having it corrected.

In the assessment phase, the healer identifies with the receiver's energy field in order to understand the nature of the imbalance. In the treatment phase, therapists use their own healthy self as a model to repattern the receiver's energy. Studies in energetics have shown that energy naturally flows from the top of the head down to the feet; therefore, a Therapeutic Touch treatment flows in the same pattern.

To treat an imbalance, one hand is placed directly over the site of dysfunction and the other hand is placed above but not on the opposite area. Again, the hands are hovering near the body, but not making contact (Figure 10-3). Energy is then directed from one hand through the body to the other hand. If the opposite side is not accessible, the other hand can be placed anywhere else on the receiver's energy field. Treatment should not be conducted mechanically. Each action should be performed as a specific response to specific cues. To ensure that treatment is being performed according to the exact and often changing needs of the recipient, the energy field is periodically reassessed.

Unlike modalities like tuina or Swedish massage where the body is worked globally first and then the focus is honed down to the small details, Therapeutic Touch starts by attending to the specific sites of dysfunction and then the therapist works at the end to synchronize, balance, and integrate the body as a whole.

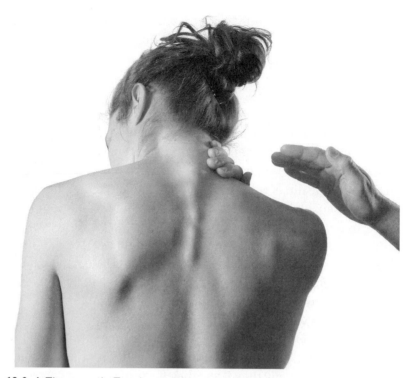

Figure 10-3 A Therapeutic Touch practitioner holding his hand over a specific area of shoulder pain in the client. *Image copyright 2009, Yanik Chauvin. Used under license from shutterstock.com.*

A Therapeutic Touch session normally does not last beyond 20 to 25 minutes. Beyond this time frame the receiver may suffer energy overload and become restless, anxious, irritable, or even hostile. In Therapeutic Touch it is better to underdo rather than overdo. Overdoing can cause harm and discomfort to both the patient and the relationship. If underdoing, it is always possible to come back later for another session. Following the session, the recipient is allowed to rest for 10 to 15 minutes in order for energy to ground and stabilize.

Patients have reported many feelings during treatment ranging from tingling, warmth, increased circulation, a gentle bursting of effervescent bubbles, to a general sense of calmness. In the case of energetic breakthroughs during which longstanding stagnations have suddenly been released, patients may feel a sort of "jump" or a sudden boost in their body.

Practitioners describe the feeling of treating as being immersed in new surroundings. Their awareness and emotions subtly but distinctly shift from "normal" everyday existence. Some describe sensations of peace, quiet, and calmness. Others describe a kind of "hyperawareness" with a crispness of memory, thought, and concentration that they normally don't have. Still others describe a quiet joy that can't quite be called happiness. It is described as a state more grounded than happiness and less fleeting. Time seems to slow down and the moments seem to fill with greater vividness, imagery, experience, and energy. Although the treatment is meant for the other person, the practitioners, too, often feel more balanced in process.

Benefits

- Decreases anxiety before surgery
- Improves recovery from surgery
- Helps the dying find peace, acceptance, and understanding
- Reduces chronic pain or makes it manageable
- Releases endorphins to promote better quality of emotions
- Balances fluid electrolytes
- Improves healing time for injuries
- Boosts the immune system
- Promotes feelings of peace and well-being

Contraindications

- Pregnancy—near term

Precautions

- Cranial injuries
- Burns and other sensitive areas
- Recent injuries

Training of a Practitioner

There are several levels at which Therapeutic Touch can be practiced. A basic, introductory workshop plus a five-day mentorship program can help a newcomer grasp the foundations of Therapeutic Touch and feel comfortable enough to treat friends and family. For those who want to take their work to the next levels, intermediate-stage workshops and mentorship programs are available that provide more intense and focused training. Completions of these levels allow one to comfortably treat others. An advanced course can only be taken after at least three years of Therapeutic Touch practice.[5]

Often, those who seek training in Therapeutic Touch are health care professionals looking to supplement their practice. The nursing field especially has embraced Therapeutic Touch as an adjunct modality and offers continuing education credits for its study and training.

REIKI

The details of the origins of Reiki as practiced today continue to change as new and more information comes to light from Japan. As often is the case, because there is a lack of documentation left behind by those involved, particularly the founders themselves, histories often have to be pieced together by those who come after. That can make for some stark and interesting differences, as well as great difficulty in deciphering the true findings and versions of the facts. However, one thing that is generally agreed upon is that **Reiki**, as known today, was at some time a Tibetan ancient healing art and made its recent comeback through a rediscovery. From that point on there are many versions regarding the specifics of Reiki history. What is told here follows one of the more common accounts by Mrs. Hawayo Takata who studied and practiced Reiki from 1936–1980. It is what she taught her students when explaining how Reiki made its way to the west.

The energetic healing practice of Reiki was created by Dr. Mikao Usui. Born in 1865, Usui grew up at a time when the society and culture of Japan was going through a time of great change.[6] As a Christian minister teaching at a small university in Kyoto, Japan, Dr. Usui was challenged by some of his senior students, who questioned the reality of Christ's healing miracles. Unable to reply with definite conviction, Usui went out in search of answers—not just for the sake of his students, but for his own need to understand. As a minister of the Christian tradition, this was a question that penetrated into the core of his religious beliefs.

Usui's initial excavations into the mysterious world of Christ yielded little. His immediate impulse was to seek the information through the Christian church, but he found little that was documented. However, during his research, Usui noticed remarkable similarities between the life of Christ and the life of the Buddha, so he turned his attention to Buddhism. His studies took him to a Zen monastery in Japan where he discovered strange symbols and mantras preserved within their ancient texts. Although he couldn't decipher their meaning, something within him registered their importance. However, he couldn't uncover their meaning alone.

His considerable time spent at the monastery created the opportunity for friendship with the head abbot. The holy man directed Usui to meditate for

21 days at a nearby mountaintop. On the last day of meditation, Usui had a profound experience. In his vision, he saw a white light shooting towards him. The light shot into his forehead at the third-eye chakra and he felt his awareness grow larger and larger. In this heightened state he saw the same symbols he had seen in the scriptures, yet somehow they were no longer foreign to him. He understood. As the secrets of the symbols unraveled before him, he felt a powerful healing force being opened inside his body. Excited and energized by his profound experience, he hurried back down the mountain, but in his rush he tripped and badly injured his toe. In pain, he placed his hands over his damaged toe and to his amazement, both the pain and bleeding completely subsided.

With his newfound gift, Dr. Usui set out to heal the sick and needy. He traveled to the slums to heal the most helpless of mankind, but quickly realized that even though their bodies had been cured, their minds were still sick. They didn't reintegrate themselves back into society and didn't take steps to take care of themselves. Sadly, Usui realized that they didn't really want to be healed. They just wanted to be free from pain. It was then that Usui realized how important it is that patients not only possess a strong desire to be better but also that they become active participants in their own healing process. He also came to understand that it was necessary for them to give something in return or else they wouldn't value what they received.

With this understanding a new phase of his life began, and he set out not only to heal the way that people thought but also to teach the method of his healing. In the last few years before his death in 1926, Usui entrusted Dr. Chijiro Hayashi, a retired naval officer, as his successor. Dr. Hayashi carried on the teachings of Usui and opened a private clinic where he treated the general public and trained new practitioners. There he met Hawayo Takata. She had come from Hawaii following an inner calling to seek healing in Japan rather than have an operation for a multitude of serious, life-threatening ailments. Prior to coming to Japan, she had never heard of Reiki or Dr. Hayashi, but in the course of her journey she happened to come across Hayashi's clinic. There she was treated for several months and was completely healed.

She ended up staying for another year as a student of Hayashi's before returning to Hawaii. In 1938, Takata was initiated as a Master of the Usui system and in 1941, following Hayashi's death, she became his successor. Until 1976 Hawayo Takata was the only Reiki Master alive, but in the last few years of her life she trained 22 other Master-level Reiki practitioners.[7]

When Takata died she did not leave behind any structure or organization by which Reiki could evolve and move forward. As a result there was a split into two main lineages by her own trained Reiki masters. One was Barbara Weber

Ray who developed the Radiance Technique School and the other was Takata's granddaughter Phyllis Lei Furumoto who created the Reiki Alliance.

Today there are a variety of different forms of Reiki that are practiced—some that follow the symbols, mantras, and rituals of the original lineage and others that have developed their own customs, traditions, and characteristics. More than 1200 Reiki Masters are practicing worldwide, all of whom can trace their lineage back to Hawayo Takata.[8]

Theory and Principles

Literally translated, the word Reiki is Japanese for "spiritually guided life energy." *Rei* refers to a higher wisdom beyond that of the individual human being and *ki* refers to the universal life force that both surrounds and composes all things (Figure 10-4). Although Reiki is spiritual, it is not religious and has no dogmatic system of beliefs. In fact, its only true goal is to promote health and well-being, and it achieves this by tapping into the innate healing forces of nature by using a method once employed long ago, but just recently discovered again.[9]

The work of the Reiki practitioner is to boost the amount of life force within an individual through the use of special symbols and mantras. By increasing the

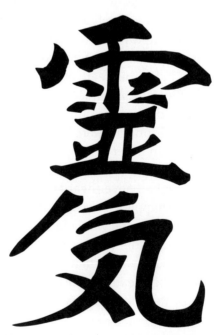

Figure 10-4 The word Reiki is made up of two Japanese words, rei, which means "universal" and ki, which means "life force energy." *Image copyright 2009, Daniela Illing. Used under license from shutterstock.com.*

amount of Ki flowing through an individual, the Reiki practitioner can dramatically improve just about every function of the body and mind. This is because Ki is a fundamental substance and is a precursor to every other form of energy such as food, water, and oxygen. If this fundamental nutrient is lacking, it will not matter how much air, water, or food a patient is given, he or she will not heal. However, if this energy is strong, it is said that it alone can sustain a patient completely.

Everyone has access to the Reiki energy, but not everyone is able to receive it in their current condition. It is said that the Reiki energy once flowed naturally through everyone, but along the course of time people's energetic pathways have become stagnant and blocked. Reiki practitioners unleash these obstructions and channel ki into the receiver by using their own body as a bridge. While this process dramatically amplifies the life energy of the recipient, providing a Reiki session is actually not at all draining. This is because practitioners are not drawing from their own wells; rather, they are simply acting as a conduit for Universal energy to flow through them. Just as a metal wire retains the heat of electricity conducted through it, Reiki practitioners are imbued with the energy that flows through them.[10]

Unlike other forms of bodywork, there is generally no assessment required in Reiki.[11] This is because the Universal energy is said to have an innate intelligence that does not require human input or direction. It is, after all, the same intelligence that created both humans and the world in which we live. Reiki energy is said to flow naturally from the chakras located in the palms of the hands, and the mere placing of the hands above or on another person with the right intent is all that is needed for the energy to correct any ailment in its path (Figure 10-5). Because it is this "higher" intelligence that guides the treatment, even new initiates with no background in energy work immediately gain the ability to "heal" others. [12]

The Three Degrees of Reiki

There are three levels at which Reiki can be practiced. Each level is called a **degree** and each degree is achieved through a series of treatments called attunements. The process of attunement is different than that of a normal Reiki session. An attunement is conducted in order to create a new Reiki practitioner. A Reiki session is conducted for the purpose of therapy. Although the Reiki energy can be utilized by anyone, an attunement can only be conducted by an experienced Reiki Master.

In the process of attunement, a permanent connection to the infinite reservoir of Universal energy becomes established and the receiver too becomes a carrier of the Reiki energy. Although this allows them to pass energy onto

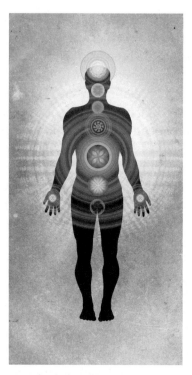

Figure 10-5 A figure of a human depicting the seven major chakras and the two lesser known chakras located in the center of the palm of each hand. *Image copyright 2009, Rgbspace. Used under license from shutterstock.com.*

others, this first level is primarily intended for self-healing. However, no matter what the usage of their new abilities, from this point on they are considered Reiki healers. For this reason, the first session is called the initiation.[13]

Although the first Reiki session takes only an hour, it will take three to four weeks for the attunement to fully run its course. During this time the receiver may feel the Reiki energy turning on and off sporadically as it sputters to life. Although the initiate may experience strong changes and gain abilities they've never before had, nothing new has been added to them. Like a lamp inside of a house already wired for electricity, the recipient has simply been "plugged in." Following the first attunement, the initiate can return to this source at any time to reconnect with the higher forces.[14]

During this process, initiates may also experience sudden onsets of tingling, intense dreaming, or spaciness. Symptoms of detoxification such as a runny nose, diarrhea, or increased urination are also common. This is the clearing process necessary before the Reiki energy can run at full force. Following the first session it is recommended that self-attunements be administered daily for a month to maximize the effects. This is the first degree of Reiki.

While the first degree allows the practitioner to perform Reiki on others through direct contact, the second degree empowers the practitioner to perform Reiki from a distance with the help of a special symbol. When working from a different location, the same energy is still being accessed but here the practitioner learns to direct it more powerfully and with greater intent.[15]

Initiation into the third degree empowers one to teach and initiate others. Here practitioners are called Reiki Masters and are entrusted with the use of new symbols. Again they receive attunements that amplify their healing abilities. This level of training can take years to develop under the proper tutelage of a seasoned Master.

The Techniques

The exact methods of the Reiki tradition, along with the symbols utilized for healing, are closely guarded and are only granted to those who have the proper training. Practitioners swear an oath to keep secret the details of their craft from the uninitiated in order to control the abuse of power that often comes from knowing just a small amount of a much larger system. As apprentices grow in their practice and training, they are entrusted with the use of more and more symbols.[16]

These symbols are carefully crafted keys that unlock specific functions of the Universal energy. Just as the vibrational qualities of different music can induce different emotions, the resonations produced by the various symbols of Reiki can create entirely different effects. Some are used to increase the body's physical energy, some are used to sedate troubled hearts and minds, some are used for protection, and some are used to promote peace and enlightenment. And as already mentioned there are even some that are used to heal from a distance.[17]

Practitioners of Reiki utilize two main modes of healing. The first method is direct healing where the giver and receiver are in the same location and are able to have physical contact. The second method is for when giver and recipient are in different locations.[18] Distance healing can be achieved by several means. The practitioner can conjure a mental image of the recipient, use a surrogate (such as a teddy-bear or a pillow), use their own body as an alternative, use a photograph, or imagine the receiver in the palm of their hands. Because ki is a universal energy that travels throughout and connects the entirety of existence, Reiki practitioners, with the use of special symbols, can "ride" these energetic "highways" in order to reach recipients no matter how distant their location.[19]

The Session

Treatments are conducted through a series of hand positions beginning from the top of the head and down either to the feet or to the pelvis. Most positions are directly on or over the seven energetic centers along the midline of the body (the chakras) and each position is held for three to five minutes (See Figure 10-5). Beginner practitioners will adhere to a prescribed course of treatment while the advanced practitioner will rely more on intuition to guide them.

A full session lasts from an hour to an hour-and-a-half. The treatment is performed on a cushioned table with the receiver fully clothed. Treatments can even be effectively administered through bandages and plaster casts. Since no part of the body is actively moved or manipulated, no oils or lotions are necessary. Although treatment is generally accomplished while the hands are either on or off specific areas of the body, in the case of burns, fractures, rashes, recent surgeries or cuts where contact is not permissible, the hands should be held a few inches away.[20]

As the energy flows out, the practitioner will feel his or her hands become hot and the receiver will often feel the energy being channeled as heat. However, if the receiver's condition is such that cold would be better for them, the energy will self-calibrate according to the specific needs of the recipient. This is a function of the energy's innate intelligence and does not require direction from the practitioner.

After the initial feeling of heat, the healer may experience other sensations, including cold, trembling, static electricity, color, sound, and, very rarely, even pain. The sensations will differ from position to position and session to session and can continue for as long as five minutes. There is no predetermined amount of time that is needed for each site and the transition from one position to another will be largely intuitive. When the receiver has had enough, the sensations will naturally cease.

Occasionally, however, the sensations can seem to go on for much longer. Often these are sites that are in extreme need of healing and may take more than one session to alleviate. Again, the best guide is the intuition. After the healer feels that they have spent adequate time in one location, he or she should move on and can always come back to it later. Some problems are years in the making and will not all go away in just one session.[21]

The experience of a Reiki session will vary from receiver to receiver. Some see pictures, some perceive colors, and some feel as if they are filled with light, peace, wonder, or love. For some it may be a strong experience, but for others it may only produce a mild, gentle sensation.[22] Benefits of treatment are sometimes not felt until days after the treatment. In some cases an entire series of treatments must be finished before the desired effects can be achieved. To enhance the power of the treatment, two or more practitioners can work together. Or, other healing therapies can be applied, including crystal, color, and sound therapies.[23]

Benefits

- Promote faster recover from surgery and chemotherapy
- Reduce side effects of medications
- Help the dying find peace before passing on
- Promote healing, wellness, and relaxation
- Develop a positive outlook on life
- Enhance personal and spiritual development
- Support of other healing therapies

Contraindications

It is said that the effects of Reiki are always positive and because Reiki is completely noninvasive and does not require physical contact, there are no dangers under any known conditions.

Training

There are no special requirements, trainings, or credentials needed to be inducted into Reiki training. Many Reiki practitioners, however, are already health care professionals who are looking to complement their existing training and practice. Unlike other forms of bodywork where the student learns much of the information in classes and lectures, the knowledge and techniques are learned in an apprenticeship format. Because of this, the techniques taught can vary greatly from teacher to teacher.

There are typically three (or sometimes four) levels or degrees of training that the Reiki trainee can pursue. Initiation into the first and second degree status can be completed over a weekend seminar or over the course of several evenings. To move on to the Master level, however, is a much more involved process that may require an extensive apprenticeship, practical demonstrations, and substantial fees. This process is designed to test the dedication and suitability of the aspirant.[24]

The laws regulating Reiki can vary widely from state to state. Because of its noninvasive nature, some states may not have any policies concerning its practice while other states, like Florida, may require that the Reiki practitioner also be a certified massage therapist.[25]

POLARITY THERAPY

Developed by Dr. Randolph Stone (1890–1981), **Polarity Therapy** is an open-armed system that utilizes whatever means necessary to establish balance and order in the human energy field. Techniques can range from bodywork, to dietary counseling, to exercises, stretches, and changes in lifestyle.

With a background in chiropractic, osteopathic, and naturopathic medicine, Dr. Stone began his developments in energy work with a firm foundation of the body's structure. His later explorations in the eastern arts of energetics, including the Ayurvedic medicine of India, traditional Chinese medicine, yoga, and **reflexology**, helped to create a form of bodywork that spans the range of different approaches from somatic to energetic.

A consummate explorer of the healing arts, his eclectic interests are reflected in the diversity of techniques employed within the generous boundaries of Polarity Therapy. Because his work draws on such a wide range of practices and philosophies, Polarity Therapy has attracted a diverse population of students and patients who have gone on to influence the fields of psychotherapy, osteopathy, chiropractic, dance, yoga, massage therapy, physical therapy, athletic training, and more. This extensive acceptance of his work, however, was no accident. Dr. Stone intentionally sought to create a universal system that integrated truth at all levels.

During his life he was respected as a hard-working doctor who garnered his knowledge from real-life experience rather than theory alone, and his seminars drew upon practitioners and lay people of all walks and professions, including doctors, psychologists, chiropractors, massage therapists, martial artists, astrologists, and many, many more.[26]

Theory and Principles

After extensive research in a variety of medical philosophies, Dr. Stone came to the realization of the existence of certain fundamental principles that tied together all fields of healing. He concluded that all of existence flows from one source and is composed of one universal substance. He then described this universal substance as being composed of three forces—the positive, the negative, and the neutral. Energy is said to pulse back and forth between these three forces in a rhythmic tide called the Polarity Principle.[27]

Dr. Stone considered the movement of energy between these three forces the pulse of life. The positive phase of the Polarity Principle represents a yang-like stage where energy expands and radiates outward. The negative, yin-like phase represents a drawing inward and contracting of this same energy. The neutral territory is the in-between phase of the two opposites.

This same dynamic is apparent in the anatomy of the atom with its positively charged protons, negatively charged electrons, and neutral neutrons. In the human being, the positive pole is represented by the head, the feet are the negative pole, and the mid-section is the neutral. The work of Polarity Therapy is to balance the fluctuation of energy from pole to pole—from yin to yang.[28]

The relationship between these three forces is represented in the ancient Greek sign of the physician—the caduceus, or the staff of Hermes (Figure 10-6). In the caduceus, the two serpents represent the interplay of positive and negative forces while the central staff, called the "Ultrasonic Core" by Dr. Stone, represents the neutral or balancing force. This central core reflects the higher vibrational aspects of each of the five elements which ultimately manifest as the spinal cord and Central Nervous System. The wings represent the two cerebral hemispheres of the brain, and the globe at the end of the shaft is the pineal gland. When the caduceus is placed over the body, the points at which the serpents cross create five interacting energy fields that represent the five lower energetic chakras. [29] Each of these chakras corresponds to one of the elemental

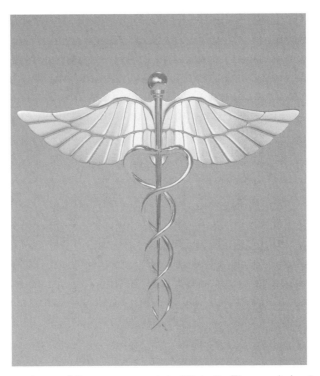

Figure 10-6 The anatomy of the energy model of Polarity Therapy is best represented by the ancient Greek symbol of the caduceus, or staff of Hermes. *Image copyright 2009, Eduard Härkönen. Used under license from shutterstock.com.*

forces of Ayurvedic medicine: earth, water, fire, air, and ether. Each element rules specific parts of the body, emotions, senses, and even astrological signs.

Techniques

Because Dr. Stone covered such a large expanse of practice and theory, treatment in Polarity Therapy can vary greatly from practitioner to practitioner. Some may involve more bodywork while others incorporate more psychology, exercise, diet, and so on. Even the boundaries of their bodywork techniques are loose and permeable, including physical manipulations, gentle stretching, light reflex contacts; and hand movements off the body. Rather than having a specific set of hand manipulations to call their own (like effleurage, petrissage, etc. of Swedish massage), the techniques of Polarity Therapy are defined by general qualities borrowed from Ayurvedic medicine.

According to the Vedic philosophy of ancient India (home to one of the oldest forms of medicine still in practice) rajas, tamas, and sattva represent three primary principles or forces of the universe. Rajas represents light, activity, and movement. Techniques described as rajasic are quick and lively. An effective way of applying these stimulating techniques is with circular pressure of the fingers and palms to activate movement. Tamas represents darkness, heaviness, and inertia; therefore, tamasic techniques are slow, deep, and penetrating. These can be done with the fingers, thumbs, knuckles, or elbows to apply a deep and sustained pressure. Sattva represents purity and stillness, and these techniques are almost entirely energetic. A light, feathery pressure is applied with just the tips of the thumbs and fingers to balance the subtle flows of energy.[31]

Assessment

Gathering the patient's history is an important step in understanding the internal dynamics of their energetic system. This examination is based on more than just what clients state. It also has to do with picking up on the tell-tale signs that are often nonverbal. By analyzing the quality of their voice, studying their stance, or observing their actions, the practitioner can decipher clients' emotional states, which in turn helps to understand which element is out of balance. Their astrological sign, too, can be used to determine their imbalance. If someone is born under the sign of Taurus, for example, it may mean that they will tend towards imbalances of the earth element.

Discovering which of the five elements is ailing tells the therapist what to treat. However, this is only half of the Polarity equation. Determining how to treat is decided by diagnosis of the patient's pulses.

Pulse evaluations are conducted at two locations—the back of the neck and inside the ankles. Here the therapist is checking the pulse's strength and balance. If the pulses at the neck differ in strength from the pulses on the ankles, this indicates a problem in the bipolar current, the current of energy that flows vertically. This type of imbalance requires a deep, Tamasic touch to penetrate the blockage and create movement in the energy current. If the left and right pulses are not in sync, then this means that the transverse current flowing from side to side is blocked. Balance of this current requires a light sattvic touch. If all the pulses are weak, this indicates weakness in the umbilical current that emanates from the belly. This is considered a condition of deficiency, so a strong, stimulating, rajasic technique is applied to enliven its flow of energy.[32]

The Session

A Polarity Therapy session will typically last 60 to 90 minutes. The work takes place with the client partially undressed or lightly clothed on a padded massage table. No oil or lotion is used during the session.

Before the session begins, the therapist gathers information about the client's medical history and current condition. By listening to their voice, observing their actions, and considering their astrological sign, the therapist can determine which element is out of balance. Although this won't tell the entire story, it will at least provide a good starting point for the treatment.

Each element will require work at its positive, negative, and neutral poles. For the Earth element, this means the neck, the bowels, and the knees. Rajasic work, used to stimulate the umbilical current, begins with the therapist at the head of the table with both hands applying a brisk, circular pressure to the neck. Rajas is a force that is creative and lively and these qualities are reflected in these strokes that circle up and down, side to side, and back and forth all around the neck to awaken the drowsy currents of energy. This is followed by a round of grasping motions that are applied with the full palms to the back of the neck while rolling the head from side to side. This is the positive pole of the earth element and work here helps to activate the entire element.

Once this area has been sufficiently activated, the focus moves to the neutral pole of the earth element—the bowels. Here the therapist uses both hands to apply layers of wide circular strokes that cover the entire abdomen from rib to pelvis. This technique helps to simulate the motion of the large intestines and improves digestion overall. This movement also mimics the umbilicus energy, which is said to spiral outward from the belly. A back-and-forth rocking motion further helps to release this area of tension and holdings followed by double-handed circular strokes applied around and around the navel center. In similar fashion, the negative poles are activated with small, swift circular strokes above, below, and to the sides of the knees to bring energy and life to the area.

Tamasic bodywork, designed to encourage the bipolar current, is deep but slow. Rather than focusing on moving the energy, as in rajasic work, the focus here is to allow. Again, starting at the positive pole, the thumbs gently press into flesh just a few inches below the ears and then the pressure gradually builds as if moving through butter. Although tamasic work is strong and deep, it is not painful or invasive. At the neutral pole, the fingers are allowed to sink into the tension at the base of the belly—again, just allowing the hands to melt into the body. The negative pole is handled in much the same way with the thumbs dissolving into the tension around the knees.

Sattvic techniques, used to strengthen the transverse current, are light and airy. To start, the therapist stands at the side of the table with the right hand resting delicately on the client's abdomen and the left hand softly cradling the back of the client's neck. With barely any pressure, these positions are held until the therapist feels the pulsation of energy moving in his or her hands—signaling that the area has freed. Moving on, both hands drift to the belly to sit side by side over the soft flesh between the ribs and pelvis. Here at the neutral pole over the bowels, the therapist again tunes in to the subtle currents beneath the hands. Once the pulsation is felt here, the right hand glides down to the negative pole of the earth energy at the knees to bring balance to the element.[33]

This bodywork portion of the Polarity treatment will often be supplemented with lifestyle coaching, nutritional guidance, exercise recommendations, and so on. However, due to the wide range of Polarity providers in existence, each practitioner's definition and design of a Polarity Therapy session may differ significantly.

Benefits

- Promotes feeling of peace and balance
- Improves digestive disorders
- Calms emotional issues
- Reduces stress
- Relieves muscle aches and body pains
- Helps alleviate acute and chronic conditions
- Improves overall quality of life
- Offers feeling of health and vitality

Contraindications

None. The wide range of Polarity techniques can be adapted for any condition. However, it is recommended that anyone with a serious medical condition consult a medical doctor before initiating Polarity Therapy treatments.

Training

An Associate Polarity Practitioner (APP) requires 155 hours of schooling while a Registered Polarity Practitioner (RPP) necessitates an additional 520 hours (totaling 675 hours of education). Full training involves clinical practice, lectures, physical anatomy, energetic anatomy, nutrition, business management, and professional ethics. In addition, the American Polarity Therapy Association (APTA) requires 15 continuing education hours to be undertaken from an approved program every two years in order to maintain practitioner status.[34]

SUMMARY

This chapter introduces the energetic approach of massage therapy and bodywork, modalities whose intent is to affect changes in the underlying energy body by primarily directly accessing and affecting the energy with little or even no direct physical contact. It includes detailed discussions of how the modalities of Therapeutic Touch, Reiki, and Polarity Therapy fit into this category, how they differ, and how they are similar to each other. A basic overview of the history, the theory and principles, and the process of assessment, as well as a description of the techniques involved, are presented for each of these modalities of the energetic approach. This chapter also acquaints the reader with what the general experience of undergoing a treatment session is like and identifies who are the best candidates to seek this form of treatment and what conditions are most benefited. Also presented is a list for each of these modalities of their general benefits, contraindications, and/or precautions. A brief discussion of training, licensing, certifications, and requirements is also included.

CHAPTER REFERENCES

1. Stein, D. (1995). *Essential reiki.* Berkeley: Crossing Press.
2. *Therapeutic touch defined.* (2004). Retrieved July 8, 2007, from http://therapeutic-touch.org/what_is_tt.html
3. Krieger, D. (1993). *Accepting your power to heal.* Sante Fe: Bear & Co.
4. Krieger, D. (1993). *Accepting your power to heal.* Sante Fe: Bear & Co.

5. *How do I become a therapeutic touch practitioner?* (2004). Retrieved July 15, 2007, from http://therapeutictouch.org/practitioner.html

6. Stein, D. (1995). *Essential reiki.* Berkeley: Crossing Press.

7. Honervogt, T. (1998). *Reiki - Healing and harmony through the hands.* United Kingdom: Simon & Schuster Ltd.

8. Claire, T. (1995). *Body work.* New York: William Morrow & Co.

9. *What is reiki.* (2007). Retrieved June 17, 2007, from http://www.reiki.org/FAQ/WhatIsReiki.html

10. Claire, T. (1995). *Body work: What kind of massage to get and how to make the most of it.* Laguna Beach, CA: Basic Health Publications, Inc.

11. Decker, G. M. (2003). *What are the distinctions between reiki and therapeutic touch.* Retrieved August 31, 2007, from http://www.ons.org/publications/journals/cjon/Volume7/Issue1/pdf/89.pdf

12. Stein, D. (1995). *Essential reiki.* Berkeley: Crossing Press.

13. Stein, D. (1995). *Essential reiki.* Berkeley: Crossing Press.

14. Stein, D. (1995). *Essential reiki.* Berkeley: Crossing Press.

15. Stein, D. (1995). *Essential reiki.* Berkeley: Crossing Press.

16. Claire, T. (1995). *Body work: What kind of massage to get and how to make the most of it.* Laguna Beach, CA: Basic Health Publications, Inc.

17. Stein, D. (1995). *Essential reiki.* Berkeley: Crossing Press.

18. Claire, T. (1995). *Body work: What kind of massage to get and how to make the most of it.* Laguna Beach, CA: Basic Health Publications, Inc.

19. Stein, D. (1995). *Essential reiki.* Berkeley: Crossing Press.

20. Claire, T. (1995). *Body work: What kind of massage to get and how to make the most of it.* Laguna Beach, CA: Basic Health Publications, Inc.

21. Stein, D. (1995). *Essential reiki.* Berkeley: Crossing Press.

22. Stein, D. (1995). *Essential reiki.* Berkeley: Crossing Press.

23. Claire, T. (1995). *Body work: What kind of massage to get and how to make the most of it.* Laguna Beach, CA: Basic Health Publications, Inc.

24. Claire, T. (1995). *Body work: What kind of massage to get and how to make the most of it.* Laguna Beach, CA: Basic Health Publications, Inc.

25. *An introduction to reiki.* (2007). Retrieved June 20, 2007, from http://nccam.nih.gov/health/reiki/#11

26. Stone, R. (1986). *Polarity therapy: The complete collected works* (Vol. 1). Summertown, TN: CRCS Wellness Books.

27. Claire, T. (1995). *Body work: What kind of massage to get and how to make the most of it.* Laguna Beach, CA: Basic Health Publications, Inc.

28. Claire, T. (1995). *Body work: What kind of massage to get and how to make the most of it.* Laguna Beach, CA: Basic Health Publications, Inc.

29. Sullivan, M. (2001). *Polarity therapy* [DVD]. Real Bodywork.

30. Sullivan, M. (2001). *Polarity therapy* [DVD]. Real Bodywork.

31. Sullivan, M. (2001). *Polarity therapy* [DVD]. Real Bodywork.

32. Sullivan, M. (2001). *Polarity therapy* [DVD]. Real Bodywork.

33. Sullivan, M. (2001). *Polarity therapy* [DVD]. Real Bodywork.

34. *Standards for practice and education and code of ethics* (4th ed.). (2006). Greensboro, NC: American Polarity Therapy Association.

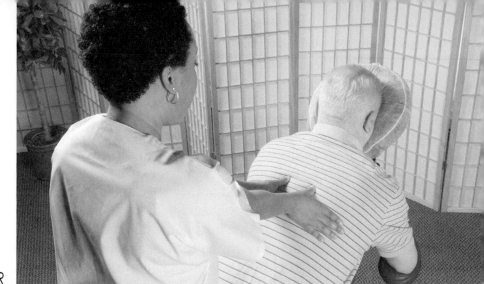

11
CHAPTER

Practice Settings: A Day in the Life of a Massage Therapist

CHAPTER GOALS

1. Become aware of the most common massage therapy and bodywork practice settings.

2. Develop an overall understanding of the need for therapist self-care.

3. Understand what is involved in a therapist's self-care, including dealing with the physical and emotional demands of a busy massage therapy career, personal grooming and hygiene, client compliance, and maintaining professional boundaries.

4. Understand the differences and similarities in the experience of a day in the life of massage therapists who work in a variety of practice settings, including private practice, a multidisciplinary clinic, spa settings, sports massage therapy environments, the business and **corporate** world, and in a hospital.

INTRODUCTION

From one perspective all massage therapists do essentially the same thing—they use their hands in a myriad of ways to manipulate the soft tissue and/or energy of the body in an effort to promote numerous positive benefits in the overall health and wellbeing of their clients and patients. As already discussed, this takes place on many levels and is determined by a range of factors including their training, education, years of committed practice, intention, attention, and compassion.

Where massage therapists choose to practice those skills is varied and will mostly be determined by the paradigm they practice from. For example, First Paradigm practitioners whose treatments focus mostly on relaxation and stress reduction may find themselves gravitating towards working in spas or in the corporate setting where stress and tension relief are badly needed and always welcome. Second Paradigm therapists whose treatments focus on remediation, therapy, and pain relief may find themselves working in a hospital, a clinical setting, with athletic trainers and with sports teams, as well as alongside other health care practitioners such as chiropractors, osteopaths, physiatrists, acupuncturists, and physical therapists. Third Paradigm practitioners, whose treatment approach often tends to be more holistic, lean towards working more in the realm of primary health care. Although they may be found working in medical and clinical settings, Third Paradigm practitioners often find those environments too specialized and restrictive of what they are allowed to do. Third paradigm practitioners most often work privately, where they can focus on a more overall approach to enhancing, balancing, and transforming the quality of life of their patients by integrating a number of approaches, modalities, and recommendations into their treatment protocols.

The purpose of this chapter is to present a brief overview of the experience of massage therapists in a variety of practice types and settings regardless of what actual form(s) of massage therapy and bodywork they practice. What is it like to be a massage therapist working in a spa verses working for a professional ball club treating athletes with sports massage? What's the difference in the day of a corporate massage therapist who works alone, and that of a practitioner who works in a multidisciplinary clinic alongside other health care practitioners?

In addition, it wouldn't be a complete picture of the daily experience of massage therapists if it didn't include a short discussion of the physical and emotional demands of treating, some of the ethical issues that frequently come up particularly with clients, the pressures of building a successful practice and dealing with money regardless of the setting.

A TYPICAL DAY IN THE LIFE OF MOST MASSAGE THERAPY AND BODYWORK PROFESSIONALS

Although there are many differences in the daily routines, responsibilities, and experiences that exist among specialists practicing in different settings and from different paradigms, there are also many similarities. In order to avoid redundancy, the general responsibilities and similarities found across the board in almost all settings will be discussed first. This will be followed by a more focused look at the practices of five different successful massage therapy and bodywork specialists in the field, including a mention of some of their main differences.

Schedule

Besides onsite practices found at sporting or special events, airport lounges, and large conventions where treatments are offered on a first-come-first-serve basis, a typical day for a massage therapist often begins with a review of the treatment schedule. The schedule generally includes prearranged appointments, scheduled breaks, personal days off, and vacations. Depending upon the arrangements of the individual practice, appointments may be booked back-to-back. There may also be empty appointment times and/or brief gaps in the schedule that the massage therapist can use to stay current with treatment notes, professional research, or work on marketing to help build the practice. Careful scheduling on the part of the therapist will also help to avoid the stress of becoming severely backlogged.

Policies

In any professional health care office or setting, a reasonable set of policies and procedures are essential for the smooth operation of the day-to-day details of the practice. These will most often include patient policies related to payment, lateness, and cancellations. There are endless possibilities as to why a patient may be late, cancel an appointment at the last minute, or even not pay for a treatment after it has been administered. However, if clear policies have been established and all patients are made aware of the minimum behavior expected of them at the time of their first booking, enormous amounts of time, energy and emotion can be saved.

Informing clients of a policy after the fact or reminding them when they have breached a policy can be a rude awakening. So the care and foresight to implement a set of policies and ensure that clients are well aware of them in advance is important and beneficial for all, even though they may be uncomfortable to enforce. As a result of setting and enforcing policy, the potential for losing clients is actually reduced. Often, just having the policy effectively communicated to clients is enough to generate adherence to the appointment schedule and serves as a gentle reminder of the professional boundaries that exist.

If the practice has a front desk with reception, then the enforcement of the policy is taken out of the therapist-patient relationship. Keeping the therapeutic relationship separate from business concerns is beneficial for obvious reasons. In cases where the practitioner is functioning without the aid of a staffed front desk, then the ability to exercise diplomacy can go a long way to enforcing these needed policies.

The best practice is to have the policies posted conspicuously so that they are quietly reinforced. It is also useful to include a form that specifically states the policies and which the client signs, so that a clear message is sent that policies will be enforced. Leniency is generally expected in extenuating circumstances and may be advisable in the case of a rare infraction from an otherwise consistent client.

Patient Records

The patient files for the day are reviewed to familiarize the therapist with the condition, treatment, special needs, and history of progress for each client. Although variations abound, these files usually contain information that includes a client or patient's full contact information, medical history, informed consent, relevant medical records and tests, release forms, and **SOAP notes** (described below) for each treatment visit.

Before the workday begins, intake and medical case history forms may be readied as well for new clients and patients that are scheduled. Patient notes are an invaluable asset, particularly for Second and Third Paradigm practitioners since they will usually be dealing with people who have more serious problems and will return for treatment on a consistent basis. Besides helping therapists to maintain a consistent treatment plan from one session to the next, notes also aide them in assessing the condition and provide a useful reference should a past condition resurface. Practices focusing on treating medical conditions, physical disabilities, and the like will have more paperwork inherent than would be found in most onsite or spa settings. Patient charting is not just a good idea, but a legal necessity in many states. In fact, there are laws regarding the formulation, use, storage, and distribution of these records.

The most often utilized form for client and patient charting is the SOAP notes (Figures 11-1 and 11-2). SOAP is an acronym which stands for subjective, objective, assessment, and plan/protocol and represents the four sections of a typical treatment record that needs to be documented after each treatment.

INITIAL INFORMATION

Name _____ Date _____

S Subjective
_____

(Symptoms, frequency, duration, intensity, how it started, aggravating/relieving activities, etc.)

Client's experience, expectations, and goals:

O Objective
_____

Observations, tests, and results:

Treatment goals:

A Assessment & Applications
_____

Massage treatment given:

Changes due to massage:

P Planning
_____

Homework:

Plan for next session:

Long-range plans and goals:

Figure 11-1 SOAP notes is probably the most used method of charting patient finding. The form shown here is used for recording findings during the initial consultation and treatment.

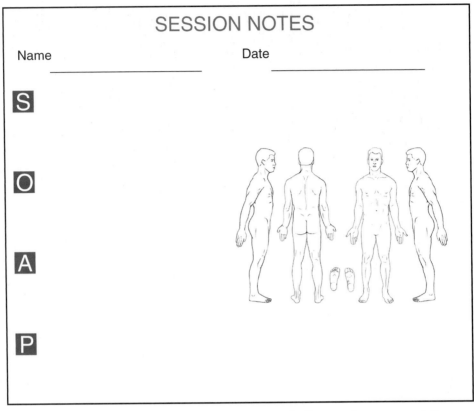

SESSION NOTES

Name _____   Date _____

S

O

A

P

Figure 11-2 SOAP notes form for updating treatment findings and recommendations.

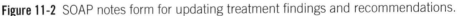

Purpose and Importance of SOAP notes:

- Legally required in most states
- Enables the therapist to monitor on an ongoing basis the patient's treatment plan and health
- Assists the therapist to continually tweak and evolve the treatment plan over the course of time
- Provides a clinical picture that the patient may wish to share with another health care provider
- Patients/clients or their attorneys may request notes to submit in the case of litigation

Treatment Room Preparation

At the beginning of the working day or shift, a therapist will inspect the treatment room to be sure that the needs of the day will be met. This includes all bolsters, linens, oils, and products that clients will need (Figure 11-3).

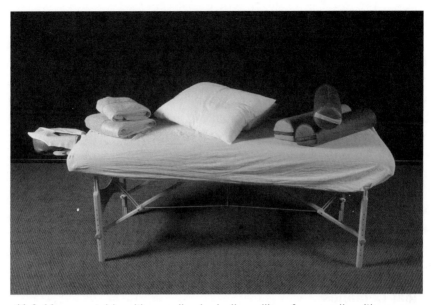

Figure 11-3 Massage table with supplies including pillow, face cradle with cover, draping towels, and bolsters for positioning.

The cleanliness and tidiness go a long way to creating a safe, welcoming, and professional atmosphere.

Also, having the room at a comfortable temperature with soft music and subdued lighting helps to create a soothing ambience that the client will appreciate. The relative tranquility of the room also makes the work of a massage therapist easier as it primes the client's mind, muscles, and fascia to release built-up stress and tension.

Most practitioners will utilize some if not all of the following supplies:

- Sheets
- Towels
- Oil
- Lotion
- Liniment
- Table cleaner
- Paper towels
- Bolsters
- Face-rest covers
- Gowns
- Music CDs or a digital music player

THERAPIST SELF-CARE

The job of a massage therapist is not only demanding physically, but emotionally and mentally as well. Boredom and emotional burnout are just as common a malady for a massage therapist as physical aches and pains. As such, therapists often spend some time on a consistent basis training not only their physical body, but emotional and intellectual capacities as well. The purpose of this training is as much for the client as it is for the therapist. If a therapist is encumbered by physical pain, burdened by emotional upset, or unable to focus beyond the enumerable distractions and daydreams that arise out of personal conflict and boredom, the patient's treatment will invariably suffer. If patients detect that they are not the focus of the treatment, they may seek treatment elsewhere.

Thus, adequate training and preparation on the part of therapists to be able to leave such issues at the treatment room door or set them aside as they arise while treating, enables them to be in a better place to handle another's care.

Physical Demands

The job of a massage therapist can be physically demanding because he or she is continually utilizing the same bodily postures and repetitive motions many times over in a given day. Hence, acquiring techniques that take advantage of gravity, using larger muscle groups and harnessing the strength inherent in good body mechanics are integral parts of massage therapists' education. Additionally, having the massage table at the right height for the therapist is crucial for remaining injury free.

However, simply adjusting the table and employing these techniques does not ensure that the therapist will be able to handle the physical demands of this profession over the course of hours, days, weeks, and years. Therapists who wish to remain injury free and continue to treat for many years will do well to consistently eat healthy foods, get plenty of restful sleep, and exercise regularly to stay in shape. To this effect, disciplines such as weight training, stretching, yoga, tai chi chuan, martial arts, and the like should be employed as part of an overall program for maintaining the necessary physical condition for a long career. This is in addition to more specific stretches and exercises for the fingers, hands, and forearms, the parts of the body that obviously take the most direct and consistent physical abuse.

Emotional Demands

Emotions are a large part of what massage therapists deal with on a day-to-day and moment-to-moment basis—their own, as well as their patients'. For our purposes here, we will focus more exclusively on the emotional states and experience of the massage therapist.

Some therapists become interested in massage therapy simply because Aunt Millie complimented them on their wonderful hands after a back rub. However, there is a vast difference between rubbing a friend or relative's back for 15 minutes, and treating many clients in a row, some for up to 90 minutes. Add to this the potential for sexual attractions, repulsions, a client's poor hygiene, physical discomforts, fatigue, hunger, and boredom and it can wind up being a very uncomfortable and disagreeable scenario. It is exactly in these kinds of circumstances when a massage therapist's emotional discipline, self-control, maturity, and training must come to the fore. With some patients it may take all of one's will to smile and set aside personal reactions and continue forth with the best treatment possible. Developing strong, long-term relationships is not only the path to becoming a successful therapist; it is also a hallmark of a mature and skilled professional.

The massage therapist, of course, may always redirect conversation if it is particularly counterproductive to the treatment and/or distracting to the therapist. For example, if a client begins to indulge in very negative and angry states related to his or her personal life it may be reinforcing the physical tensions already present in the patient's body and making it more difficult for the practitioner to obtain the goals of the treatment. In other circumstances, it may be to the benefit of the patient to allow the venting to occur.

Additional difficulties that a therapist may expect to face include clients and patients who

- do not follow guidelines and recommendations.
- talk down to the therapist.
- just never stop talking.
- consistently cancel appointments without notice.
- stop coming in even if they were getting good results.
- make unreasonable demands such as expecting treatment on the therapist's day off.

Also, it is not uncommon for patients to get up from the table feeling in no better shape than when they came in. Sometimes they may even feel worse directly after the treatment, later that day or even the next day. Generally this is not an indictment of the quality of the therapist's work at all, but most often a necessary part of the therapeutic treatment process in which it may take some time for the positive benefits to kick in. Since this can be very upsetting to patients, they should of course be forewarned of this very real possibility. In some cases as a client or patient begins to relax and really let go, emotional issues that have been long pushed away may rise to the surface. At these times it may be necessary for the therapist to refer out to a psychological counselor or to a health care practitioner better suited to treat what has newly emerged as a result of the massage therapist's work.

Here is a brief list of ways in which practitioners can actively pursue their own emotional development:

- Professional peer groups
- Counseling/psychotherapy
- Biofeedback
- Stress management techniques
- Meditation
- Martial arts
- Qi gong and tai chi
- Spiritual retreats
- Religion
- Prayer
- Yoga

Developing Rapport and Patient/Client Compliance

Rapport, a quality of immense importance when looking to develop a strong patient-therapist relationship, begins the moment the two meet, whether in person or on the phone. This first contact must be warm and professional in order to develop the layers of trust that are necessary for successful care of the patient. This is actually the first stage of the therapeutic process. The therapist's job here is to make the patient feel welcome, cared for, and understood (Figure 11-4). Patients must also get a sense that the therapist is capable of managing their concerns, and this must be conveyed early on in the professional relationship. However, the knowledge of the therapist is only useful if it can be transferred to the patient. Since different people take in information differently, the therapist must be versatile enough to cater to the learning styles of a wide range of people. Some patients digest information best visually, others need to hear it, and still others need to be part of the experience to understand it.

An unfortunate outcome of low rapport is the lack of patient compliance. Without rapport and trust, the patient may not heed the recommendations or

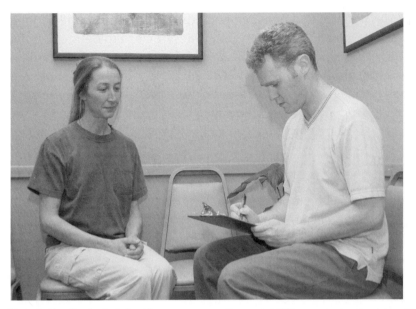

Figure 11-4 Patient's first visit with a massage therapist filling out a patient health history form.

warnings of the therapist, leading to poor treatment results. Bodywork, dietary changes, exercise, and other lifestyle recommendations can transform a patient, but the patient must first be "opened" so that the therapist's full range of skills and knowledge can be taken in and applied.

Professional Boundaries

Given the private setting and intimate nature of massage, patients often naturally begin to confide in their massage therapist. In relating personal matters usually reserved for close friends and family, the line between a therapeutic relationship and a personal relationship can become blurry. This is known as **transference**—when attitudes, feelings, and habits from one relationship are transferred on to another.

As a result of this misunderstood relationship and these misplaced emotions, patients may begin to unwittingly make unreasonable demands on their practitioners. Sometimes practitioners cross the boundary-line as well and become too friendly with their patients. This can lead to a variety of unhealthy results including loss of purpose and focus, poor treatments, and an overall reduction in the kind of care and attention the client should be receiving. In order to ensure the highest levels of therapeutic care, clear professional boundaries must be outlined and maintained. But because the boundaries of a professional relationship can sometimes be hard to define and maintain with some clients and patients, massage therapists can and should refer to various social organizations, mental health professionals, and support groups, who may be better equipped to handle these trickier situations, for guidance and advice. And at the least it may also be appropriate to refer the client to another massage therapist.

Professionalism, Personal Grooming, and Hygiene

If you asked people in general if they would like to lie down on a table, partially disrobe, and be touched by a complete stranger, do you think they'd jump at the chance? So what then makes them more or less willing to do this? The answer lies mostly in the professional image of massage therapists. The public's image of what a massage therapist is has come a very long way. No longer is a career in massage therapy and bodywork a fringe pursuit, and today it can be argued that it isn't really even "alternative." There are now many large national and state professional massage therapy and bodywork associations, state-accredited massage programs, schools and colleges, state licensing boards, and national certification exams, and there is also quite a bit of ongoing media exposure. All of this has aided massage therapists in elevating the prestige of the profession while at the same time educating the general public. Yet still the social stigma of massage remains somewhat of a hurdle.

Appearance, grooming, and hygiene are important tools for distinguishing oneself as a professional. The therapist will encounter a wide range of divergent personalities and as such it is necessary to tailor one's grooming to be as neutral and professional as possible while retaining the ability to communicate with warmth and compassion. Fingernails should be kept short, hair should be pulled back (if long), and clothing should be simple, without loud colors or designs. The therapist should also refrain from using perfumes and colognes because many patients have sensitivities and allergies that can be triggered by synthetic chemicals. Hands should be clean and washed before and after every treatment and fresh breath is a must for working in close proximity.

FORMULATING THE TREATMENT PLAN

Once in a more private area such as a consultation room or the treatment room itself, the patient's condition is discussed. Simply asking a patient how they feel is effective in starting the more objective and difficult task of understanding their condition. While they are answering, a therapist is usually not just hearing what is said, but also looking for nonverbal clues. This may be the tone of the skin, the posture of the body, or some other sign or symptom that is readily discernable to a trained therapist. In this way, further questions may be fine-tuned and any contraindications to treatment may be discerned. Finally, palpation where applicable may yield both new clues and confirm previous insights. From this information, a treatment protocol is tailored to meet the specific needs of the individual patient.

PRE-TREATMENT COMMUNICATION

The specific treatment protocol is explained to the patient in a digestible format, often beginning with a brief explanation of the particular modality, what it does for the condition, and how it may feel. This is followed by a brief explanation of the more immediate goals of the treatment and the necessity of follow-up visits when applicable. The massage therapist alerts the client in regard to products such as oils and liniments that will be used during the treatment. This is done to assure safety and comfort since individual patients may have specific allergies, sensitivities, or requests. Previous history of surgery and serious injury, particularly if recent, must be discussed in addition to any pre-existing or previous medical conditions. And finally, explanations, instructions, and inquiries regarding bolstering, positioning, and draping to ensure that the patient's individual issues such as postural difficulties and modesty are taken into account and addressed.

ALTRUISM AND MAKING A LIVING

Just because massage therapy is **altruistic** in nature does not mean that concerns for income can just be thrown out the window. In fact, because of a tendency to focus on the altruistic nature of massage and healing through touch, massage therapists often experience guilt over such things as charging for their sessions, selling therapeutic products, encouraging people to try massage therapy, and even asking their clients and patients who have been coming and getting good results to continue on with their sessions for maintenance. Yet in spite of this, massage therapy remains an altruistic business pursuit.

Therapists want to help people, but need to earn a living. At the same time there are millions of people ready and willing to pay to not only reduce or resolve their conditions, but to relax, unwind, and harmonize their mind, emotions, body, and energies as well. There is truly nothing wrong with charging good money for massage therapists' time, focused attention, skills, and effort. Likewise, selling products that aid and support treatment makes good sense, and also makes for good business.

GENERATING AN INCOME

Without a strong sense of direction and at least some business knowledge and skills, some therapists enter the profession and flounder or even fail. Perhaps the number one mistake of budding massage therapists is to make a simple mathematical equation and ignore what it takes to make that equation a reality. The simplistic equation goes something like this, "Let's see, 7 hours a day times 5 days a week times $75 an hour equals . . . I'm rich!" Here's another one, "3 treatment rooms, filled 6 hours of the day times $40 per session (what I would get after I pay the therapist) equals . . . early retirement!"

Massage education and repayment of student loans is a financial burden that must be met on top of the always increasing cost of living. Add to that the generally slow building process involved in developing a strong practice, the reduction in income incurred either by working for someone else or from the overhead of having a private massage studio ("with three rooms"), and suddenly that six-figure income is quite a bit less, although still attainable with patience and determination, the right attitude, skills and effort.

Simply having a sign out front, a pretty business card, and telling everyone you know is not nearly enough effort to generate a useful income. The truth is that even having a private practice requires quite a bit of business sense, sly logic, strong interpersonal skills, and consistent marketing. Opening and managing a multiroom facility requires a lot more of the same to be successful. Interpersonal skills are critical, even as an employee. It is the rare spa or massage therapy clinic that can keep a practitioner busy every shift. In fact, many employers may ask a therapist to do some introductory massages at a reduced rate in the interest of generating business. It is not uncommon for massage therapists to be found working in two or even more practice settings during a regular workweek to get their practices up to full-time status.

Wise money management is another necessary skill for all massage therapists as income may fluctuate week-to-week and season-to-season, often depending on the kind of practice. Additionally, for most massage therapists, there aren't any juicy company retirement plans, employer-sponsored health insurance, disability, and the like.

Marketing

Because it is outside the scope of this book and as volumes have been written on the subject of marketing and salesmanship, only a very brief review of the most common marketing venues for massage and bodywork therapists are listed here. For a more in-depth study of what is involved in the marketing of a massage therapy practice and business see the bibliography at the end of this book.

The message by now should be clear. Massage therapy is not an automatic cash cow. It takes diligence, patience, and steadfast adherence to sound business and career goals to produce a meaningful income, let alone enough for an early retirement. Those who can achieve this will find the path of massage therapy to be wonderfully rewarding both personally and financially—but also more challenging than they ever anticipated.

Listed below are popular and effective ways a massage therapist can promote and market his or her services.

- Joint marketing ventures
- Free or reduced-rate treatments, treatment packs (e.g., 10 for the price of 9)
- Public-speaking events
- Public events: street fairs, malls, health-related store openings
- Direct mailing/emailing: birthday cards, newsletters
- Networking with other health care professionals: introducing your skills through letters and free lunches
- Targeting specific demographics through speaking engagements and doing onsite treatments
- Print Advertising: ads in local papers, ads in the yellow pages, direct mailing ads

A DAY IN THE LIFE OF FIVE MASSAGE THERAPY SPECIALISTS

While the previous sections explored the common grounds shared by all massage therapists, the following provides a glimpse into their differences. These scenarios are straight out of the life of five very successful massage therapists who work in very different practice settings including a spa, a multidisciplinary clinic, with professional athletes, in a corporate office, and a hospital.

The Spa Environment

Diane is a massage therapist who works in a day spa. Working in a facility where the focus is on relaxation and beautification treatments really appeals to her. Although the schedule can be demanding, she derives satisfaction in being a part of a team whose job it is to help people find a brief respite from the stresses of life.

One of her latest clients is Kelly, an executive and mother of two young children. Although Kelly was enjoying her career, the rigors of the office and home had been catching up with her. She found that in the rush of life, her own sense of self was becoming lost. Going for treatments at the day spa gives her a chance to let go. For her, it is a world without phones, email, kids yelling, and deadlines. In fact, the kindness and sincere attention she had been given at the day spa has had positive repercussions in her life. And that change has not been lost on her husband who initially thought her forays to the day spa an unnecessary extravagance, but who is now a regular at the spa himself.

Kelly's treatments begin, in her own words, "the moment I book the appointment. Just knowing I have that to look forward to has been a tremendous help!" She arrives for her appointment 10 minutes early, as recommended by the spa, to give her a chance to leave the outside world behind. Kelly is greeted at the reception desk, discusses her desired treatment with the staff, and then takes a seat in the waiting area and casually leafs through a magazine.

At her appointed time, a spa attendant arrives with a robe and slippers and guides Kelly to a locker room where she puts her clothing and personal affects. Then she takes a brief shower and enters the sauna. This softens her muscles and prepares her skin for the treatments to come. Donning her robe, she emerges from the sauna and is greeted by her massage therapist, Diane, who has just finished reviewing Kelly's file to be sure the treatment Kelly chose is appropriate for her skin and constitution.

Diane and Kelly chat on the way to the wet room, where Kelly's treatment begins. While Kelly is getting on the table, Diane gathers a few supplies for the treatment. Returning, Diane first applies a mud that Kelly had picked out earlier, the specific ingredients of which are tailored to Kelly's particular skin type. Then Diane wraps her to encapsulate the product on her skin. Diane then begins to prepare the oil she will use for Kelly's Swedish massage. The essential oil blend is specifically tailored for Kelly's mood and constitution.

Soon it is time to rinse the mud product off, and while many spas require the client to shower again, this spa has the luxury of a **wet room** which is essentially a waterproofed room that is tiled with a drain in the floor. It also has a waterproof table and a Vichy shower used when exotic mud wraps, herbal wraps, salts, or sugar exfoliation scrubs cover the skin and need to be washed off (Figure 11-5). Once the entire product has been removed, the massage begins. Diane begins by gently massaging Kelly's face and continues on to the rest of the body, utilizing the essential oil blend. It's a gentle treatment that

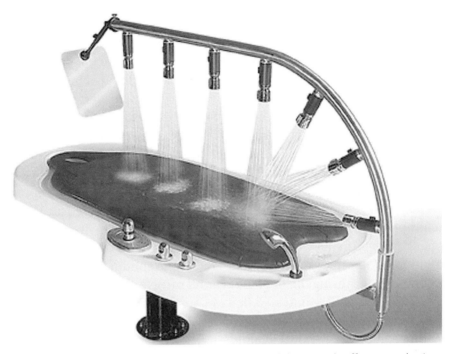

Figure 11-5 Vichy shower with a wet table is used mainly to wash off spa products used in various types of wraps and exfoliation skin treatments.

helps circulate blood and lymph while promoting relaxation and improving skin tone.

At the conclusion of the treatment, Diane tells Kelly that she should remain on the table for another 10 minutes to nap or just focus on her breathing. Soon, Diane reappears and assists Kelly getting up off of the table with her towel wrapped around her. When Diane leaves, Kelly puts her robe on and returns to the locker room to dress.

Diane gathers some products from the shelves in the lobby that would benefit Kelly for use at home. Diane really enjoys selling products to clients because of the results that correctly chosen products can produce as well as the added income their sale generates. Kelly emerges looking fresh and at peace. Diane begins to walk Kelly through the products she has chosen to help her maintain her radiance in between visits. Diane deftly discusses Kelly's skin type and explains the properties of the products to help her skin retain its elasticity, clarity, and tone. Finally, Kelly lounges for a little while sipping tea before it is time to go for her facial, manicure, and paraffin hand dip, a hot wax treatment that's soothing and relaxing. Diane prepares the room for her next client.

Multidisciplinary Clinic

Doug is a massage therapist who works in a multidisciplinary clinic. Working alongside other health care providers, including a chiropractor, physical therapist, and acupuncturist, provides him with a greater level of insight into his patients' conditions. For instance, in the clinic Doug was alerted that he was being referred a patient, Julia, who had been in a recent automobile accident. The accident resulted in very bad neck pain radiating down her right arm. In addition, Julia is experiencing mid-back pain along both sides of her spine and lower-back pain that radiates down both legs. She had recently visited a medical doctor who prescribed a course of treatment including chiropractic, physical therapy, and massage therapy. The doctor also ordered an MRI and the chiropractor took his own set of X-rays. In conferring with the various practitioners involved in her care, Doug learned that she had suffered several disc herniations of the spine, which constricted nerve conduction and was likely one component causing the ongoing painful muscle spasms she was experiencing. The X-rays also indicated that her spine had a reversed curvature in her neck and that her pelvis had shifted out of place.

Doug conducted his own evaluation based on the principles of assessment from a massage therapy perspective. This helped to further develop the emerging clinical picture of her trauma and most importantly to decide on the best protocol and techniques for her various problems. After reviewing her detailed case history, medical records, and various test reports, Doug assessed her postural alignment and then did some muscle testing, asking her to push in various directions against resistance that he provided (Figure 11-6). By doing this he could determine more precisely which muscles were damaged or weak. Doug then palpated the associated musculature and checked for swelling, "knots," temperature changes, and other signs of dysfunction. Then, based on her history, medical records, input from her other health care practitioners, and his initial observations and assessment, Doug explained to Julia what he would be seeking to accomplish with this first massage and the initial protocol he would be following. Notably, he told her that her body has just suffered a tremendous strain. In just a moment, during the car crash, her body was very forcibly jolted. He explained to her that as a result, there are likely to be countless micro-tears in the muscles and that her body would be laying down scar tissue like a fishnet over those areas that could lead to some restriction in movement. He also explained that some of her pain appeared to be related to the chronic muscle spasms due to the shock and jolt of the accident. Doug instructed her that massage would

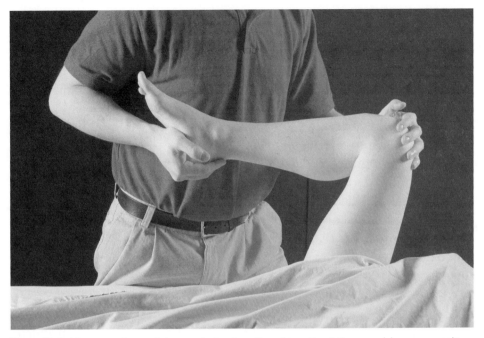

Figure 11-6 Massage therapist muscle testing the strength of the quadriceps muscle on a patient.

help to align those torn muscle fibers so that the tissue can properly heal and return to maximum strength and mobility and would also help to release the spasms by relaxing the muscles.

Leaving the room to let Julia change into a gown and lie face down on the table, Doug took another look at the intake form to further mentally delineate his treatment approach. Then, after a gentle knock, he reentered the room, made sure that she was as comfortable as possible and proceeded with the treatment.

Walking into the room, Doug first noticed that the muscles alongside her spine were swollen. Doug considered that this may be a sign of a lot of metabolic wastes caught up in the tissue. He palpated the area carefully, knowing that if it is in severe spasm, moderate pressure can be excruciating. Doug then checked other muscles in her lower back, hip, neck, and shoulder regions. Each area yielded another clue to add to the clinical picture of how to begin to unwind the spasms that had emerged and would prevent her from achieving sustainable proper skeletal alignment.

By the end of the full-body deeptissue treatment Doug provided, there was a discernable, overall improvement in Julia's body. She also reported feeling much less pain and tightness than when she first came in. Although the treatment was a success, Doug reminded her that in the case of automobile accidents, patients often have recurring symptoms. Because of this, they will have to work together to reach a complete and lasting resolution. He will need her to be diligent in her diet, stretches, and continued treatments or else things could backslide and the intensity of her pain could easily reappear. They decide that it would be best to come in three times a week for now and taper off as her condition improves.

Afterwards, Doug reviewed his findings with other members of his health care team. Julia was also scheduled to come back for chiropractic and physical therapy later in the week, and it was important that they were made aware of any significant discoveries during his treatment. Then, after entering his SOAP notes into Julia's file, Doug quickly moved on to his next patient, John, whom he has been treating with deep tissue massage for an injury to his right shoulder.

Sports Massage Therapy

Linda is a sports massage therapist who has been treating professional athletes for seven years. During this time she has worked with numerous players and professional ball clubs including the NHL: Islanders, Dallas Stars; the NFL: Jets, Giants, Washington Redskins, Philadelphia Eagles, St. Louis Rams, and New York Dragons (Arena Football); the Olympic Soccer Team; the New York Power Professional Soccer Women's Team; and the Roughriders (men). Linda decided to pursue this specialty discipline of massage therapy because she was an athlete herself and had a great love and appreciation of sports. She was also drawn to the excitement of working with celebrities and the potential perks, like great seats at the games.

When Linda first began the pursuit of seeking employment specifically in the sports massage arena, she was sometimes interviewed by the athletic trainers of these teams; but most often she would sit down with the team coaches. These coaches, who asked her about her education and training qualifications, were mostly interested in her level of experience and her Second Paradigm expertise in evaluating and treating various injuries such as tendonitis, bursitis, rotator cuff strains, chondromalacia (runner's knee), calf strain and pain (Figure 11-7). They also wanted to make sure that she was well versed in pre- and post-event sports massage therapy treatment, stretching, and hydrotherapy. In addition, a question she was always asked during her interviews was how she felt about working long hours because that was certainly going to be a requirement. Depending on the season, Linda works

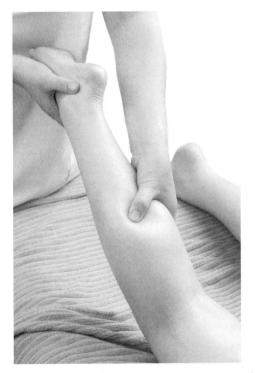

Figure 11-7 Massage therapist performing sports massage to an athlete's calf muscles.
Image copyright 2009, Iofoto. Used under license from shutterstock.com.

35 to 40 hours per week and takes her vacations during the off-season periods in order to maintain her own health and vitality.

Over the years Linda has practiced in a variety of different athletic treatment environments, depending on the particular job. Most of the time, however, she has worked in a private treatment room reserved for the athletes' therapy sessions. At other times, treating was done in a more open physical therapy setting or training-room environment, sometimes alongside other practitioners. Linda has also maintained a private office so athlete clients can also make visits to her. There, Linda can also maintain her private practice for regular clients. Although she would never turn down someone in need, overall she tries to keep her private practice focused on those clients seeking sports massage therapy. At other times, when athletes require it, she visits them at their homes.

Some sports massage therapists are hired specifically to travel with their teams. Linda, however, chose not to since she preferred the freedom to work in a variety of different venues within the specialty of practicing sports massage. In the sports business, athletes are traded on and off teams every year so she does lose some good friends and opportunities when they leave, but come next season, Linda always meets new people. One of the most exciting things for Linda is watching her own "work" play well on TV. She loves to see her team win and her athletes achieve their goals by overcoming the very injuries that she has helped to heal. She experiences the most satisfaction when her professional athlete clients give her credit, thank her, and tell her how well they played because of her treatments.

The role of a sports massage therapist working with professional athletes can be very stressful given the potential severity of even a minor injury on both the performance and career of the athlete. So in many ways there is a lot riding on the hands of a sports massage therapist. One advantage, however, is that when Linda is working with a team she has the opportunity to see and treat her clients more regularly, thus helping to heal injuries, reduce pain, and improve range of motion faster and more effectively.

Generally, when working in a team environment, all the health care staff conference with each other to exchange ideas and talk about treatment options. Various techniques are discussed and opinions are voiced concerning an athlete's health and wellbeing. Some of the most common athletic injuries and conditions that Linda treats are

- Knee sprains
- Chondromalacia
- Iliotibial band syndrome
- Sore muscles
- Calf strain
- Muscle strains and spasms
- Ankle sprains
- Tendonitis and bursistis
- Pinched nerve
- Sciatica
- Thoracic outlet syndrome
- Stiff neck and back
- Rotator cuff strains and tears

Linda treats these injuries using a combination of basic moves including effleurage, petrissage, tapotement, muscle stripping, friction, and stretching, as well as some of the more advanced and deeper-working techniques such as myofascial release and trigger point therapy. Her treatment plans vary significantly depending upon the athlete and the nature of the injury.

When Linda is working with teams, she does a lot of pre-event treatment that prepares athletes for the games. For example, when working for a professional soccer team she can often see all 20 players for 10 to 15 minutes before and after a game. With hockey, most of the players are treated right before they get on to the ice.

An average, long work day for Linda can go something like this: She prepares by eating a big breakfast and staying hydrated by drinking lots of fluids in order to ready herself for the players after they have finished their practice sessions. She begins with about four hours of treating, usually 1 to 1½ hours per player depending on his or her size and the injury being treated. After lunch, she treats four or five more athletes and then after dinner, she often has one last treatment. For peace of mind, health, and much needed rest, Linda always tries to keep one day for herself where she will take no appointments. On non-treating days she can also catch up with her paperwork and may even get to watch a game.

Although Linda prefers to have a balanced schedule, it's not really possible when working with athletic teams. Her hours must be accommodating because most of her work comes just a day or two prior to game day. Often during these times an entire week's workload is crammed into just a few days and she'll have to work around practices, workouts, and events. Although it's a lot to take on, to Linda, it's completely worth it in the end.

In the course of her practice, Linda herself has also suffered some injuries from treating. She has strained her wrists and experienced **tendonitis** of her elbows, as well as some standard neck, back, and shoulder pain. Her legs and feet also can get sore from standing for long periods—all part of the occupational hazards of not only being a massage therapist but also a sports massage therapist whose average clients range in size from very large to even much larger.

In Linda's case, she books her own appointments and is paid either by the athlete, by the athlete's insurance coverage, or by the team owner. If a player sets up the appointment, it is usually paid for by the player. If the organization or trainer sets up the appointments, the team (organization) will compensate her. She works primarily as an independent contractor because it allows her to enjoy the freedom of coming and going as she pleases. If she were on contract she would be bound to treat anyone at any time or else the team would quickly find a replacement. Working as an independent contractor, without an employee contract, Linda is still able to keep all her other clients so she can still be earning a living when the sports season is over. That said, the advantage of being contracted by a sports club is a steady paycheck and, often, benefits. But that means as an employee you are on call every day, will have to travel with the team and may not work with opposing teams. So in the end it boils down to a personal decision for the sports massage therapist.

Corporate Massage Therapy

If ever there was a health profession that crossed over into many arenas and fulfilled an unspoken need in all of them, massage therapy is it. And given today's insanely fast-paced work and highly stressed corporate environment, companies and their employees are certainly another clientele that can benefit greatly from implementing an in-house corporate massage therapy program.

In today's corporate environment, emotional stress is the basis for the majority of costly absenteeism. Office-bound occupations are also physically stressful due to the harmful effects of repetitive motions coupled with a sedentary desk job. At the very least, these physical strains lead to reduced work performance, and at their worst they are debilitating. The cumulative effects of this emotional and physical stress build over a period of time until a breaking point is reached. Indeed the stressful, static, and sedentary work of the corporate employee is the "silent killer" of employee productivity and thereby corporate profitability. By and large, corporate massage therapy programs offering regular treatments to their employees help them to pay attention to their work and not on their worries or aches and pains.

Gary is a massage therapist whose primary practice is in the corporate environment. When he began seeking to develop a practice within corporations he did so by contacting the human resources directors, managers, or owners of prospective companies in which he wanted to work. Armed with useful information regarding the point and purpose of massage therapy in the corporate world and important statistics about the benefits for the company, Gary made his pitches. He soon found out that if there was sufficient understanding as to the positive benefits for the employees and ultimately the company, then all that remained was negotiating the terms and conditions of the contract. The times when there were any doubts on the part of a prospective employer, a trial visit by Gary for a day or even a week was generally enough to satisfactorily answer any remaining questions, such as, "Will the employees of this company be interested in this?" "Will employees get any benefit from these treatments?" And, "What value will it provide the company?" Clearly, one week is hardly enough to demonstrate and document to everyone the real value of implementing a corporate massage therapy program. However, because Gary is so very good at what he does, it always seems to be enough to garner an over-whelmingly positive response in favor of return visits leading to some form of regular employment for him.

During the course of his professional practice as a corporate massage ther-apist, Gary has been hired by companies looking to do anything from providing an ongoing tangible perk for their overworked staff to functioning as a public relations medium at corporate sponsored events. The thing that Gary appre-ciates the most about corporate massage is the results, both for the company and those he has the pleasure to treat.

When it comes to public relations work, Gary has done treatments for an international banking institution that sought better ways to market to the public. In this instance he was hired to treat at local home, auto, and boat expos in which the bank had its own booth. There, people who had never had massage therapy before received treatment onsite and gained some insight into their own bodies as well. Then, emerging deeply relaxed and often pain free, they would be in a much more receptive mood to hear what the salespeople were offering. Everybody benefited.

In another, perhaps more extreme experience, Gary treated on 8th Avenue in NYC in front of the post office at an event sponsored by a major online ser-vice seeking to increase brand awareness. After a brief intake, anybody walking by on the street that day could receive massage therapy either on a massage chair or table. What really made this event so successful were the media who just ate it up.

However, most of Gary's corporate work involves providing the more cus-tomary in-house treatments for the company staff. Given the numerous dif-ferent companies Gary has worked in as a corporate massage therapist, he never experienced an employee that couldn't use massage therapy, didn't benefit from it, or wasn't enthusiastic about receiving regular massage therapy treatment.

Often, in those environments, Gary is asked how he manages to keep up his energy levels and deal with his own physical stress given that he has to do so many treatments in a row day in and day out. He actually likes answering that question because he feels that it gives him the opportunity to engage the company's employees in beneficial conversations about the importance of stretching, massage therapy, and a healthy diet and exercise. In that discussion Gary also expresses that to him, of all the jobs he has ever had, working in an office was by far the most stressful physically and mentally.

These massage therapy treatments and health-oriented conversations of-ten result in more educated, clearer-thinking employees who begin to make positive changes in their lives and become less prone to being plagued by stress. As a result they begin to lead more productive workdays and carry less of the office home with them. Gary has witnessed the dynamics of tension-filled offices do a 180-degree turnaround following three months of massage therapy offered to employees once a week. He finds that it's thrilling to be the catalyst for something like that while doing something he loves. With emotional and physical health issues an eventuality in any business, it quickly becomes apparent that overlooking employee health care can result in greater turnover, hardship, and financial burden for all involved. Massage therapy not only creates a stopgap between injurious levels of stress and status quo productivity, but excels at boosting productivity.

In a corporate office environment a specific schedule for treatments can be difficult to adhere to as employee workloads, demands, and meetings commonly overlap and fluctuate. So in these settings Gary schedules open hours when treatments are rendered on a first-come, first-served basis. He tries to accommodate most employees' needs by scheduling these open times during different parts of the day. Treatments are often performed on a massage chair specifically designed for this purpose and which may be used in lieu of a massage table (Figure 11-8). In massage chairs, employees can sit comfortably in an upright posture, making it preferable for those who feel uncomfortable lying prone on a table, particularly in more open environments where there is a lack of privacy. In other corporate settings, Gary has been provided with a private treatment room, which helps to give it all a much more professional and serious feel for the employee.

Payment arrangements for Gary's work have varied, depending mostly upon the company and the kind of program being implemented. At times, Gary's treatments have been either subsidized or paid for in full by the company. At other times the treatments were paid for by the employees who were simply given the time off to be treated.

As for how much to charge, there are also many options. Gary has been hired as a full-time massage therapist and for a time worked solely for one company as part of its corporate-wide fitness program. There he was on salary, received benefits, and actually became one of the employees of the corporation. In other work experiences, Gary has been paid per treatment and/or by the hour according to the number of treatments or amount of time spent at the company. He has also charged daily rates in which he was paid a set fee per day regardless of how many treatments he rendered. On other occasions, Gary has arranged to rent space in the company as part a work agreement, and yet at other times the space was given to him free by the

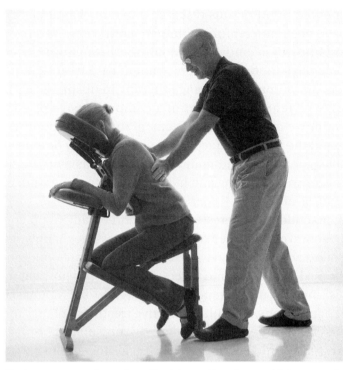

Figure 11-8 Chair massage allows the client to easily relax and let go comfortably while maintaining an upright posture, making it preferable in the corporate settings where it can even be done in an employee's office. *Image copyright 2009, lofoto. Used under license from shutterstock.com.*

company because his presence and the benefits he brought to the company were valued.

Some of the larger companies Gary has worked for have an intranet where the massage therapist's in-house services are advertised to all employees. Smaller companies generally get the word out with company-wide emails. The bottom line is, however, that arranging advertising of onsite massage therapy treatments to corporate employees is yet another piece of the collective agreement and is necessary for running a successful corporate massage therapy program.

Hospital-Based Massage Therapy

Of all the different therapies and modalities considered part of complementary and alternative medicine (CAM), massage therapy is now the most common one offered in United States hospitals. Because its effectiveness in reducing and relieving the symptoms of many medical conditions has been documented in numerous research and clinical studies, medical institutions have been much more willing to embrace it. As a result, a growing number of hospitals and medical clinics throughout the country are integrating massage therapy into their patient care treatment plans. Some of the most common uses of massage therapy in hospitals are in pre- and post-operative patient care; as part of a comprehensive physical therapy regimen to improve mobility and movement; helping patients to cope with pain, stress, and the anxiety of facing life-altering injury or illness; as a therapeutic service for cancer and maternity patients; as a method to help reduce swelling; providing loving and healing touch to premature infants; and hospice or end-of-life care.

Massage practitioners interested in a Second Paradigm practice focusing on these ameliorative and remedial benefits of massage therapy seek employment in hospitals where they have the wonderful and rare opportunity to treat the very sick and dying. In order to successfully work in a hospital setting, massage therapists need to understand how to develop assessment skills for specific patient populations, formulate effective treatment plans, apply various modified massage techniques on hospital patients suffering with chronic and progressive diseases, and recommend strategies for supporting patient self-care.

Anthony is a licensed massage therapist working in a hospital rehabilitation clinic alongside two other full-time therapists. There he treats patients mostly referred by doctors, as well as some who are self-referred. The patients come from diverse departments of the hospital such as oncology, the general public health clinic, physical therapy, cardiology, geriatrics, obstetrics, perinatal, psychiatric, and, of course, rehabilitation departments.

Anthony always knew he wanted to work in a clinical setting. He began his career doing massage therapy in a chiropractic office. There he gained a great deal of experience treating musculoskeletal conditions of the back, neck, and shoulders. After a while he began volunteering at a local hospital a few days a month to gain exposure to patients with more serious conditions and the terminally ill. While there he began reading medical texts recommended to him by hospital staff so that he could gain more insight into different patient's conditions and treatments. Anthony had always attended continuing education classes in advanced forms of massage and bodywork, including seminars in hospital-based massage therapy specifically for the seriously ill and dying. When a position opened up for a licensed massage therapist in the hospital's rehab clinic, he jumped at the chance and was hired.

A hospital is a challenging environment to work in. There are always new medical treatments coming out that Anthony must become aware of, particularly regarding possible contraindications to massage. There is also always an inexhaustible supply of patients in need of physical relief and whose conditions are quite diverse. Though for Anthony, perhaps the most challenging aspect of working at the hospital is dealing with his emotional reactions to the sad stories and debilitated physical states of so many patients. And when one of his patients' passes, that takes a terrific emotional toll. For many patients in the hospital, Anthony is a beacon of hope as they anxiously look forward to receiving their next treatments from him.

Anthony's treatments are carefully administered with great skill and compassion. Whether the treatment involves carefully applied friction to break up adhesions after knee or shoulder surgery or gentle relaxing effleurage with acupressure points to tonify a cancer patient, Anthony puts a friendly, warm, human face on the often sterile, and lonely persona of hospital care for all of his patients.

For those patients hospitalized for extended periods, there is often a severe disruption in their normal social life. Visiting hours are usually very short and allow too few visitors. In cases where terminal illness is involved, both friends and family may tend to avoid contact because they don't know what to say, or because they mistakenly believe that they could catch a noncommunicable disease. For these patients, massage therapy is a priceless gift. In some hospitals, including the one Anthony works in, it is even possible for friends, relatives, and co-workers to purchase gift certificates on a website in the patient's name, provided of course that the doctor approves.

Anthony, along with other therapists, are always meeting with doctors and other health care practitioners involved in their patient's cases to discuss care, as well as forwarding their client progress notes. Communication amongst the various medical personnel involved in a patient's care is crucial as health conditions can change rapidly. Without effective and timely updates, a practitioner may unwittingly perform treatments that are contraindicated or unnecessary. On a more positive note, clients benefit greatly whenever a conscientious team of professionals jointly discuss patient care routinely. With each practitioner adding something from his or her area of expertise the resultant diagnoses and treatment principles become better defined. Accordingly, the whole becomes greater than the sum of its constituent parts.

For those hospitals offering massage therapy, it's a win-win scenario. Patients' overall satisfaction with hospital care increases when massage therapy is part of their treatment program. This enhances the patient's compliance level to follow-up treatment protocols. Additionally, it often reduces the duration of hospital stays, freeing up beds for new patients. Finally, in hospitals where massage therapy is offered to the staff, employee-employer relations are enhanced. And once the staff experiences professional massage therapy treatment, it increases the likelihood that they will recommend massage therapy for their patients.

At the end of the day, Anthony leaves feeling exhausted from meeting the physical, intellectual, and emotional demands the position requires. However, he also leaves feeling that he is making a difference in the lives of many people, perhaps when they need it most.

SUMMARY

The purpose of this chapter is to bring awareness of a typical day in the life of most massage therapy and bodywork professionals. In order to accomplish this, the chapter first looks at the basic similarities in the daily routines, responsibilities, and experiences that exist among all massage and bodywork therapists. It then proceeds to take an in-depth look at the differences that exist in the working day life of five massage therapy specialists working in different settings and the various forms of massage therapy and bodywork they practice. These settings include a multidisciplinary clinic, a day spa, sports massage therapy environments, corporations, and a hospital.

The chapter also discusses and emphasizes an understanding of the need for therapist's self-care and what it involves, including dealing with the very real and often intense physical and emotional demands of a busy massage therapy career. Personal grooming and hygiene, client compliance, and maintaining professional boundaries are also covered and their importance emphasized.

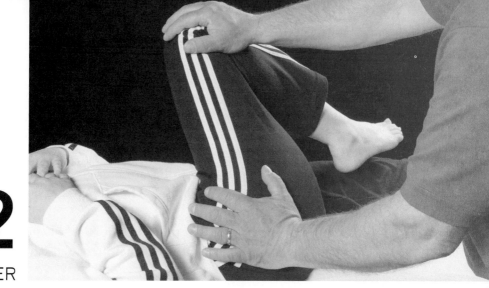

12
CHAPTER

Massage Therapy within the Larger Healthcare/Well Being Team

CHAPTER GOALS

1. Develop an overall understanding of the role that massage therapy plays within the larger health care and wellbeing team.

2. Become aware of the huge demand for massage therapy throughout the United States.

3. Become aware that 43 states and the District of Columbia currently regulate and/or license massage therapists.

4. Understand the difference between National Certification and State Licensure.

5. Understand the difference between the National Certification Board for Therapeutic Massage and Bodywork (NCBTMB) and The Federation of State Massage Therapy Boards (FSMTB).

6. Become aware of the job outlook and trends for the profession of massage therapy.

7. Become aware of the major role of baby boomers in forcing market growth.

8. Recognize the important role the spa industry plays as this profession's largest employer.

9. Become knowledgeable of the fact that over the last decade major research universities and medical institutions across the country have begun to embrace and integrate alternative practices into mainstream medicine.

10. Become aware of the existence of the National Center for Complementary and Alternative Medicine (NCCAM), the United States Government's lead agency for scientific research on complementary and alternative medicine (CAM), including massage and bodywork therapy.

11. Become aware that job opportunities for massage and bodywork practitioners exist in a variety of settings and locations as well as in a variety of contractual arrangements.

12. Develop an understanding of the relationship between the massage and bodywork therapist and the other members of the health care team, including:
    - The patient
    - The family/significant others
    - Physicians
    - Nurses
    - Acupuncturists
    - Chiropractors
    - Physical therapists
    - Psychiatrists/psychologists

INTRODUCTION

Not long ago, the field of massage and bodywork therapy was considered to be "underground mainstream." When it was finally surveyed, it was discovered that tens of millions of massage and bodywork therapy treatments were being administered by professionals all over the country. Willing consumers, mostly paying one hundred percent out of pocket for these services, were lining up for treatment, and virtually no one was aware of it! These trends have grown stronger still and all the numbers indicate continued unprecedented growth. Today, it is clear and no longer any secret that massage therapy and bodywork have come out from the underground and have stepped proudly into the mainstream of this nation's health care system as one of the fastest growing professions in America.

REGULATION ACROSS THE USA: NATIONAL CERTIFICATION AND STATE LICENSURE

National Certification and Licensing

With the creation in 1992 of the National Certification Board for Therapeutic Massage and Bodywork (NCBTMB), an independent, private, nonprofit organization, massage therapy and bodywork have gained rapid and increased acceptance and respect as a health care profession. The NCBTMB was the first professional organization to develop a recognized credentialing program for the profession of therapeutic massage and bodywork. Although there are different levels and definitions of the term "certification," the highest and most accepted one means that a practitioner has met the requirements of a federally approved organization such as NCBTMB that tests eligible graduates of schools and programs on a specific core body of knowledge—in this case massage therapy and bodywork.

Although it is often the case that certification examinations offered by a federally approved certifying body such as NCBTMB are adopted by states to be used as their licensing exam, certification and licensure should not be confused. Licensure is something that is only granted by a governmental agency such as the state department of education. Licensure, from a state's point of view, is not a measure of a practitioner's expertise but rather a measure of "minimal competence." In other words, a state's concern is to ensure that whoever is issued a license to practice is competent enough to not harm the public. It is the job of certifying bodies, not state licensing boards, to measure expertise and even test and certify professionals in more advanced specialties of the field.

State licensing is a state-by-state issue and each state has its own set of rules, regulations, and academic requirements. Since its inception, NCBTMB examinations have become accepted or recognized by statute or rule in 33 states and the District of Columbia. There are currently more than 90,000 professionals with NCBTMB certification.[1] In cases in which states choose to adopt the NCBTMB examination as their licensing exam, it serves as both certification and licensure. However, national certification for a successful candidate is awarded by the certifying agency (NCBTMB) only after the candidate has filed and paid for the appropriate fees, while state licensure for the same candidate is awarded once all state requirements have been met, including passing the exam. Today some states still choose to use their own separate licensing examination. In those cases, if a person so chooses and desires to become nationally certified, he or she must sit for the separate National Certification Exam in Therapeutic Massage and Bodywork. The NCBTMB credentialing program has been accredited by the National Commission for Certifying Agencies.

In total, 43 states and the District of Columbia currently regulate and/or license massage therapists.[2] An interesting fact one observes when looking at the list of states and dates of massage legislation enactment is that at least two-thirds or more of these laws were implemented by their state education departments only in the last 15 years, underscoring the rapid development, spread, and regulation of this health care profession and the impact that national certification has had, intended or not, on moving states towards developing licensing laws throughout the country.

Federation of State Massage Therapy Boards (FSMTB)

In 2005, a move to bring together massage regulators nationwide took place. After much discussion and agreement, this group recognized the need for an organization to formally bring the regulatory community of state massage boards together. They formed the Federation of State Massage Therapy Boards (FSMTB), whose primary mission is to support its member boards to ensure that the practice of massage therapy is provided to the public in a safe and effective manner. Part of carrying out this mission involves providing a valid, reliable licensing examination to determine entry-level competence. The examination developed by the FSMTB on behalf of its member boards is known as the Massage & Bodywork Licensing Examination (MBLEx).

At this time, 18 member state boards of its 30 members which includes Puerto Rico, have voted to accept the FSMTB MBLEx. In many of these states, graduates of approved programs will now have a choice between the NCBTMB or the MBLEx test for licensure. There are a number of other states that are in process of considering adopting the MBLEx and there are also several others that presently administer their own licensing exams apart from both NCBTMB and FSMTB, such as New York and Ohio.[3]

ACCREDITATION

The goal of accreditation is to ensure that education provided by institutions of higher learning meets acceptable levels of quality. Accrediting agencies, which are private educational associations of regional or national scope, must be recognized by the U.S. Secretary of Education as reliable authorities concerning the quality of education or training offered by the institutions or programs of higher education they accredit. Accrediting agencies develop evaluation criteria and conduct peer evaluations to assess whether or not those criteria are met. The process requires that an educational institution or program seeking accreditation complete an extensive Self Evaluation Report (SER) documenting the compliance with the accrediting body's standards. The SER is then followed by a rigorous on-site visit to the school by trained accreditation site-evaluators whose job is to verify that the SER report accurately reflects the school's operation. Institutions and/or programs that request an agency's evaluation and that meet an agency's criteria are then "accredited" by that agency.[4] Final accreditation approval enables the institution to establish eligibility to participate in the Federal student financial aid programs administered by the US Department of Education under Title IV of the Higher Education Act of 1965.[5]

In 1982, The American Massage Therapy Association (AMTA) formed the AMTA Council of Schools COS. Over the next many years, massage educators and activists from the COS played a pivotal role in working to form an independent government-recognized accrediting agency and finally in 1989 the Commission on Massage Therapy Accreditation (COMTA) was born. In 2002, COMTA was recognized by the U.S. Department of Education as a specialized accrediting agency, an acknowledgement of its expertise in ensuring quality education and allowing programs to access federal student aid funds.[6]

In addition to COMTA, other accrediting agencies recognized by the U.S. Department of Education exist that also offer a pathway to federal financial aid to schools and programs of massage therapy. These include:

- Accrediting Bureau of Health Education Schools (ABHES)
- Accrediting Commission of Career Schools and Colleges of Technology (ACCSCT)
- Accrediting Council for Continuing Education and Training (ACCET)
- Accrediting Council for Independent Colleges and Schools (ACICS)
- Council on Occupational Education (COE)
- National Accrediting Commission of Cosmetology Arts and Sciences (NACCAS)

RESEARCH AND MEDICINE

Over the last decade, major research universities and medical institutions across the country have begun to embrace and integrate alternative practices into mainstream medicine. Practice, research, and courses in these therapies, including massage therapy, are being conducted and taught at institutions such as Columbia University's Center for Complementary and Alternative Medicine, Harvard Medical School, Beth Israel Hospital, Kessler Institute for Rehabilitation, Stanford University, Johns Hopkins University, and Stonybrook University. Through its National Center for Complementary and Alternative Medicine (NCCAM), even the National Institutes of Heath (NIH) has recognized massage therapy as an important noninvasive form of treatment.

The NCCAM is the United States government's lead agency for scientific research on **complementary and alternative medicine (CAM)**. The NCCAM is one of the 27 institutes and centers that comprise the NIH within the U.S. Department of Health and Human Services.

> The mission of the National Center for Complementary and Alternative Medicine is to
>
> - explore complementary and alternative healing practices in the context of rigorous science.
> - train complementary and alternative medicine researchers.
> - disseminate authoritative information to the public and professionals.

NCCAM studies CAM using scientific methods and technologies. The NCCAM defines CAM as "a group of diverse medical and health care systems, practices, and products that are not presently considered to be part of conventional medicine." Massage and bodywork therapy are included in CAM. **Conventional medicine** is defined as medicine practiced by medical doctors (MDs), doctors of osteopathy (DOs), and by other related allied health care professionals including physical therapists, psychologists, and registered nurses.[7]

DEMAND FOR MASSAGE THERAPY

Throughout the United States people are turning to complementary and alternative health therapies. Hospitals are opening alternative health care clinics as growing numbers of clinical studies validate the effectiveness of these methods, including massage therapy.

In two recent documents entitled "2009 Massage Therapy Industry Fact Sheet" and "Massage Therapy: Not Just a Trend," based on annual surveys and published by the American Massage Therapy Association (AMTA), this country's largest professional organization, many important statistics about the continued growth of the massage therapy profession over the last several years were cited. Following are some of the most significant points:

- Thirty-nine million American adults—more than one out of every 6—get massage annually.[8]
- 26 percent of Americans integrate massage into their health care routines with relaxation as a strong motive; 30 percent are using massage therapy for medical purposes such as injury recovery, pain reduction, headache control, and for overall health and wellness.[9]

- Doctors and consumers are turning more and more to massage as an adjunct to regular health practices. Because of the trust that most patients have for their doctors' opinions, when doctors begin embracing massage therapy as an adjunct to their patient's health care choices, it creates a huge demand for properly trained massage therapists. Nine million more people discussed massage therapy with their doctors or health care providers in 2006 as compared to five years earlier. Almost twice as many doctors recommended it to their patients in 2006 as compared to five years earlier.[10]

- More than half of massage therapists (69%) indicate that they receive referrals from health care professionals.[11]

- Over half of adult Americans (60%) would like to have their insurance health plans cover massage therapy.[12]

- Of the hospitals that have massage therapy programs, 71 percent indicate that they offer massage for patient stress management and comfort, while more than two-thirds (67%) use massage therapy for pain management and pain relief.[13]

- One of the major explanations for the continued explosion experienced in this field is attributed at least partly to the aging baby boomer population and their growing awareness of the impact that stress has on the body and the powerful and beneficial physiological effects of massage therapy. Baby boomers aged 55 and older have tripled their use of massage therapy over the past 10 years.[14]

- One of the reasons that the use of massage therapy is on the rise is its use by Americans aged 18 to 34, among whom there is a high level of agreement that massage is more beneficial to one's health than it is a luxury.[15]

- In 2005, massage therapy was projected to be a $6 billion- to $11 billion-a-year industry.[16]

- According to the U.S. Department of Labor, from 2006 through 2016 massage therapists are likely to see a 20 percent increase in job opportunities, faster than average for all occupations.[17]

Health and health care delivery paradigms are dramatically shifting and emphasizing a more integrated and mutlidisciplinary approach, addressing the connection of the body, mind, and sprit. As clearly demonstrated from the above statistics, public interest and demand for alternative and complementary approaches to health care, particularly massage therapy, has resulted in more research validating the various benefits of massage therapy; inclusion into health insurance plans all over the country, including Oxford, Aetna/US Health Care, Mutual of Omaha and HIP; and increased acceptance by traditional medical practitioners.

Another important sector of this rapidly expanding profession is the spa industry. It is important to recognize and understand the interrelatedness and growing interdependences between the spa industry and the massage therapy profession because spas are one of the largest employers of massage therapists.

SPA INDUSTRY

Employment in resort spas, destination spas, medical spas, and day spas, incorporating various modalities in massage therapy, has become an avenue of practice that has soared over the last several years. In 2000, the International SPA Association (ISPA) engaged PricewaterhouseCoopers to conduct the inaugural Spa Industry Study. It was the first study to provide a research-based profile of the industry, including industry size and growth. Recognizing the need for current information, ISPA continues to conduct comprehensive surveys to update the findings from earlier years. The 2007 study develops a current profile of the industry in the United States and Canada. The key findings from the 2007 study are highlighted below and answer the question, "How big is the spa industry?"

Spa Locations and Visits

As of 2007 there were an estimated 14,615 spas throughout the United States and an estimated 2800 spas in Canada. The largest spa category, accounting for over three-quarters of locations, is day spas. Resort/hotel spas are the second largest group, followed by club spas, mineral springs spas, medical spas, and destination spas. Geographically, the distribution of spas in the United States generally reflects the distribution of the population. There were approximately 110 million spa visits made in the United States in 2006. Most of these were to day spas. Resort/hotel spas and club spas received the next largest numbers of spa visits.[18] This all translates into the need for more education and training opportunities in massage therapy.

JOB OUTLOOK AND TRENDS

All of the statistics clearly demonstrate that the market for massage therapy continues to experience rapid growth. The American Massage Therapy Association (AMTA), founded in 1943, represents almost 60,000 massage therapists and has chapters in all 50 states, the District of Columbia, and the U.S. Virgin Islands. In 1990, the AMTA had a membership of 12,000 members.

Upon graduation, most massage therapists start their own practices. In fact, working for oneself is often a big motivating factor for getting into this profession to begin with. Generally speaking, massage therapists who have the marketing and business skills can often do better financially when working on their own compared to working for someone else.

It is also not uncommon to find private practicing massage therapists working part time in one or several different types of employment settings at the same time. It offers a way to make an income while building a private practice; provides a broader type of patient base, which helps build important experience; and presents numerous invaluable opportunities to work alongside, and network with, other health care professionals.

The most common employment settings are

- medical and day spas.
- hotels, resorts, cruise ships.
- along with other health care providers including chiropractors, naturopaths, medical doctors, acupuncturists, and in holistic and/or multi-disciplinary clinics.
- large clinics specializing in massage including franchises such as Massage Envy, Elements, Massage Heights, etc.
- hospitals, hospice facilities, and nursing homes.
- health and wellness centers.
- hospitals, clinics, and doctor's offices.
- fitness centers or spas within fitness centers.
- professional sports organizations.
- fortune 500 corporations.

According to the U.S. Department of Labor, Bureau of Labor Statistics, between 2006 and 2016 the demand for licensed massage therapists will increase 18 to 26 percent.[19] This means the demand for massage therapy is growing at an ever-increasing rate, particularly as more and more people learn the many benefits of massage therapy.

Increased interest in massage therapy means great personal and professional growth opportunities for massage therapists. According to the results from the 2007 AMTA Survey, 33 percent of massage therapists polled reported working from home (often cited as a big factor for getting into this field), but employment in spas/salons, private offices outside of home, and health care settings has grown in importance from previous surveys. In addition, the survey reported that on average massage therapists are working in 1.6 employment settings, a confirmation that many therapists are working in multiple settings.[20]

BABY BOOMERS FORCE MARKET GROWTH

The 76 million boomers born between 1946 and 1964 have begun aging. As this aging population continues to grow and chronic illness increases, regular treatment and prevention programs utilizing massage therapy will become a greater focus of health care, and this noninvasive therapy will be increasingly utilized.

As a result, more massage therapists than ever will be needed to provide various levels of professional health care and treatment to boomers to help them stay more fit and pain and stress free. In a certain way, baby boomers will become one of the major driving forces of the massage therapy market. Interestingly, Generations X and Y, having grown up watching their parents take care of their minds and bodies, can also be expected, and already have begun, to become part of the expanding market of the massage therapy industry (Figure 12-1).

THE BIGGER PICTURE

In the last 30 years, the role of the massage therapist has undergone a drastic change. Once known only as a "masseur" or "masseuse" and usually associated with the image of some huge muscle-bound man or large beefy European woman vigorously kneading and slapping their clients' backs in a gym or the association of sexual favors with massage, one can certainly say that massage has evolved. More accurately, massage has returned to its original roots as a therapeutic modality and an integral part of a complete approach to health care.

The view of massage has changed along with the change in the health care system. Thousands of years ago, in numerous cultures from the days of Hippocrates to the Taoist monks of China, massage was considered a necessary treatment for a wide range of illnesses, as well as prevention of disease, and played an essential role in health care. With the advent of western science and technology, the importance of touch was superceded by the focus on materialism and structure as applied to the human body and disease. The idea that massage therapy could

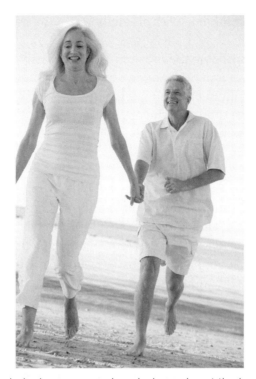

Figure 12-1 A healthy baby boomer couple enjoying a day at the beach. *Image copyright 2009, Monkey Business Images. Used under license from shutterstock.com.*

be therapeutic was dismissed as the emphasis moved to using surgery, drugs, and pharmaceuticals as if they were the cure for every possible illness.

For a long time, massage was consigned to gyms and "massage parlors," so that its public image became tainted and unsavory. In the 1970s, massage practitioners began working hard to dispel such images and in the last decades such pictures have disappeared to a large degree. However, among many physicians and insurance companies, massage is often still not viewed as the wonderful adjunct to a multidisciplinary team that it truly is but rather as some superficial technique only useful for relaxation. Nothing could be further from the truth— skilled massage therapists, especially those practicing from the Second and Third Paradigms, can and should be equal members of a health care team. So despite all the growth that has taken place in this field, massage therapists still have a lot of work to do in order to educate other health professionals as to the great benefits of massage therapy and bodywork to an individual's health.

Every patient should be entitled to the benefits of their health care practitioners working in concert, with the patient's health the priority. Patient care should be "patient-centered," with all members of the health care team contributing their area of expertise with the goal of bringing the patient to a state of optimum health utilizing the most minimally invasive approaches. Every therapist should have a network of health care providers to whom they can refer their clients/patients if need be. Ideally, the network should be made up of health care practitioners who are interested in advancing patient care through a multidisciplinary approach.

THE PATIENT

As strange as it may sound, the patient is often the most overlooked person in the health care team. Often, patients are ill-informed about their condition, their medications, the tests they need to take, their diagnosis, and their prognosis. The two patient populations most in need of an advocate to help them navigate through the labyrinth of the modern health care system are children and the elderly. All massage therapists should have an up-to-date medical history on their clients/patients and have in their possession the necessary drug and pharmaceutical texts and/or computer programs to check the medications of the people they are treating and to be aware of the potential side effects of such drugs, which can affect their treatments. Sometimes massage therapists, who spend significant amounts of time with the same patients on a regular basis, may find that they need to be referred to another member of the health care team, or that they need help in interacting with their physician, to know what questions to ask regarding tests, medications, diagnosis, and prognosis of their condition. The massage therapist can take the role of advocate on patients' behalf and help them to have input into their health and the kind of care they wish to receive. The massage therapist should also be able to communicate with other members of the health care team and answer any questions they may have that could potentially impact the kind of treatments rendered. All communications must be documented in the patient's chart, whether it is in person, by phone, or in writing. Not only will this help the massage therapist to remember the important aspects of the communication, it is also necessary for legal purposes (Figure 12-2).

THE FAMILY/SIGNIFICANT OTHERS

The family and significant others play a vital role in the health of clients with serious illnesses, who require not just treatments but perhaps medication regimens, dietary changes, surgery, or debilitating treatments such

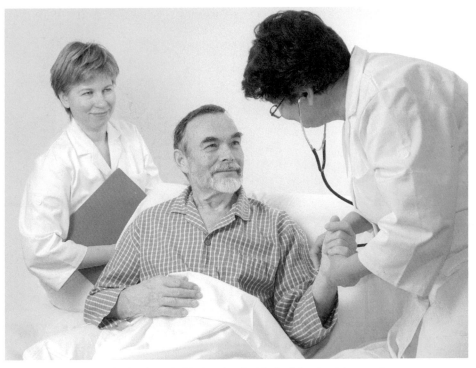

Figure 12-2 A patient in the hospital being tended to by his physician and a nurse. *Image copyright 2009, Alexander Raths. Used under license from shutterstock.com.*

as chemotherapy and radiation. These patient support members must be educated along with the patient as to the overall health care program. Often, members of the family know as little as the patient or less. They are confused by medical language, may be intimidated by medical practitioners and afraid to ask questions. Often their fears are well founded because many western medical practitioners dismiss family members and treat them like second-class citizens along with the patient. Since the relationship of the patient with the massage therapist is often open and trusting, the massage therapist is in a position to help the family as well as the patient understand the medical terminology, encourage them to ask questions, and generally help them to help the patient. Although most well-trained massage therapy practitioners may be able to do this, it's really practitioners of the Third Paradigm who are in the best position to make the commitment to take on this level of patient responsibility. It certainly is not a requirement of any massage therapist but rather an individual choice for those willing practitioners competent and knowledgeable enough to step into this often-needed role (Figure 12-3).

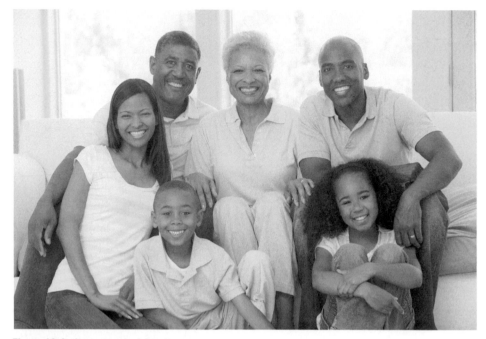

Figure 12-3 An extended family. *Image copyright 2009, Monkey Business Images. Used under license from shutterstock.com.*

THE PHYSICIAN

At one time, the physician was the most prominent person on the health care team—in fact he or she was often the only health care provider available to the patient. In the days of the general, or "family," doctor, the physician was the primary person that people turned to when they were ill. However, with the advent of the reductionist view of medicine leading to a growing number of specialties, people often don't know which doctor they should see. And with the emphasis on managed care, people are often forced to abide by the decisions of the primary care physician (PCP), who acts as a gatekeeper for their medical needs and determines which specialized services they may need. Although many physicians still do not regard massage therapy as a therapeutic modality, it is more common today for a physician to recommend massage therapy, usually when there is a musculoskeletal problem, such as low-back pain or some soft tissue injury. Most clients find their way to massage practitioners on their own or by word of mouth. In either case, if the patient has medical issues that the massage therapist will be addressing in one form or another during treatment, the massage therapist must be prepared to contact the physician, either by phone or in writing, when there are questions or concerns regarding the patient's overall health care program (Figure 12-4).

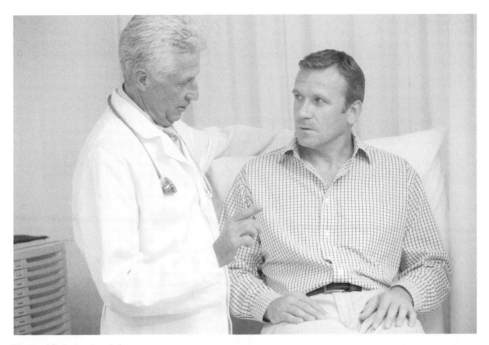

Figure 12-4 A physician.   *Image copyright 2009, Monkey Business Images. Used under license from shutterstock.com.*

NURSES

Nurses are often the health care practitioners most open to integrative and complementary medicine. They have traditionally been trained in hands-on therapy and are no strangers to physical contact with patients. Some even enroll in massage schools to add massage therapy to their list of skills and techniques, because they value the need for touch and physical contact with their patients. Sometimes massage therapists may find themselves interacting with nursing staff rather than the physician. The massage therapist must be prepared to communicate in the requisite medical language and can often enlist the nurse in assisting with questions and test interpretations (Figure 12-5).

ACUPUNCTURISTS

As more Americans are discovering that western medicine alone does not always work, they are turning to acupuncture as a natural way to heal without the side effects of many drugs and chemicals prescribed by western medical practitioners.

Acupuncture is an ancient Chinese healing art that has helped literally billions of people. The essentially painless technique employs the insertion of

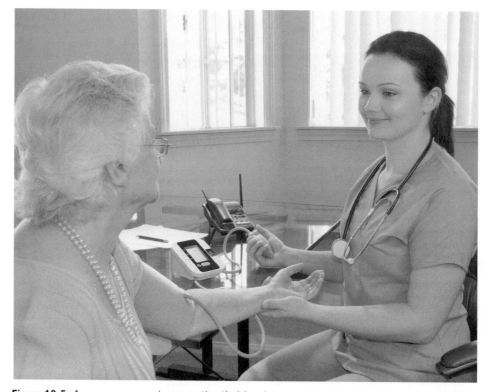

Figure 12-5 A nurse measuring a patient's blood pressure. *Image copyright 2009, Mikhail Tchkheidze. Used under license from shutterstock.com.*

fine, sterile, disposable needles into specific points on the body to manipulate the flow of energy or 'qi', thereby restoring balance, removing blockages, and generating energy where necessary. Acupuncture points, which lie on energy channels, are directly related to specific organs and physiological functions. This principle has been confirmed by research in which obvious physiological changes were observed through the manipulation of specific acupuncture points.

Acupuncture has been widely used for anesthesia and is growing in use not only to treat and heal various conditions but also to maintain good health. It has been shown to be effective in both children and adults—treating disorders such as asthma, arthritis, palsy, impotence, sciatica, chronic or acute back and neck pain, headaches, ulcers, diabetes, colitis, gastrointestinal problems, genito-urinary conditions, cancer, and the common cold. Acupuncture is also capable of inducing deep relaxation, and is an extremely useful modality for prevention of illness as well as for treatment of disease. Many massage

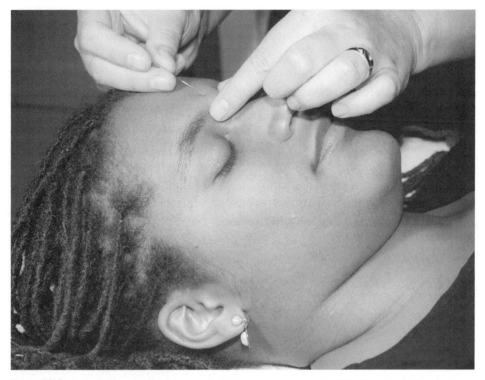

Figure 12-6 A woman receiving acupuncture. *Image copyright 2009, Cora Reed. Used under license from shutterstock.com.*

therapists, particularly those trained in Asian bodywork techniques, work together with acupuncturists for the benefit of the patient. Massage therapists often share office space with acupuncturists because the two modalities work hand-in-hand especially to help clients suffering from neck and back pain, sports injuries, stress and anxiety, hypertension, arthritic changes, and a whole host of other medical problems (Figure 12-6).

CHIROPRACTORS

Chiropractic is a modality that treats the musculoskeletal system, focusing mainly on the proper alignment of the spine and the effects of misalignment on the body. Since ancient times, "bone setting" has been practiced, not only by the Greeks and Romans but also by Asian cultures as well. However, it wasn't until 1895 when Daniel David Palmer cured Harvey Lillard of deafness after 17 years of being unable to hear, that chiropractic was born. Palmer used a spinal manipulation after Lillard declared that his deafness occurred when he felt something "give" in his back. While traditional physicians considered chiropractic quackery, its popularity continued to grow and today it is regarded as one of the largest health care professions in the world.

Chiropractic is very complementary to massage therapy, and many chiropractors employ massage therapists in their practices. Chiropractors find that after a patient has a massage therapy treatment, they are able to adjust the spine with greater ease and effectiveness. While many think that chiropractors only treat back problems, skilled chiropractors can act as adjunctive therapists for a wide range of physical disorders. The spinal cord is surrounded by the spinal column and, with the brain, comprises the central nervous system. It is easy to see how any misalignment (subluxation) of the spine can affect many areas of the body. Chiropractors often recommend specific exercises to their patients and often recommend massage therapy as well. It is helpful for a massage therapist to network with several chiropractors and be able to communicate with them about patient care (Figure 12-7). Chiropractic is not an appropriate treatment for people with osteoporosis, brittle bones, or patients with bone disease or bone cancer.

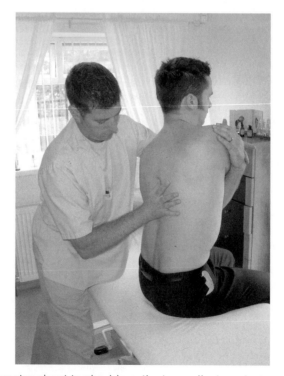

Figure 12-7 A chiropractor about to give his patient an adjustment. *Image copyright 2009, Terry Walsh. Used under license from shutterstock.com.*

PHYSICAL THERAPISTS

Physical therapists help patients regain normal function after they have suffered an injury or a disease. Their expertise is in developing individualized treatment programs for patients, teaching them how to prevent further injury or to slow the progression of disease and its effects on their movements and functions. People are recommended to physical therapists by their physicians and often seek out physical therapy as an alternative to surgery or medication. While there are many types of physical therapy, in general physical therapists utilize exercise, heat, cold, electrical stimulation, and ultrasound to treat their patients and help them improve their use of their bones, muscles, and joints. People often seek physical therapy for many of the same reasons that they seek massage therapy: neck and back pain, shoulder, arm, elbow, or wrist pain, arthritic pain, knee and ankle pain, post-surgical healing, strains, sprains, postural problems, and balance and coordination problems. The physical therapist excels at helping patients to implement the proper exercises and helping them with daily living tasks, putting the affected area(s) through the movements and exercises that patients often neglect or can't do for themselves. Massage therapists will often see patients who are also undergoing physical therapy, and the massage therapist needs to be clear on what the physical therapist is doing so that they can work together on the patient's behalf (Figure 12-8).

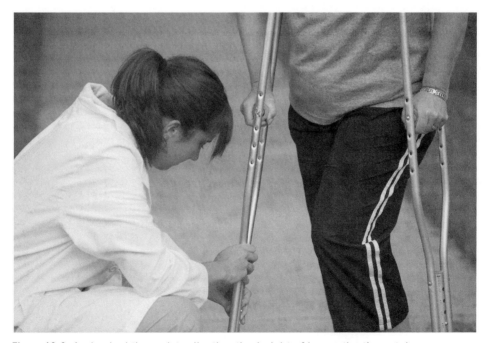

Figure 12-8 A physical therapist adjusting the height of her patient's crutches. *Image copyright 2009, Salamanderman. Used under license from shutterstock.com.*

PSYCHIATRISTS/PSYCHOLOGISTS

Often patients are on medications for stress, anxiety, depression, and other emotional problems. These medications should be prescribed by a psychiatrist who is knowledgeable about their purposes and side effects and not by a general physician. Many of these medications have serious side effects, so the massage therapist should investigate these medications and may need to communicate with the psychiatrist if he or she suspects that the drugs are causing the patient serious injury. Psychologists do not prescribe medication but rather try to help the client solely through counseling. Psychologists in the health care provider field offer mental health care in clinics, schools, private settings, or in hospitals. They may offer individual, family, or group psychotherapy sessions and may create behavior modification programs for their patients. Some clinical psychologists cooperate with physicians and other health care providers, including massage therapists, to develop and implement treatment and intervention programs. All massage therapists should have a psychologist who they can refer their clients to if necessary and they should be able to communicate with that psychologist about their patient's issues when they are seriously concerned. Serious massage practitioners should also be able to clearly convey the benefits that massage therapy can have for the

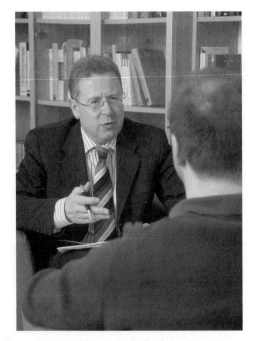

Figure 12-9 A counseling session with a psychologist. *Image copyright 2009, Gina Sanders. Used under license from shutterstock.com.*

patients of any psychologist in aiding the progress of emotional healing and in overall health development (Figure 12-9).

SUMMARY

This chapter describes the unprecedented growth of the massage therapy profession that has taken and continues to take place in the country. This chapter also looks at the role of the massage therapist as an integral part of the health care team and describes the relationship between massage therapists and the various health care professionals with whom they work closely including: physicians, nurses, acupuncturists, chiropractors, physical therapists and psychiatrists/psychologists. A description of each of these professions is also presented.

A very important concept presented in this chapter is that the patient's care should be patient-centered, and that the patient and his or her family are very important members of the health care team and should always have a major role in the direction of the patient's treatment and therapy. The world of health care can be confusing, frustrating, and difficult to navigate for the average patient. Therefore, growing numbers of Second and Third Paradigm massage therapists have the opportunity to act as a liaison between patient and doctor, helping to ensure that both parties gain a more complete and accurate understanding of the patient's current state of health, treatment results, and other treatment options that they may want to explore.

CHAPTER REFERENCES

1. The National Certification Board for Therapeutic Massage and Bodywork (NCBTMB). Retrieved March 30, 2009, from http://www.ncbtmb.org/about_required_states.php.
2. American Massage Therapy Association Website (AMTA). Retrieved March 30, 2009, from http://www.amtamassage.org/about/lawstate.html
3. Federation of State Boards of Massage Therapy (FSBMT). Retrieved March 30, 2009, from http://fsmtb.com/html/licensing/mblex.html
4. The US Department of Education Database of Postsecondary Institutions and Programs. Retrieved March, 30th, 2009, from http://ope.ed.gov/accreditation/
5. *ED.Gov: US Department of Education.* Retrieved March, 30, 2009, from http://www.ed.gov/admins/finaid/accred/accreditation_pg10.html#TitleIVRecognition
6. Commission on Massage Therapy Accreditation (COMTA). Retrieved March 30, 2009, from http://www.comta.org/about_introduction.php
7. The National Center for Complementary and Alternative Medicine (NCCAM) of the National Institutes of Health (NIH). Retrieved March 30, 2009, from http://nccam.nih.gov/about/ataglance/

8. "Massage Therapy: Not Just a Trend" Opinion Research Corporation International. (August 2006).

9. "Massage Therapy: Not Just a Trend" Opinion Research Corporation International. (August 2006).

10. "Massage Therapy: Not Just a Trend" Opinion Research Corporation International. (August 2006).

11. "2009 Massage Therapy Industry Fact Sheet," American Massage Therapy Association. (January, 2008).

12. "2009 Massage Therapy Industry Fact Sheet," American Massage Therapy Association. (January, 2008).

13. "2009 Massage Therapy Industry Fact Sheet," American Massage Therapy Association. (January, 2008).

14. "Massage Therapy: Not Just a Trend" Opinion Research Corporation International. (August 2006).

15. "Massage Therapy: Not Just a Trend" Opinion Research Corporation International. (August 2006).

16. "2009 Massage Therapy Industry Fact Sheet," American Massage Therapy Association. (January, 2008).

17. "Massage Therapy: Not Just a Trend" Opinion research corporation international. (August 2006).

18. International SPA Association (ISPA) Survey. (2007).

19. Bureau of Labor Statistics, U.S. Department of Labor. *Occupational outlook handbook, 2008-09 edition,* Massage Therapists. Retrieved August 06, 2008, from http://www.bls.gov/oco/ocos295.htm

20. American Massage Therapy Industry Survey. 2007.

Appendix:
Reference List, Bibliography and Additional Resources

1. American Massage Therapy Association (2008). *The business of massage.* Chicago, IL: Author.
2. Ashley, M. (1998). *Massage: A career at your fingertips.* (3rd ed.). Barrytown, New York: Station Hill Press.
3. Beck, M.F. (2006). *Theory and practice of therapeutic massage.* (4th ed.). Baltimore, MD: Lippincott, Williams and Wilkins.
4. Benjamin, B., & Sohnen-Moe, C. (2004). *The ethics of touch: The hands-on practitioner's guide to creating a professional, safe and enduring practice.* Tucson, AZ: Sohnen-Moe Associates, Inc.
5. Benjamin, P., & Lamp, S. (2005). *Understanding sports massage.* (2nd ed). Champaign, IL: Human Kinetics.
6. Benjamin, P., & Tappan, F.M. (2005). *Tappan's handbook of healing massage techniques: classic, holistic and emerging methods.* (4th ed.). Upper Saddle River, NJ: Prentice Hall.
7. Beresford-Cooke, C. (2003). *Shiatsu theory and practice: A comprehensive test for the student professional.* (2nd ed.). New York: Churchill Livingstone.
8. Biel, A. (2005). *Trail guide to the body.* (3rd ed.). Boulder, CO: Books of Discovery.
9. Braun, M.B., & Simonson, S. (2005). *Introduction to massage therapy.* Baltimore, MD: Lippincott, Williams and Wilkins.
10. Calvert, R. (2002). *The history of massage.* Rochester, VT: Healing Arts Press.
11. Capellini, S. (2006). *Massage therapy career guide for hands-on success.* (2nd ed.). Albany, New York: Thomson Delmar Learning.
12. Changye, L. (1992). *Concise tuina therapy.* Jinan, China: Shendong Science & Technology Press.
13. Chow K.T., & Moody, E. (2006). *Thai yoga therapy for your body type: An ayurvedic tradition.* Rochester, VT: Healing Arts Press.
14. Claire, T. (1995). *Body work: What kind of massage to get and how to make the most of it.* Laguna Beach, CA: Basic Health Publications, Inc.
15. Douillard, J. (2004). *The Encyclopedia of Ayurvedic massage.* Berkeley, CA: North Atlantic Books.
16. Dubitsky, C. (1997). *Bodywork shiatsu.* Rochester, VT: Healing Arts Press.
17. Finando, D., & Finando S. (2005). *Trigger point therapy for myofascial pain.* Rochester, VT: Healing Arts Press.
18. Fritz, S. (2004). *Mosby's fundamentals of therapeutic massage.* (3rd ed). St. Louis: Mosby/Elsevier.

19. Fritz, S., & Grosenbach, J.M. (2004). *Mosby's essential sciences for therapeutic massage: anatomy, physiology, biomechanics and pathology.* (2nd ed.). St. Louis: Mosby/Elsevier.
20. Gelb, M.J. (1996). *Body learning: An introduction to the Alexander Technique.* (2nd ed.). New York: Henry Holt and Co.
21. Johnson, J. (1995). *Healing art of sports massage.* Emmaus, PA: Rodale Press Inc.
22. Juhan, D. (2002). *Job's body: A handbook for bodyworkers.* (3rd ed.). Barrytown, New York: Station Hill Press.
23. Kaptchuck, T.J. (2000). *The Web That Has No Weaver: Understanding Chinese medicine.* (2nd ed.). New York: McGraw-Hill.
24. Kendall, F., & Kendall, E. (1993) *Muscles: testing and function.* (4th ed.). Baltimore, MD: Williams and Wilkins.
25. Knaster, M. (1996). *Discovering the body's wisdom.* New York: Bantam Books.
26. Krieger, D. (1993). *Accepting your power to heal: The personal practice of therapeutic touch.* Santa Fe, NM: Bear and Company.
27. Levine A, Levine V. (1999). *Bodywork and massage sourcebook.* Los Angeles, CA: Lowell House.
28. Lowe, W. (2006). *Orthopedic assessment in massage therapy.* Oregon: David Scott.
29. Lundburg, P. (2003). *The book of shiatsu: A complete guide to using hand pressure and gentle manipulation.* New York: Fireside.
30. Maciocia, G. (1989). *The foundations of Chinese medicine.* New York: Churchill Livingstone.
31. McIntosh, N. (2004). *The educated heart: professional boundaries for massage therapists, bodyworkers and movement teachers.* (2nd ed.). Baltimore, MD: Lippincott, Williams and Wilkins.
32. Miller, E. (1993). *Day spa operations.* Albany, New York: Milady.
33. Miller, E. (1993). *Day spa techniques.* Albany, New York: Milady.
34. Mitchell, S. (2000). *The complete illustrated guide to massage: A step-by-step approach to the healing art of touch.* Shaftesbury, Dorset, UK: Element Books Ltd.
35. Montagu, A. (1971). *Touching: The human significance of the skin.* New York: Harper and Row.
36. Mumford, S. (1998). *The healing massage: A practical guide to relaxation and well-being.* USA: Plume.
37. Neighbors, M., & Tannehill-Jones, R. (2005). *Human diseases.* Albany, New York: Thompson Delmar Learning.
38. Premkumar, K. (2004) *The massage connection: anatomy and physiology.* (2nd ed). Baltimore, MD: Lippincott, Williams and Wilkins.
39. Pritchard, S. (1999). *The Chinese massage manual: The healing art of tuina.* New York: Sterling Publications.
40. Rattray, F., & Ludwig, L. (2000) *Clinical massage therapy: understanding, assessing and treating over 70 conditions.* Ontario: Talus, Inc.
41. Rogoff, J.B. (1980). *Manipulation, traction and massage.* Baltimore, MD: William and Wilkins.
42. Roseberry, M. (2006). *Marketing massage: From first job to dream practice.* (2nd ed.). Albany, New York: Thompson Delmar Learning.

43. Salvo, S.G. (2003) *Massage therapy principles and practice.* (3rd ed.). St. Louis: Saunders/Elsevier.

44. Scheumann, D. (2002). *The balanced body: A guide to deep tissue and neuromuscular therapy. (*2nd ed.). Baltimore: Lippincott Williams and Wilkins.

45. Sohn, T., & Sohn, R. (1996). *Amma therapy: A complete textbook of oriental bodywork and medical principles.* Rochester, VT: Healing Arts Press.

46. Sohnen-Moe, C. (2003). *Business mastery.* (3rd ed.). Tucson: Sohnen-Moe Associates Inc.

47. Stein, D. (1995). *Essential Reiki.* Berkeley: Crossing Press.

48. Stone, R. (1999). *Polarity therapy: The complete collected works, Vol 1.* Summertown, TN: Book Publishing Company.

49. Teeguarden, I. (1999). *Acupressure way of health: Jin shin do.* Tokyo, Japan: Japan Publications.

50. Thibodeau, G.A. (2004). *Structure & function of the body.* (12th ed.). St. Louis: Mosby/Elsevier.

51. Thomas, C.I. (2001). *Taber's cyclopedic medical dictionary.* (19th ed.). Philadelphia, PA: Davis Co.

52. Tortora, G. & Grabowski, S.R. (2004). *Principles of anatomy and physiology.* (10th ed.). New York: Harper and Collins Publishers, Inc.

53. Upledger, J. (1997). *Your inner physician & you.* Berkeley, CA: North Atlantic Books.

54. Werner, R. (2005) *A massage therapist's guide to pathology.* (3rd ed). Baltimore: Lippincott, Williams and Wilkins.

55. Wittlinger, G. & Wittlinger, H. (2004). *Textbook of Dr. Vodder's manual lymph drainage, Vol 1.* (7th Ed.). Stuttgart: Thieme

WEBSITE LINKS

The following links provide useful information regarding the many facets of the massage therapy and bodywork profession. They include professional membership organizations; certifying and accrediting bodies; and magazines, journals, and research institutions where current research in massage and bodywork therapy can be obtained. The list below also includes links for complementary, alternative, and integrative medicine research sources, many of which contain information about massage and bodywork therapy. Also included are some links for seeking useful employment and practice information; information regarding schools, programs, and courses in massage therapy and professional continuing education; general online resource sites for product and practice information; and sites that offer employment opportunities and information on community, county, and state regulations.

MASSAGE THERAPY & BODYWORK MEMBERSHIP, CERTIFYING & ACCREDITING BODIES

1. **American Massage Therapy Association:** http://www.amtamassage.org

    The American Massage Therapy Association (AMTA), which represents more than 58,000 massage therapists, is a national professional membership organization with chapters in all 50 states. AMTA works to establish massage therapy as integral to the maintenance of good health and complementary to other therapeutic processes and to advance the profession through ethics and standards, continuing education, professional publications, legislative efforts, public education, and fostering the development of members.

2. **American Medical Massage Association:** http://www.americanmedical massage.com

    The American Medical Massage Association (AMMA) was specifically created to represent the image, growth, and protection of medical massage therapists. The AMMA seeks to promote medical massage therapy as an allied health care profession while encouraging unity within the massage profession. This goal is achieved through professional standards, education, and testing and by offering a wide array of services for its members.

3. **American Organization for Bodywork Therapies of Asia:** http://www. aobta.org

    American Organization for Bodywork Therapies of Asia (AOBTA) is a non-profit, professional membership organization representing instructors, practitioners, schools, and programs, as well as students of the various forms of Asian bodywork therapy (ABT).

4. **American Society for the Alexander Technique:** http://www.amsat.ws

    The American Society for the Alexander Technique is the professional association for certified Alexander Technique teachers in the United States. The Alexander Technique is a proven, effective way to promote wellness and optimize functioning by eliminating body misuse in everyday activities. AmSAT's mission is to define, maintain, and promote the Alexander Technique at its highest standard of professional practice and conduct.

5. **Associated Bodywork and Massage Professionals:** http://www.abmp.com

    Associated Bodywork & Massage Professionals (ABMP) is a national membership association that provides comprehensive liability insurance and practice support for massage therapy and bodywork practitioners, students, and schools and programs.

6. **Commission on Massage Therapy Accreditation:** http://www.comta.org

   The Commission on Massage Therapy Accreditation (COMTA) accredits both educational institutions and programs offering instruction in massage therapy and bodywork. The organization was formed to establish and maintain the quality and integrity of the profession. In 2002, COMTA was recognized by the U.S. Department of Education as a specialized accrediting agency, an acknowledgement of its expertise in ensuring quality education and allowing programs to access federal student aid funds.

7. **Federation of State Massage Therapy Boards:** http://www.fsmtb.org

   The mission of the Federation of State Massage Therapy Boards (FSMTB) is to support its member boards in their work to ensure that the practice of massage therapy is provided to the public in a safe and effective manner. In carrying out this mission, the Federation ensures the provision of a valid, reliable licensing examination to determine entry-level competence.

8. **Federation of Therapeutic Massage, Bodywork & Somatic Practice Organizations:** http://www.federationmbs.org

   The Federation is a forum for building community and communication among nonprofit membership organizations representing massage, bodywork, or somatic practices and facilitating readiness to respond to issues that affect their values. By serving as a vehicle for building bridges and breaking down barriers between groups, the Federation promotes understanding, cooperation, and respect between its member organizations.

9. **Feldenkrais Guild® of North America:** http://www.feldenkrais.com

   The Feldenkrais Guild is a professional membership organization representing instructors, practitioners, schools and programs, and students of The Feldenkrais Method of Somatic Education.

10. **Hospital-based Massage Network:** http//:www.hbmn.com

    The Hospital-Based Massage Network (HBMN) supports massage and touch therapists pursuing skilled touch for the ill, recovering, and elderly and the dying in hospitals, medical centers and nursing homes.

11. **International Organization of Structural Integrators:** http://www.structuralintegration.org

    The International Association of Structural Integrators (IASI) is the professional membership organization for Structural Integration. Founded in 2002, IASI sprang up as a grassroots organization from within the profession to set standards, move towards certification, ensure continuation of a professional identity, and promote Structural Integration's continued growth as a respected profession in the health care field.

12. **International Somatic Movement Education & Therapy Association:** http://www.ismeta.org

    The International Somatic Movement Education & Therapy Association (ISMETA) promotes a high level of standards and professionalism in the field of somatic movement education and therapy through advocacy and maintainance of a registry of professional practitioners.

13. **The International SPA Association:** http://www.experienceispa.com

    Since 1991, the International SPA Association (ISPA) has been recognized worldwide as the professional organization and voice of the spa industry, representing more than 3,200 health and wellness facilities and providers in 83 countries. Members encompass the entire arena of the spa experience, from resort/hotel, destination, mineral springs, medical, cruise ship, club and day spas to service providers such as physicians, wellness instructors, nutritionists, massage therapists, and product suppliers. ISPA advances the spa industry by providing educational and networking opportunities, promoting the value of the spa experience, and speaking as the authoritative voice to foster professionalism and growth.

14. **National Certification Board for Therapeutic Massage & Bodywork:** http://www.ncbtmb.com

    The National Certification Board for Therapeutic Massage & Bodywork (NCBTMB) was founded in 1992 to establish a certification program and uphold a national standard of excellence. Today, the independent, private, nonprofit organization has certified more than 91,000 massage therapists and bodyworkers, who safely and competently serve millions of Americans each year. The site also includes a resource for locating certified practitioners.

15. **The Rolf Institute®:** http://www.rolf.org

    Rolf Institute of Structural Integration was founded by Ida P. Rolf in 1971. The Institute headquarters in Boulder, Colorado and its international offices in Europe, Brazil, Australia, and Japan are the only schools that certify Rolfers® and Rolf Movement Practitioners™.

16. **United States Trager® Association:** http://www.tragerus.org

    The United States Trager Association (USTA) represents and supports Trager psychophysical integration and Mentastics® movement education, the innovative approach to movement education developed by Milton Trager, M.D. The USTA is a member of Trager International, a worldwide international organization dedicated to the growth and support of the Trager Approach and also represents instructors, practitioners, programs, and students of The Trager Approach.

MAGAZINES, JOURNALS & RESEARCH SITES

1. **Centers for Disease Control:** http://www.cdc.gov/

   CDC.gov is the Centers For Disease Control and Prevention's (CDC) primary online communication channel. CDC.gov provides users with credible, reliable health information on data and statistics, diseases and conditions, emergencies and disasters, environmental health, healthy living, injury, violence and safety, life stages and populations, travelers' health, workplace safety and health, and more.

2. **Integrated Healthcare Policy Consortium:** http://ihpc.info

   The Integrated Healthcare Policy Consortium (IHPC) is a broad coalition of health care professionals and organizations driving public policy to assure all Americans access to safe, high quality, integrated health care. The Academic Consortium for Complementary and Alternative Health Care (which includes the field of massage therapy and bodywork) is a project of the Integrated Healthcare Policy Consortium (IHPC) and can be viewed at http://ihpc.info/accahc/accahc.shtml.

3. **Massage & Bodywork:** http://www.Massageandbodywork.com

   Massage & Bodywork magazine is a bimonthly journal for an international audience of licensed massage, bodywork, somatic, and skin care professionals. Each issue offers in-depth articles on subjects that impact both the practicing professional and the lay person and incorporates the latest research, historical perspectives, massage techniques, business information, and trends in the profession.

4. **Massage Therapy Foundation:** http://www.massagetherapyfoundation.org

   The Massage Therapy Foundation was founded by the American Massage Therapy Association in 1990 with the mission of bringing the benefits of massage therapy to the broadest spectrum of society through the generation, dissemination, and application of knowledge in this field.

The Massage Therapy Foundation advances the knowledge and practice of massage therapy by supporting scientific research, education, and community service.

5. **Massage Magazine:** http://www.massagemag.com

   Massage magazine is a paid monthly subscription that has been a leading massage publication since 1985 and is probably the most well-known magazine in the industry. Readers pay for this magazine rather than receiving it free as a benefit of belonging to one of the national membership organizations. Massage Magazine integrated print with the web when it formed www.massagemag.com, a fully interactive multimedia platform with expert blogs, streaming videos, reader polls, and podcasts, as well as massage news, press releases, business tips, health news, and much more.

6. **Massage Therapy Journal:** http://www.amtamassage.org/journal/home.html

   The Massage Therapy Journal is a quarterly, award winning publication of the American Massage Therapy Association. Members of the association receive the journal as part of a package of benefits that comes with joining.

7. **Massage Today:** http://www.massagetoday.com

   Massage Today is a monthly trade journal provided free of charge to licensed or practicing (if not residing in a regulated state) massage therapists and bodyworkers, and massage suppliers. The paper covers current news and techniques and includes current issue and archives, regular columns, directory of therapists, calendar, and more.

8. **Massage Therapy Research Consortium:** http://www.mtrc.info

   The Massage Therapy Research Consortium is a voluntary collaboration of massage schools that are interested in enhancing their own understanding of and participation in research on therapeutic massage. They have banded together to provide mutual support and to pool resources for joint educational and research activities.

9. **MEDLINE Medical Library maintained by the NIH:** http://www.pubmed.org

   PubMed is a service of the U.S. National Library of Medicine that includes over 18 million citations from MEDLINE and other life science journals for biomedical articles since 1948. PubMed includes links to full-text articles and other related resources.

10. **National Library of Medicine:** http://www.nlm.nih.gov

    www.nlm.nih.gov is the web site for the National Library of Medicine (NLM), which is on the campus of the National Institutes of Health in Bethesda, Maryland, and is the world's largest medical library. The library collects materials and provides information and research services in all areas of biomedicine and health care.

11. **National Center for Complementary Medicine:** http://nccam.nih.gov

    The National Center for Complementary and Alternative Medicine (NCCAM) is the Federal Government's lead agency for scientific research on complementary and alternative medicine (CAM), which includes massage therapy. The NCCAM is one of the 27 institutes and centers that make up the National Institutes of Health (NIH) within the U.S. Department of Health and Human Services.

12. **Natural Solutions Magazine:** http://www.naturalsolutionsmag.com

    Alternative Medicine magazine has changed its name. The trusted voice and magazine of the complementary and alternative medicine field now known as Natural Solutions magazine provides natural remedies and healthy solutions for the most pressing health concerns as well as practical strategies for self-care and prevention.

13. **Touch Research Institute:** http://www.miami.edu/touch-research

    The Touch Research Institute (TRI) is dedicated to studying the effects of touch therapy. The TRI has researched the effects of massage therapy at all stages of life, from newborns to senior citizens. In these studies the TRI has shown that touch therapy has many positive effects.

COMPLEMENTARY, ALTERNATIVE, & INTEGRATIVE MEDICINE RESEARCH SOURCES

1. **American Association of Integrative Medicine:** http://www.aaimedicine.com/main.php

   American Association of Integrative Medicine (AAIM) is a network of related integrative health care providers that disseminates information, fosters closer relationships among all health care providers, educates the public about the benefits and advantages of integrative medical approaches, advocates for higher standards of quality in the profession, and recognizes the contributions and professionalism of its members.

2. **American Holistic Health Association:** http://www.ahha.org

   The American Holistic Health Association (AHHA) encourages health care physicians and practitioners to incorporate holistic principles into their practices and sees the need for this organization to educate the public on the power of the holistic approach. AHHA offers free information about health and wellness resources to help people better cope with an illness or disease, or to enhance their health. Resources include offerings in both conventional and alternative medicine

3. **American Holistic Medical Association:** http://www.holisticmedicine.org

   The American Holistic Medical Association (AHMA) serves as the leading advocate for the use of holistic and integrative medicine by all licensed healthcare providers. AHMA embraces integrative, complementary, and alternative medicine techniques; holds on to what is helpful in allopathic medicine; and understands that healing includes one's body, mind, emotions, and spirit. The AHMA is committed to increasing awareness and understanding of the natural healing tenets of holistic medicine and to linking together those who wish to utilize and promote a holistic approach to conventional and integrative medicine.

4. **Rosenthal Center for Complementary & Alternative Medicine, Columbia University:** http://www.rosenthal.hs.columbia.edu

   Based at Columbia University's College of Physicians & Surgeons, Department of Rehabilitation Medicine, the Rosenthal Center is one of the first comprehensive programs at a major medical center to examine alternative therapies with an academic focus and scientific rigor. The Rosenthal Center's mission is to contribute to the informed research and practice of complementary and alternative medicine and to foster the development of a more comprehensive and inclusive medical system.

JOB, BUSINESS, MARKETING & PRODUCT SITES

1. **Biotone:** http://www.biotone.com

   Biotone professional massage and spa therapy products include a wide variety of massage oils, crèmes, essential oils, books, music, videos, and spa treatment products. Biotone products are used by massage schools, massage therapists, chiropractors, physical therapists, hospitals, and spas.

2. **Bureau of Labor Statistics, U.S. Department of Labor, Occupational Outlook Handbook:** http://www.bls.gov/oco/ocos295.htm

   Occupational Outlook Handbook (OOH), 2008–09 edition, is sought out for accurate information and statistics on hundreds of different types of jobs such as teacher, lawyer, nurse, and massage therapist. The OOH provides information on the training and education needed for specific occupations, earnings, expected job prospects, what workers do on the job, and working conditions.

3. **Massagetherapy.com:** http://www.massagetherapy.com/home/index.php

   Massagetherapy.com is a public education site owned and operated by Associated Bodywork & Massage Professionals (ABMP). It offers information about massage and on becoming a massage therapist, as well as a directory for finding a therapist practicing specific modalities.

4. **Massage Newsletters:** http://www.massagenewsletters.com

   Massage Newsletters specializes in creating client education newsletters for massage and bodywork therapists. The purpose of the newsletter is to raise client awareness and understanding of the actual benefits received through regular massage sessions. The newsletters keep health issues, massage benefits, and the practitioner on the client's mind. In 2003, the owners of Massage Newsletters teamed with a partner and launched Massage On The Web (http://www.massageontheweb.com), a company that creates esthetic web sites specifically for massage and bodywork therapists.

5. **Massage Warehouse, A Scrip Company:** http://www.massageware house.com

   A 2006 merger created the largest single source supplier for chiropractic, massage, and day spa products when Scrip Chiropractic Supply joined forces with Massage Warehouse and Day Spa Warehouse. In addition, they pass along educational information to massage therapists to help keep them well informed and knowledgeable.

6. **Natural Healers:** http://www.naturalhealers.com

   Natural Healers is the number one education resource for people pursuing careers in the natural healing arts. Natural Healers is a complete alternative medicine and holistic health school directory and career center that includes information about massage therapy schools, natural health degree schools, acupuncture schools, personal training certification, and chiropractic colleges.

7. **Natural Touch Marketing for the Healing Arts:** http://www.naturaltouch marketing.com

   Natural Touch Marketing for the Healing (NTMHA) offers a large selection of professional marketing tools and supplies available for massage therapists, bodyworkers, and other healing arts practitioners to help build their businesses.

8. **Spa Jobs:** http://www.spa-jobs.com

   Spa-Jobs.com is the specialist spa recruitment site for the international spa industry—a place where spa job seekers and spa employers meet. This site is dedicated to those who want to develop their careers in the spa industry and to the spas worldwide who are looking for qualified spa personnel, including massage therapists.

9. **The Bodyworker.com:** http://www.thebodyworker.com

   The Bodyworker.com is a very broad resource site for massage therapy students, massage therapists, and massage instructors, as well as the lay person interested in either entering the profession of learning more about the field and seeking information about possible massage therapy treatment. It also provides a great deal of useful information for those massage practitioners interested in building a rewarding massage therapy practice and successful career.

10. **Work.com:** http://www.work.com

    Work.com is a new service from Business.com, the largest business-to-business search engine and directory. Business.com and Work.com help small business decision makers solve their most pressing business problems. They make it easy to find the most useful business websites, products, and services, saving users time and money.

Glossary

Active trigger points those that radiate pain without being touched.

Acupressure Treatment having its roots in traditional Chinese medicine in which physical pressure is applied to specific points along the body's meridians for therapeutic or relaxation purposes.

Acupuncture health care modality using fine needles to stimulate or sedate specific energy points along the body's meridians in order to balance the energy system and assist the body'self-healing processes. A part of traditional Chinese medicine.

Adjunctive therapies Treatments connected to but not part of the primary health care treatment being used.

Allopathic medicine A system of medicine, often applied to western or modern medicine, distinguished from homeopathic medicine in that the treatment seeks to produce effects that are different to the symptoms of the disease being treated.

Alternative health care Any health care modality not considered part of conventional medical treatment and used in place of it.

Amma a form of massage originating in China that uses acupuncture points and manipulation of the energy channels of the body.

AMMA Therapy® blend of ancient amma massage techniques and modern western techniques created by Tina Sohn.

Aromatherapy treatment in which essential oils having specific effects on the person are used for therapeutic purposes or to affect mood.

Asian bodywork forms of massage therapy and bodywork that focus on treating the bioenergetic layer (energy system) of the human being through the manipulation of the soft tissue.

Autonomic nervous system the part of the nervous system that governs automatic functions and consists of the sympathetic and parasympathetic nervous systems.

Ayurveda Indian system of medicine meaning "science of life." Diagnosis is primarily through reading of pulses and dosha analysis. Ayurveda seeks to balance the three doshas and bring the individual into harmony with life using diet, herbs, and lifestyle modifications, including yoga practices, as well as the marma points and cleansing practices such as *pancha karma*. Considered to be the "sister science" of yoga.

Bach Flower Remedies developed by Dr. Edward Bach, uses the inherent energies of flower essences as a natural therapy to restore emotional and physical balance.

Bindegewebe massage "soft" form of myofascial release therapy.

Bioenergetic level or layer a massage or other techniques are used at this level to affect or treat the energetic system or "energy body" through manipulation of the physical body, for example, shiatsu, amma, tuina, acupressure.

Biofeedback technique that increases patients' self-awareness through use of mechanical feedback of their physiological state and helps them to improve their emotional and physiological balance through the mind-body connection.

Bodywork any modality involving the physical manipulation of the body for therapeutic purposes.

Case history notes on the progress and outcome of a client's treatment from initial interview to end of treatment, useful for the massage therapist in evaluating the effectiveness of treatment protocols and as a reference for future cases.

Chair massage massage treatment using specially designed chairs (ergonomic) that support the body in a way that is comfortable to the client and allows the massage therapist access to the client's body. The client is clothed and the treatment is adjusted accordingly. Usually offered in semi-public settings such as offices, malls, hospitals, and gyms.

Chakras Sanskrit word meaning "wheel" or "disc" referring to seven or eight energy centers found in the subtle energetic body possessing certain characteristics affecting the body-mind-spirit complex in specific ways. The chakras can be influenced by various healing modalities and spiritual practices.

Chiropractic CAM profession that focuses on correcting disorders of the musculoskeletal system, thought to affect general health, most often through spinal manipulation or "adjustments."

Chronic stress (long-term stress) state in which the stress response is continually activated and the body cannot return to parasympathetic functioning required for relaxing the body. Whether the threat is real or perceived the effect is the same; chronic stress is disruptive to all systems in the body and manifests in a host of conditions from immune system dysfunction, heart problems, to a sense of anxiety and unease in life.

Circulatory system whole body system consisting of arteries (taking blood away from heart), veins (returning blood back to the heart), and capillaries (delivering nutrients, metabolites, and gases into the interstitial spaces) that transport blood throughout the body through the pumping action of the heart.

Collagen fibrous protein that is the chief constituent of connective tissue.

Compassion the ability to feel another's suffering usually accompanied by the desire to alleviate it.

Compensation the process by which the body or mind adjusts itself in an attempt to correct an imbalance.

Complementary and alternative medicine (CAM) a term adopted by the National Institutes of Health to describe forms of health care that are not considered part of the conventional medical system but which are recognized as valid healing modalities.

Complementary health care any health care modality that works with conventional medical treatment rather than in place of it, as in alternative health care.

Connective tissue a tissue consisting of interlacing fibers that supports and connects other tissues, i.e. joints.

Continuum of practice range of possibilities for massage therapy not necessarily implying hierarchy of importance. At one end basic level of touch and the other end the most comprehensive treatment including holistic health care and life transformation.

Contraindications conditions that suggest a treatment, including massage, should not be performed, for example, an injury or sickness that could be made worse by the treatment.

Conventional medicine typically the term applied to western or "modern" medicine in which the treatment seeks to alleviate symptoms of disease rather than assess the whole person.

Cranial osteopathy a term coined by Dr. William Sutherland in the 1900s, the first person to discover cranial bone mobility and the therapeutic potential of manipulating the cranial bones.

Craniosacral rhythm systemic pulsation caused by the filling and emptying of the craniosacral fluid first discovered by Dr. John Upledger in the 1970s.

Craniosacral therapy form of bodywork having its roots in osteopathy in which the practitioner subtly manipulates skeletal structures of the spine, sacrum, pelvis, neck, and cranial bones to unlock restrictions and restore mobility and full function of the craniosacral system and the craniosacral rhythm.

Cross-handed stretches technique used in myofascial therapy to soften and release fascia along specific lines in the body.

Deep tissue-style massage sometimes considered a natural advancement of Swedish massage, uses deep pressure and manipulation of the physical body to restore suppleness and original form to chronically tight muscles

Differentiation one of the major aims of Rolfing, to restore individual functioning of muscles in order to realize their full potential.

Directed attention state in which the massage therapist's attention is focused and intentional. Produces a calm and expansive ability to attend to the aim of the treatment. It can be cultivated by meditative practices, including yoga, tai chi, and qi gong. This quality of attention is useful at any level of practice but is required for practice at the third level.

Doshas described by the Ayurvedic system, these three fundamental energies of *vata, pitta, and kapha* exist in various combinations in each human being and need to be in balance for optimal health and well-being.

Drawn attention state in which the mind is less scattered than in zero attention. Attention is pulled towards objects or intense feelings and may appear to be focused but is still without the conscious direction of the massage therapist.

Effleurage a long, sweeping stroke associated with Swedish massage whose name means "touching lightly."

Elastin protein in connective tissue that allows tissues to resume their shape after being stretched.

Empathy the ability to vicariously feel another's feelings, thoughts, or experience without necessarily implying a desire for action.

Energetic level modalities are used to directly affect and balance the energy system or energy body with little or no physical contact, for example, Reiki, therapeutic touch, polarity therapy.

Energy system a level of human functioning connected to and animating the physical body that can become imbalanced and cause physical dysfunction or disease and that can be rebalanced by energetic bodywork techniques as well as disciplines such as yoga, tai chi, and qi gong.

Ergonomic massage chair see "Seated massage"

Fascia soft tissue part of connective tissue that is found throughout the entire body providing a covering or connecting and supportive web for all structures in the body, such as muscles, organs, nerves, bones.

First Paradigm Fundamental practices of massage education and training, skills, knowledge, and abilities. The aim and scope of massage therapy in this paradigm is relaxation and stress reduction and the beneficial effects of nurturing touch. It does not include the intention of healing specific conditions or recommending lifestyle changes to the client. Is most often the paradigm practiced in spas, massage therapy clinics, and corporate or other semi-public settings.

Five elements principle of traditional Chinese medicine in which the universal energy is seen to consist of the five fundamental qualities of wood, fire, earth, metal, and water, which create and permeate all things and can be balanced in the individual through TCM.

Five Approaches a grouping of massage therapy modalities resulting from in-depth analysis during Job Analysis Advisory Committee meetings of the National Certification program in the 1990s: 1) traditional massage; 2) contemporary western massage and bodywork; 3) structural/functional/movement/integration modalities; 4) Asian bodywork; and 5) energetic bodywork.

Fight-or-flight response of the sympathetic nervous system to a perceived threat. Heightened physiological arousal readies the body to engage in combat or run away from danger. Elevated blood pressure, stress hormones, blood flow moves to periphery.

Four Levels of Massage evolution of the Five Approaches, categorizes massage therapy into four levels: 1) somatic, 2) somato-psychic, 3) bioenergetic, and 4) energetic

Friction the deepest work of Swedish massage, involves slow, circular, or transverse strokes applied with fingers, thumbs, or elbows to a concentrated area to soften adhesions and bring mobility to locked or limited areas of the body resulting from, for example, old patterns of muscular tension, or injury.

Functional integration concept of bodywork similar in its goals to structural integration but extends the therapy to correcting the body in motion, such as habits of misuse.

Ground substance clear fluid that surrounds cells of the body and lubricates tissues.

Hara diagnosis in Zen shiatsu, palpatory evaluation of the hara energy center in the lower abdomen.

Healing sensitive person whose heightened sensitivity allows them to accurately perceive illness and distress in others and through this direct insight may offer appropriate treatment and healing.

Hellerwork founded by Joseph Heller in the mid-nineteenth century, a somato-psychic bodywork modality that incorporates both structural and functional integration principles in its multisession approach and which encourages client's self-reflection as part of the healing process.

Herbalism widespread traditional treatment using herbs to alleviate symptoms of disease and to increase health and well-being. Remedies may be in the form of dried or fresh herb; pills, powders or capsules; teas or infusions; or topical applications.

Hilot system of deep tissue massage and body manipulation from the Philippines that can include the use of herbs.

Holistic health care based on the concept that the mind, body, and spirit are interconnected and are all taken into consideration during treatment of the whole person. A.K.A.: Wholistic.

Holistic practitioner practices from the holistic health care perspective and generally offers clients/patients a comprehensive treatment plan in addition to massage therapy, often including diet and lifestyle recommendations.

Homeopathy a CAM therapy discovered by Dr. Samuel Hahnemann (who also coined the term "allopathic" to distinguish it from homeopathic) in the nineteenth century, based on the principle that "like cures like," meaning that small doses of substances that in large quantities cause symptoms of disease can stimulate the body's own healing mechanisms. Generally considered to be safe because the substances are diluted to the extent that only the "energy imprint" of the molecule is said to be remaining.

Humours described by ancient Greeks as four basic substances of the body—black bile, yellow bile, phlegm, and blood—that need to be in harmony in order for the human being to be healthy.

Hypnotherapy treatment in which various levels of hypnotic trance are induced in the client, a state of relaxation and focused attention in which healing and positive suggestions for change can more easily be received.

Intake form a comprehensive form filled out during the initial interview with a client that notes anything that might pertain to the effectiveness of massage therapy. Will vary with paradigm level being practiced.

Integrative medicine an approach to medical care that uses conventional medicine in combination with other mind-body therapies to treat the whole person.

Intuition the ability to directly achieve insight through focused contemplation

Jin Shin Do. meaning "the way of the compassionate spirit," Japanese bodywork style developed in the early twentieth century by Jiro Murai and later developed by Iona Teeguarden, who gave it its name and expanded it to include western theories and healing techniques, including acupressure, channeling ki, breathing, meditation, movements, and diet to help the individual achieve balance and stillness.

Jitsu in **shiatsu**, refers to energetic "fullness" or **yang** quality.

Ki vital energy or life force (Japanese)

Kyo in **shiatsu**, refers to energetic "emptiness" or **yin** quality.

Latent trigger points those that radiate pain only when touched or pressed.

Li underlying idea or notion of anything that precedes and reflects the physical manifestation of it, and which is animated by qi.

Lomi-lomi Hawaiian massage characterized by long flowing strokes, fluid rhythmic patterns, and use of the forearms, aiming to restore balance and spiritual harmony through the loving touch and presence of the practitioner.

Long-term stress see "Chronic stress"

Lymph fluid clear fluid similar to plasma that bathes the tissues of an organism via the interstitial spaces acting as an intermediary between the blood and tissues in the exchange of nutrients, metabolites, and waste products.

Lymph node small, bean-shaped nodules that are found throughout the human body; contain the white blood cells of the immune system and filter lymph by removing foreign cells and circulatory debris.

Lymphatic system a network of vessels, organs, ducts, and nodes that transports lymph fluid throughout the body. It has no pumping system of its own and it relies on muscular contraction for circulation of lymph fluid.

Manual lymphatic drainage essentially involves lightly and rhythmically massaging the lymph nodes to increase the flow of lymph fluid throughout the system.

Marma points vital points that lie on energy channels of the subtle anatomy, some of which are similar in location to those in acupuncture meridians and are manipulated for healing in Thai massage.

Meridians channels or lines of energy in the human body relating to organ systems along which lie points that are stimulated or sedated in acupuncture or acupressure treatments for therapeutic or relaxation purposes.

Mind-body-emotion-spirit complex model from the holistic viewpoint that the various levels of the human being are interconnected.

Modulation in **therapeutic touch**, the modification of the client's energy.

Moxibustion direct or indirect application of heat to acupuncture points, generally involving the use of the mugwort herb.

Myofascial release system that uses sustained pressure to unblock restrictions in the myofascial (muscles and fascia) system to alleviate pain and discomfort and restore normal range of motion.

Naturopathy holistic system of medicine based on the healing power of nature and the use of natural therapies for healing and wellness, such as nutrition, herbal medicine, homeopathy, and acupuncture.

Neuromuscular therapy (NMT) a form of bodywork that uses static pressure to treat soft tissues at specific points, often trigger points, to balance the nervous and musculoskeletal systems.

Nutraceuticals a combination of the words *nutrition* and *pharmaceutical* referring to food extracts considered to have medicinal and/or healing benefits, dietary supplements, vitamins, minerals, herbs and other substances such as antioxidants and amino acids. Can be taken in the form of capsules, powder, juices or other food medium such as yogurt.

Orthopedic massage a recently developed form of massage therapy that uses techniques from different modalities to treat soft tissue pain and injuries. It includes training in the anatomy, physiology and pathology of pain and injury conditions and their treatment.

Osteopathy founded in the nineteenth century by Dr. Andrew Still, a health care profession that uses spinal manipulation to correct structural dysfunction to improve overall health and well-being.

Palpatory diagnosis examination of the body through touch

Paradigm a framework or model containing examples of a specific concept or theory

Parasympathetic nervous system branch of the autonomic nervous system regulating "rest and digest" functions and the relaxation response.

Petrissage in the Swedish system, the second layer of touch, after **effleurage**, in which the pace and pressure of strokes is deeper and includes squeezing, rolling, and kneading of specific muscles using the hands, thumbs, and fingers.

Polarity therapy energetic healing technique developed by Dr. Randolph Stone involving manipulations, light stretching and hand movements, as well as lifestyle modifications, to move and balance the body's energy.

Psychoneuroimmunology field of science describing and investigating the connections between the mind and emotions, the brain, and the functioning of the immune system.

Qi literally, "breath," the life force or vital energy that supports physical manifestation. Similar to *prana* (Sanskrit) and *spirit* (from the Latin *spiritus*)

Qi gong ancient Chinese martial art that focuses on energy generation and balance through a series of exercises using intention, breath and movement.

Random body state in which the body does not function coherently and in a unified fashion due to muscular imbalance and tension and which results in inefficient and inappropriate use of energy.

Range-of motion-assessment client performs a series of actions directed by the therapist to determine the extent of joint mobility and to reveal any limitations such as those resulting from muscle tension or injury.

Rapport establishment of a trusting and communicative professional relationship with the client.

Rebalancing in therapeutic touch, the intention to create symmetry and equilibrium in the client's energy system.

Reiki meaning "spiritually guided life energy" in Japanese, an energetic healing practice created by Dr. Mikao Usuii in the mid-1800s in which practitioners, through their own contact with the universal life force (**ki**), unblock and boost the life force flowing through the client, thereby promoting health and well-being as well as spiritual development. Can be done directly or from a distance.

Relaxation response originally named by Herbert Benson, MD, the relaxation response is the counterpart of the stress response that brings about decreased muscle tension, lowered heart rate and blood pressure. Can be facilitated by all levels of massage therapy, yoga, stress-reduction techniques, meditation, tai chi, qi gong. Etc.

Release of Medical Information form completed by the patient, gives the practitioner the permission to share patient information with other health professionals or other interested party such as an insurance company.

Rolfing "hard" style of myofascial release pioneered by Ida Rolf in the 1960s and 1970s, also known as Structural Integration. Deep tissue massage techniques unify the **random body**, correcting postural distortions and allowing **differentiation of muscles** as well as restoring optimal energy use and balance in the body-mind.

Scope of practice term that defines by law the specific practices and services a health care professional may provide. Intended to ensure that health care is safe and effective and that the provider has appropriate training.

Seated massage see "Chair massage"

Second Paradigm model of massage therapy in which the aim is remediation, therapy, and pain relief. Includes the previous paradigm of relaxation and stress reduction but also includes specific aim of correcting physical dysfunction and alleviating pain for a broad range of conditions. Additional training is needed for this paradigm, particularly a more in-depth knowledge of anatomy and physiology, and more advanced training in the modality being offered as well as knowledge of adjunctive therapies such as meditation, nutritional counseling, and exercise. Involves increased record-keeping and greater responsibility for well-being of client/patient along with deeper and ongoing therapeutic relationships. Second Paradigm practitioners may practice as part of a clinical team with allied health care professionals such as chiropractors, physical therapists, and acupuncturists. They may also practice as sports massage therapists.

Self-cultivation or self-development important for massage therapists at all levels but essential for practicing in the Third Pardigm is to apply to oneself techniques and methods that increase self-awareness, self-discipline, and overall health and well-being with the goal of being a more focused, compassionate, and effective health care provider and role model.

Shiatsu meaning "finger pressure," a Japanese bioenergic bodywork modality having its roots in China whose predominant aim is to balance the energy channels. The main forms being practiced today are Namikoshi and Zen shiatsu.

Short-term stress normal activation of the stress response to deal with an appropriate threat followed by deactivation and return to parasympathetic activation and the relaxation response.

Skin-rolling technique used in myofascial release involving grasping and rolling of skin between the fingers to release tensions and adhesions.

SOAP notes stand for subjective, objective, assessment, and plan/protocol. Written out at every session by the massage therapist, these notes help to monitor the patient, chart the course of treatment, provide information for the patient's other health care providers or insurance company, and may help to protect the therapist in case of litigation.

Soma neuromuscular integration a somato-psychic modality that uses a 10-session format to affect both neurological and structural systems through deep manipulation of the myofascial system and self-investigation to bring about balance in the body-mind.

Somagraphy a method of reading the body used in Soma neuromuscular integration.

Somassage a type of massage used in Soma neuromuscular integration.

Somatic education also known as "body learning," a principle of the Feldenkrais method in which the individual learns to explore and fully understand the physical body and its full capacity for movement.

Somatic level or layer massage therapies dealing primarily with the treatment of the physical body, for example, Swedish massage, neuromuscular therapy, myofascial release, sports massage, trigger point therapy.

Somato-psychic level or layer massage therapies with the aim of affecting both body and mind, for example, Rolfing, Soma Neuromuscular Integration, Hellerwork, the Alexander and Feldenkrais techniques, craniosacral therapy.

Sports massage used to increase athletic performance, prevent injury, and assist in recovery from injury. Sports massage therapists are often considered part of the team and travel with athletes to events, treating them pre-event, during the event, post-event, and during rehabilitation from an injury. Techniques include those from the Swedish, neuromuscular, orthopedic, and myofascial release therapies, as well as body mobilizations.

Strange flows the eight meridians or channels of Jin Shin Do.*

Stress experience of challenges in life, often including a perception that threat exists (distress), that requires action and is accompanied by heightened physiological arousal.

Stress response the body's normal response to the perception of stress, the activation of the sympathetic nervous system to provide extra energy and alertness to help in self-protection.

Structural integration concept of bodywork using deep manipulation to correct the form of the physical body and restore proper alignment and range of motion.

Swedish massage Classic system of massage originated by Per Henrik Ling in the eighteenth century serving as a foundation for many current styles of massage, the primary function of which is relaxation and release from muscular tension. Involves manipulation of the physical body and promotes circulation of vital fluids; although not directly intended to address specific illnesses, its effect is inherently therapeutic due to its deep relaxing and nourishing effects.

Sympathetic nervous system branch of the autonomic nervous system activating the "flight-or-fight" or stress response.

Tai Chi Chuan ancient Chinese martial art sometimes called "moving mediation" that improves vitality, balance, and overall functioning through the daily practice of a set series of slow, continuous, relaxed movements that are done with great detail and attention.

Taoism ancient Chinese philosophy, loosely translates as "the way" offers teachings of how to live harmoniously with the flow of life.

Tapotement percussive stroke in Swedish massage performed with fists, cupped hands, or fingers in "karate chop" position to either stimulate or relax muscles, depending on how it is applied.

Thai massage massage therapy technique from Thailand in which the practitioner moves the client's body into positions that often resemble yoga poses to promote greater flexibility and range of motion as well as to balance the doshas and energy lines in the body.

The Alexander Technique developed by F. M. Alexander in the late 1890, a technique focusing on correcting faulty movement habits and restoring freedom of motion and balance.

The Feldenkrais method developed by Moshe Feldenkrais in the 1970s, a method aimed at freeing the body from old patterns as a medium for personal liberty and the realization of one's full human potential through deep investigation of the body in movement.

Therapeutic touch developed in the 1970s by Dora Kuntz and Delores Krieger, a simple energetic bodywork technique of balancing the human energy field through intentional movements of the hands off the body using three main processes: rebalancing, modulation, and unruffling.

Third Paradigm holistic integration level of massage therapy practice. The perspective expands to include the overall health care of the patient, including a toolbox of adjunctive therapies and techniques such as nutritional counseling, herbal medicine and lifestyle transformation practices, for example, meditation and yoga. Requires advanced training and greater experience on the part of therapists, a deeper level of commitment to their own self development, competence and focus of awareness, greater degree of responsibility to the patient, and a greater degree of embodiment of the principles of the paradigm.

Three Levels of Competence describe the levels of skill and ability brought to the practice of massage therapy by practitioners, dependent upon their quality of personal effort, ability to focus attention as well as degree of training.

Three Paradigms of practice models that describe the degree of education, training, and focus of practice in massage therapy.

Tissue memory concept that unexpressed or unacknowledged feelings become chemically stored in the body's tissues and can be released through bodywork or activities such as yoga and tai chi.

Traditional Chinese medicine (TCM) ancient system of medicine consisting of five main branches 1) massage and bodywork, 2) acupuncture, 3) herbalism, 4) diet and nutrition, and 5) exercise with the underlying philosophy of a unifying universal energy. Pulse and tongue diagnosis are the predominant means of assessment.

Transference in the therapeutic relationship, when the client transfers feelings and beliefs associated with another person or situation to the therapist.

Trigger points hyper-sensitive points in a skeletal muscle, palpable and often referred to as a "knot," that can cause local or radiating pain, limited mobility, and hinder everyday activities and which can often be relieved through the application of deep, static, pressure as in trigger point or neuromuscular therapy.

Tsubo traditional Japanese manual therapy that works by stimulating or sedating vital energy points in the body.

Tuina Chinese massage originally known as "ammo" that includes a variety of techniques including stroking, kneading, pressing, and tapotement, as well as the therapist moving the client's limbs to free the joints.

Unruffling in therapeutic touch, the clearing of disruptive energies in the client.

Vibration Swedish massage technique of vibrating or shaking an area of the body to stimulate hypotonic muscle or desensitize a hyperactive nerve.

Western medical paradigm typically focuses on the relief of disease symptoms through drugs or surgery as well as some lifestyle modification recommendations. May also be seen as having three paradigms within it according to the level of education and training of the practitioner.

Yin and **Yang** Chinese name for two primary and complementary energies that are always in dynamic interplay in the ongoing creation and destruction of the physical and energetic manifestions of the world.

Yoga Loosely translated as "union," a comprehensive philosophy and system of practices that support the whole person, bringing about transformation of mind and body and fostering connection to spirit. Consists of eight limbs, one of which includes the poses, or asanas, with which many people associate the practice of yoga.

Zero attention state in which the mind is unfocused and scattered. The massage therapist may be physically going through the motions but is not fully present in the moment or with the client.

Index